COLONOSCOPY AND COLORECTAL CANCER SCREENING - FUTURE DIRECTIONS

Edited by **Marco Bustamante**

Colonoscopy and Colorectal Cancer Screening - Future Directions
http://dx.doi.org/10.5772/46055
Edited by Marco Bustamante

Contributors

Muhammed Sherid, Salih Samo, Samian Sulaiman, Kenneth B. Hosie, Robert J Richards, Jerome Liang, Alberto Vannelli, Michel Zanardo, Valerio Basilico, Baldovino Griffa, Fabrizio Rossi, Massimo Buongiorno, Luigi Battaglia, Vincenzo Pruiti, Sara De Dosso, Giulio Capriata, Fritz Francois, Anjali Mone, Robert Mocharla, Allison Avery, Marco Bustamante, Paul Frederick Miskovitz, Adler, Shigeki Tomita, Sharon Zhiling Koh, Kouklakis, Carol Julyssa Cobián Malaver, Luis Bujanda Fernández De Piérola, Joaquín Cubiella Fernández, Lander Hijona, Fernando Múgica Aguinaga

Published by InTech
Janeza Trdine 9, 51000 Rijeka, Croatia

Publishing Process Manager Iva Simcic
Technical Editor InTech DTP team
Cover InTech Design team

Additional hard copies can be obtained from orders@intechopen.com

Colonoscopy and Colorectal Cancer Screening - Future Directions, Edited by Marco Bustamante
p. cm.
ISBN 978-953-51-0949-5

For EU product safety concerns:
IN TECH d.o.o., Prolaz Marije Krucifikse Kozulić 3, 51000 Rijeka, Croatia,
info@intechopen.com or visit our website at intechopen.com.

Meet the editor

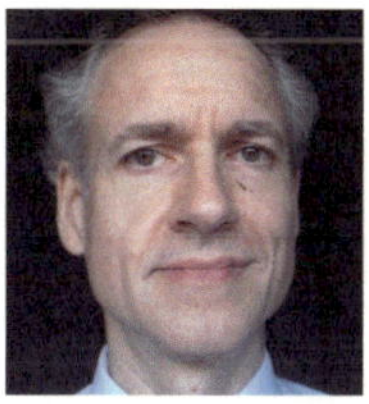

Dr. Marco Bustamante is a staff member of the Endoscopy Unit of the University Hospital La Fe, a tertiary referral center in Valencia (Spain). Devoted to endoscopy since the end of his fellowship, his main interests are the use of endoscopy to early detection of neoplastic lesions and the utility of endoscopic resection techniques as an alternative to surgery as a treatment for early cancers of the gastrointestinal tract. He has published several studies on the use of imaging enhancing technologies to improve detection and diagnosis of colon adenomas mainly with the use of chromoendoscopy and narrow band imaging.

Contents

Preface IX

Section 1 Overview of Colorectal Cancer. Implementation of Colorectal Cancer Screening Programs 1

Chapter 1 **Colorectal Cancer 3**
Kouklakis S. Georgios and Asimenia D. Bampali

Chapter 2 **Issues in Screening and Surveillance Colonoscopy 25**
Anjali Mone, Robert Mocharla, Allison Avery and Fritz Francois

Chapter 3 **The Future of Colonoscopy: The Use of Data Envelopment Analysis (DEA) for Colorectal Cancer Screening — Italian Experience 71**
Alberto Vannelli, Michel Zanardo, Valerio Basilico, Baldovino Griffa, Fabrizio Rossi, Massimo Buongiorno, Luigi Battaglia, Vincenzo Pruiti, Sara De Dosso and Giulio Capriata

Section 2 Managing Precursor Lesions: Resection Techniques and Beyond 93

Chapter 4 **Evolution and Strategy of Endoscopic Treatment for Colorectal Tumours 95**
Koh Z.L. Sharon, H. Yamamoto and Tsang B.S. Charles

Chapter 5 **Malignant Colorectal Polyps: Diagnosis, Treatment and Prognosis 123**
Luis Bujanda Fernández de Piérola, Joaquin Cubiella Fernández, Fernando Múgica Aguinaga, Lander Hijona Muruamendiaraz and Carol Julyssa Cobián Malaver

Chapter 6 **The Malignant Polyp: Polypectomy or Surgical Resection? 141**
Josef M. Taylor and Kenneth B. Hosie

Chapter 7 **Desmoplastic Reaction in Biopsy Specimens of T1 Stage Colorectal Cancer Plays a Critical Role in Defining the Level of Sub-Mucosal Invasion 161**
Shigeki Tomita, Kazuhito Ichikawa and Takahiro Fujimori

Chapter 8 **In vivo Optical Diagnosis of Polyp Histology: Can We Omit Pathological Examination of Diminutive Polyps? 177**
Marco Bustamante-Balén

Section 3 Complications of Colonoscopy: Minimizing the Risks of a Screening Tool 195

Chapter 9 **The Major Complications of Colonoscopy: Sedation-Related, Hemorrhage Associated with Polypectomy and Colonic Perforation 197**
Paul Miskovitz

Chapter 10 **Complications of Colonoscopy 215**
Muhammed Sherid, Salih Samo and Samian Sulaiman

Section 4 Colonoscopy Is Not the End of the Way: Other Screening Technologies 241

Chapter 11 **Colon Capsule Endoscopy: Quo Vadis? 243**
Samuel N. Adler and Cesare Hassan

Chapter 12 **Virtual Colonoscopy 253**
Robert J. Richards and Jerome Zhengrong Liang

Preface

Colorectal cancer (CRC) is the third more commonly diagnosed cancer in both sexes and it is also the third leading cause of cancer-related death among men and women in the United States.It represents a global public health problem and a heavy burdenfor any healthcare system. Fortunately, most CRCs originate from an adenoma, a precursor lesion that is easily accessible and removable. This is the rationale for CRC screening programs, which are aimed to diagnose CRC at an early stage or even better, to detect and resect the advanced adenoma before CRC has developed. Recent evidence suggests that colonoscopy with polypectomy is efficient in reducing the incidence of and mortality from CRC. Moreover, the CRC resection rates have recently been shown to be reduced after the implementation of colonoscopy-based screening programs. As a consequence, CRC screening programs, either directly with colonoscopy or based on fecal occult blood test, are being implemented in most countries. The physicians who are devoted to endoscopy or who are involved in CRC screening programs face several challenges. They are requested to participate in the organization of population-based CRC screening programs; screening colonoscopies have to be performed accomplishing quality standards; difficult endoscopic resections are expected because performing colonoscopy in asymptomatic individuals makes possible an early diagnosis of advanced adenomas; and finally clinical decisions have to be made based on the information provided by the number and histology of the detected adenomas.

In this background, this book providesaccurate and updated information on several topics to be faced when implementing a CRC screening program.It is divided in four sections, the first one dealing with the epidemiology of CRC and the rationale and challenges of implementing such a program both from a European and American point of view. The second section tackles the issue of managing the findings of a screening colonoscopy, commenting on the use of endoscopic submucosal dissection to resect difficult polyps, the significance and management of the malignant polyp and the possibility of using image enhancing technologies to make a presumptive histological diagnosis of diminutive polyps reducing costs without losing efficacy. The third section summarizes the main risks of diagnostic and therapeutic colonoscopy and how to manage them. And finally the last section comments on virtual colonoscopy and colon capsule endoscopy, technologies that are being developed and soon will become part of our screening armamentarium.

The relevance of the topics covered in it and the updated evidence included by the authors turns this book into a very useful tool to introduce the reader in the amazing and evolving field of colonoscopy and CRC screening.

Marco Bustamante, MD, PhD
University Hospital La Fe
Valencia, Spain

Section 1

Overview of Colorectal Cancer. Implementation of Colorectal Cancer Screening Programs

Chapter 1

Colorectal Cancer

Kouklakis S. Georgios and Asimenia D. Bampali

Additional information is available at the end of the chapter

http://dx.doi.org/10.5772/53524

1. Introduction

1.1. Epidemiology – Clinical presentation-screening

Colorectal cancer (CRC) is a common and lethal disease. The risk of developing CRC is influenced by both environmental and genetic factors. Colorectal cancer is the third most common cancer worldwide. Clinical symptoms develop late in the course of the disease, and precursor lesions (adenomas) can be easily detected and removed. The disease is a candidate for early detection and prevention by screening. The epidemiology of CRC and risk factors for its development will be discussed here.

Epidemiology — CRC incidence and mortality rates vary markedly around the world [1]. Globally, CRC is the third most commonly diagnosed cancer in males and the second in females, with over 1.2 million new cases and 608,700 deaths estimated to have occurred in 2008.Incidence and mortality rates are substantially higher in males than in females [2]. It is the fourth most common cause of cancer death after lung, stomach, and liver cancer. It is more common in developed than developing countries.

In the United States, both the incidence and mortality have been slowly but steadily decreasing. Annually approximately 143,460 new cases of large bowel cancer are diagnosed, of which 103,170 are colon and the remainder rectal cancers. Annually, approximately 51,690 Americans die of CRC, accounting for approximately 9 percent of all cancer deaths [6].

Incidence — There is significant geographical variation in age-standardized and cumulative, 0-74 year incidence and mortality rates. Globally, the incidence of CRC varies over 10-fold. The highest incidence rates are in Australia and New Zealand, Europe and North America, and the lowest rates are found in Africa and South-Central Asia [5]. The highest incidence rate of CRC is estimated in the Czech Republic [39-42]. These geographic differences appear to be attributable to differences in dietary and environmental exposures that are imposed upon a background of genetically determined susceptibility.

In Europe, the incidence of colorectal cancer is increasing, particularly in Southern and Eastern Europe, where rates were originally lower than in Western Europe [7]. In the USA, incidence rose until the mid-1980s but in the last two decades the rates have fallen for both men and women. Countries that have had a rapid 'westernization' of diet, such as Japan, have seen a rapid increase in incidence of colorectal cancer. Consumption of meat and dairy products in Japan increased tenfold between the 1950s and 1990s.

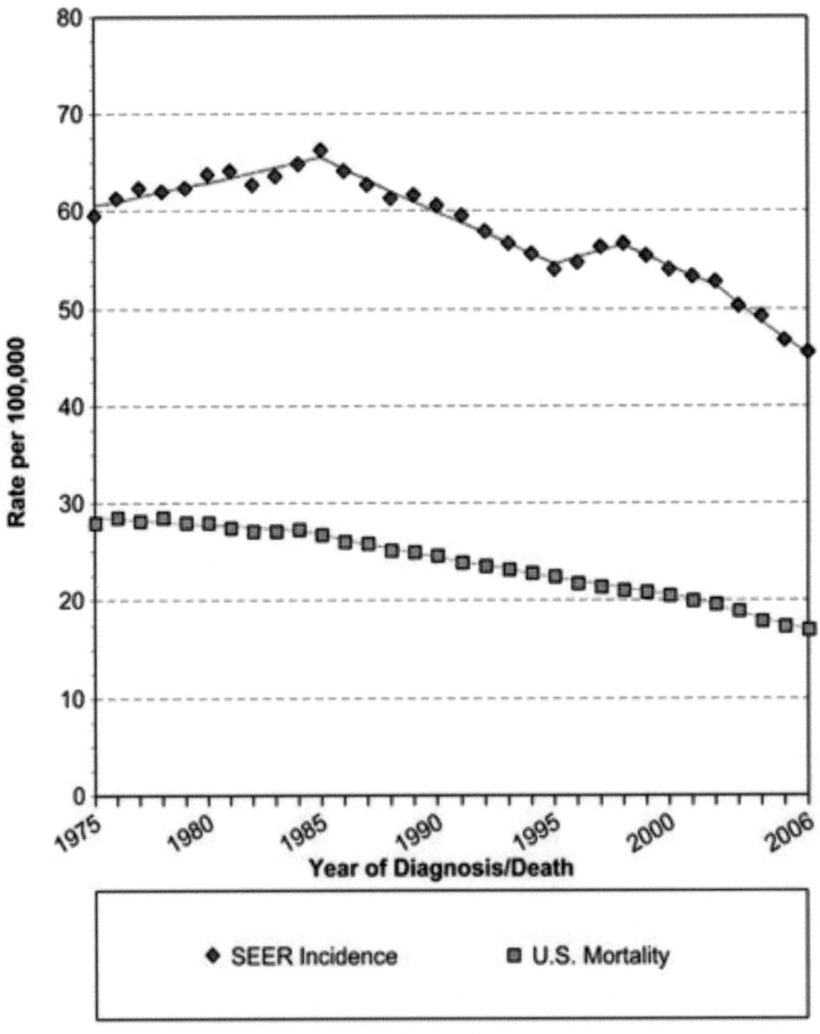

Figure 1. Age-adjusted colorectal cancer incidence and death rates in the United States 1975–2006.

Colorectal cancer (CRC) is a disease with a major worldwide burden. The worldwide incidence of CRC is increasing. In 1975, the worldwide incidence of CRC was only 500,000.In western countries, some of the increase is due to the aging of the population. However, in countries with a low baseline rate of CRC, the incidence is increasing even after age-adjustment. Prior to 1985, the age-adjusted incidence of CRC in the USA also increased (figure 1). However, since this time the rates have declined an average of −1.6% per year. In the time period 1998–2005, the rate of decline accelerated; −2.8% per year in men and −2.3% per year in women. This reduction has been mainly confined to those of white race and is largely limited to a decrease in the incidence of distal cancers. Although the cause of the decrease in incidence is unknown, and may have been influenced by many factors, it is likely that much may be attributable to screening by sigmoidoscopy and colonoscopy. In contrast, the incidence of proximal cancers has remained relatively stable over the same time period. Currently, the overall probability of an individual developing CRC in the USA over a lifetime is 5.5% in men and 5.1% in women.

From a population perspective, age is the most important risk factor for CRC. CRC is predominantly a disease of older individuals. 90% of cases are diagnosed over the age of 50. The risk of CRC continues to increase with age (Figure 2). The incidence per 100,000 people age 80–84 is over seven times the incidence in people age 50–54. However, CRC can occur at any age and the incidence of CRC occurring before age 40 may be increasing.

In the USA, the risk of CRC differs by sex. The age-adjusted incidence of CRC is over 40% higher in men than women [8]. Overall, the incidence of CRC in men is 61 per 100,000 males as compared to 45 per 100,000 females. In addition, the ratio of colon to rectal cancer differs by sex; the ratio of colon to rectal cases for women is 3:1 as compared to 2:1 for males.

Race and ethnicity influence CRC risk [20]. Ashkenazi Jewish individuals appear to be at a slightly increased risk of CRC. At least part of this increased incidence may be due to a higher prevalence of the *I1307K* mutation of the adenomatous polyposis gene (*APC*), a mutation that confers an increased risk of CRC development (18–30% lifetime risk). The *I1307K* mutation is found in 6.1% of unselected Ashkenazi Jewish individuals and 28% of Jewish individuals with CRC, while the mutation is rare in other populations. In the USA, the incidence of CRC is higher in African Americans of either sex as compared to white Americans. Asian American/Pacific Islanders, Native Americans, and Hispanic Americans experience a lower incidence of CRC than Caucasians (Table 1).African Americans have not experienced the substantial reduction in incidence of CRC found to have occurred in whites; prior to 1980 incidence in African Americans was actually lower than in white Americans. In African Americans, the increased rate of cancer is predominantly due to a higher rate of proximal cancers.

There is substantial geographic variation in the incidence of CRC, with relatively high rates in North America, Western Europe, and Australia and relatively low rates in Africa and Asia (Figure 3) Such observations led to Burkitt's hypothesis; that dietary differences, specifically fiber and fat intake, between populations were responsible for the marked variation in rates of CRC found around the world. Burkitt observed that populations in low-risk areas of the third world had greater stool bulk, a faster colonic transit time, and higher dietary fiber intake

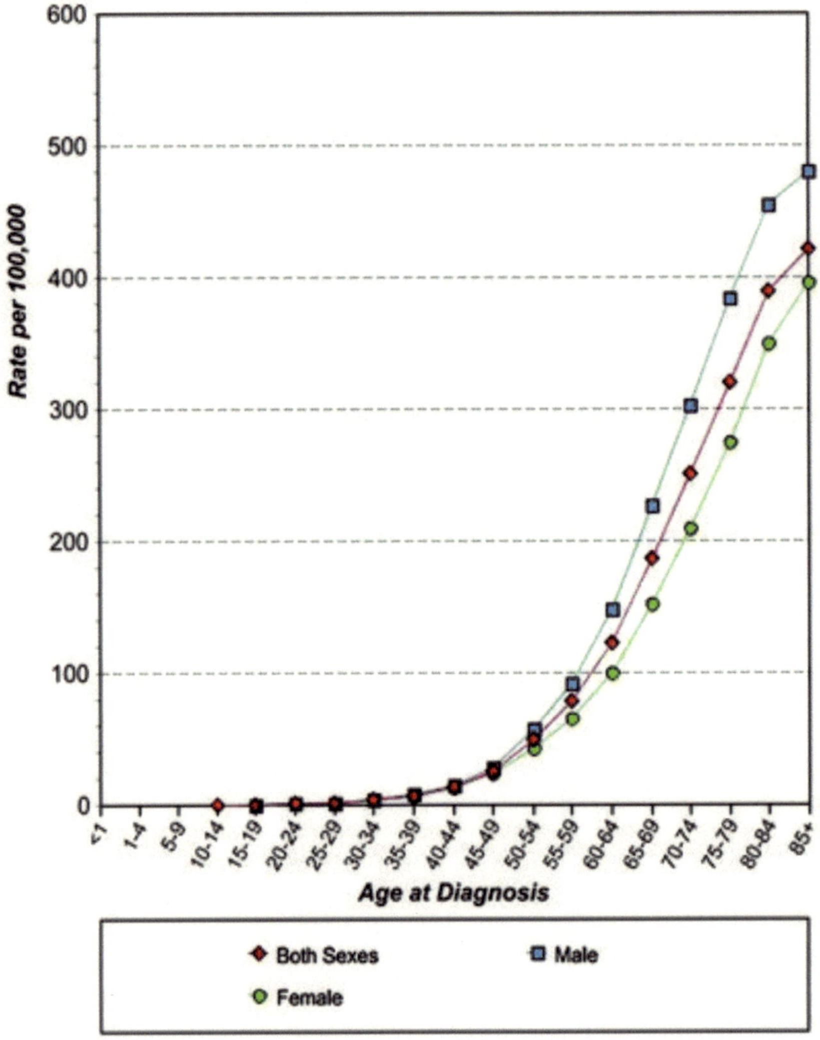

Figure 2. Age-specific SEER incidence rates in the United States 1992–2006.

		White	African American	Asian American and Pacific Islander	American Indian/ Alaska Native	Hispanic/ Latino
Incidence	Male	58.9	71.2	48.0	46.0	47.3
	Female	43.2	54.5	35.4	41.2	32.8
Mortality	Male	22.1	31.8	14.4	20.5	16.5
	Female	15.3	22.4	10.2	14.2	10.8

*per 100,000 age-adjusted to the 2000 US standard population

Table 1. Incidence and mortality rates* for CRC by site, race and ethnicity, US 2001–2005

than populations in high-risk, westernized regions. Although such ecological studies are confounded by numerous factors (for example, variations in average life expectancy, cancer detection methods, etc.), environmental factors (most prominently dietary factors) are still considered to have a major role in this disease. This is supported by studies of migrants from low prevalence areas to high prevalence areas. Such studies generally demonstrate that the incidence of CRC in the migrants increases rapidly to become similar and in some cases to exceed the incidence of the high-risk area. Interestingly, there is less variation in the incidence of rectal cancer between countries as compared to the incidence of colon cancer.

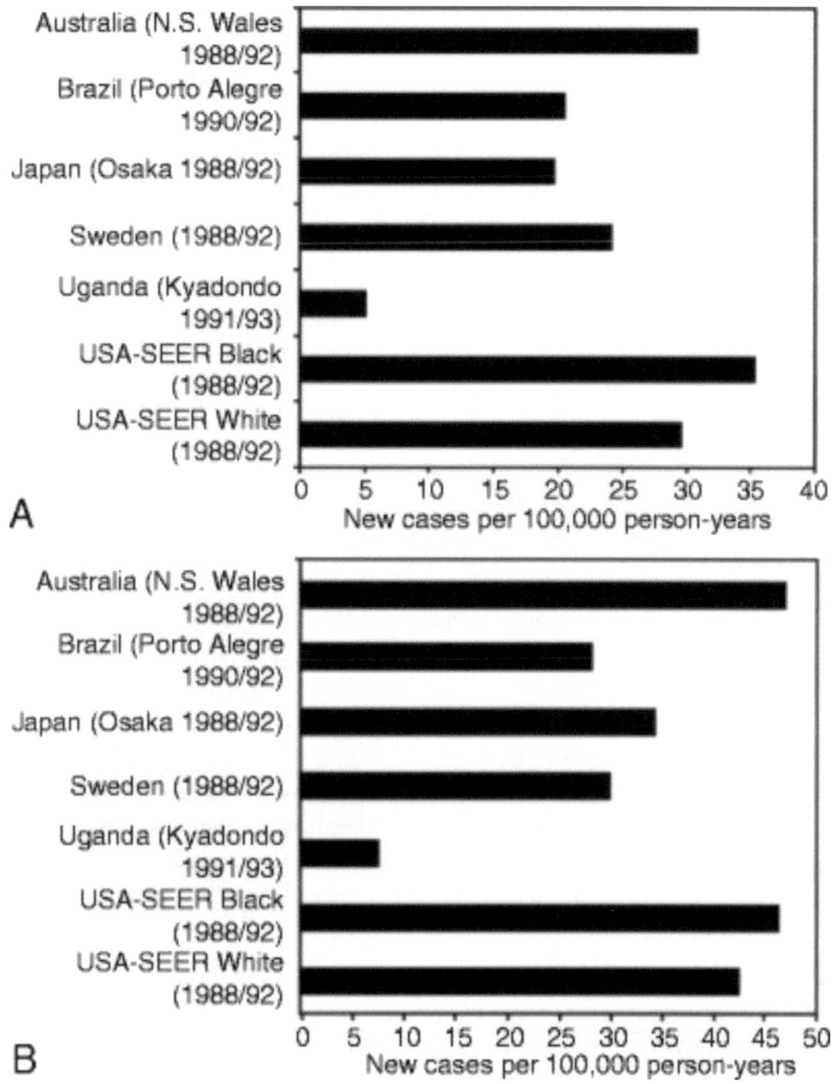

Figure 3. A Age-Standardized (to the world population) incidence rates of cancer of the large bowel among females, B Age-standardized (to the world population) incidence rates of cancer of the large bowel among males

The lifetime incidence of CRC in patients at average risk is about 5 percent, with 90 percent of cases occurring after age 50. In the US, CRC incidence is about 25 percent higher in men than in women and is about 20 percent higher in African Americans than in whites. The incidence is higher in patients with specific inherited conditions that predispose them to the development of CRC.

Mortality — Death rates from CRC have declined progressively since the mid-1980s in the United States and in many other western countries. This improvement in outcome can be attributed, at least in part, to detection and removal of colonic polyps, detection of CRCs at an earlier stage, and more effective treatments, particularly adjuvant therapy. Globally, the United States has one of the highest survival rates from CRC. However, mortality rates continue to increase in many countries with more limited resources and health infrastructure, particularly in Central and South America and Eastern Europe [43-44]. African Americans suffer the highest mortality rate from CRC in the USA (Table 1).The reasons for the higher mortality rate are likely multifactorial, including the higher incidence of CRC, and the differences in stage distribution. Differences in incidence, stage distribution and survival of CRC between white and African Americans are in part due to differences in socioeconomic status, screening rates and treatment. However, the differences may also be due to genetic and environmental factors that have yet to be elucidated. The highest mortality rates in both sexes are estimated in Central Europe (20.3/100000 for male patients, 12.1/100000 for female patients), and the lowest in the Middle Africa (3.5 and 2.7 respectively). The majority of deaths of CRC occur in older people, around 80% in people aged 65 and above and almost two-fifths of deaths appear in the group with age over 80.

Because CRC is a survivable cancer, with a 5-year survival rates adjusted for life expectancy of 64% the prevalence of people living with a diagnosis of CRC in the population is substantial.

Factors that may have contributed to the worldwide variation in colorectal cancer incidence patterns include differences in the prevalence of risk factors and screening practices. Established and suspected modifiable risk factors for colorectal cancer, including obesity, physical inactivity, smoking, heavy alcohol consumption, a diet high in red or processed meats, and inadequate consumption of fruits and vegetables, are also factors associated with economic development or westernization [35]·This partially explains the historically high albeit decreasing colorectal cancer incidence rates observed in long-standing developed countries such as the United States, Canada, and New Zealand over the past several years [36]. Colorectal cancer screening can also influence colorectal cancer incidence rates. All screening tests including stool blood tests (e.g. fecal occult blood test) and structural screening tests (e.g. sigmoidoscopy and colonoscopy) may increase colorectal cancer incidence rates initially as they detect previously undiagnosed cases.

Riskfactors-Although the exact cause for the development of colorectal cancer is not known, there are factors that increase risk for developing adenomas, polyps and cancer. These include numerous suspect factors.

Environmental and genetic factors can increase the likelihood of developing CRC. Although inherited susceptibility results in the most striking increases in risk, the majority of CRCs are sporadic rather than familial. These include:

http://dx.doi.org/10.5772/53524

1. **HereditaryCRCsyndromes** such as: Familial adenomatous polyposis (FAP) and Lynch Syndrome (hereditary nonpolyposis colorectal cancer (HNPCC)) which are the most common of the familial colon cancer syndromes, but together these two conditions account for only about 5 percent of CRC cases.

a. **Familialadenomatouspolyposis(FAP)** and its variants (Gardner's syndrome, Turcot's syndrome, and attenuated adenomatous polyposis coli) account for less than 1 percent of colorectal cancers. In typical FAP, numerous colonic adenomas appear during childhood. Symptoms appear at an average age of approximately 16 years and colonic cancer occurs in 90 percent of untreated individuals by age 45. An attenuated form of APC (AAPC) carries a similarly high risk of colon cancer but is characterized by fewer adenomas and an older average age of cancer diagnosis of 54 years.

FAP is caused by germline mutations in the adenomatous polyposis coli (APC) gene which is located on chromosome 5. The same gene is involved in the attenuated form of FAP, but the sites of the APC gene mutations are different.

b. **Lynchsyndrome** — Lynch syndrome is an autosomal dominant syndrome, which is more common than FAP, and accounts for approximately 3 to 5 percent of all colonic adenocarcinomas. The name Lynch syndrome honors the pioneering work of Dr. Henry Lynch in drawing attention to the syndrome. The term Lynch syndrome is now commonly used for families who have been genetically determined to have a disease-causing defect in one of the mismatch repair genes, most commonly hMLH1, hMSH2, hMSH6, or PMS2. As a general rule, patients with Lynch syndrome have a germline mutation in one allele of a MMR gene and the second allele is inactivated in the colorectal cancers by somatic mutation, loss of heterozygosity, or epigenetic silencing by promoter hypermethylation.

The colorectal tumors that develop in patients with Lynch syndrome are characterized by early age of onset and predominance of right-sided lesions [21]. The mean age at initial cancer diagnosis is 48 years, with some patients presenting in their 20s. Nearly 70 percent of first lesions arise proximal to the splenic flexure, and approximately 10 percent will have synchronous (simultaneous onset of two or more distinct tumors separated by normal bowel) or metachronous cancers (non-anastomotic new tumors developing at least six months after the initial diagnosis).

Extracolonic cancers are very common in Lynch syndrome, particularly endometrial carcinoma, which may occur in up to 60 percent of female mutation carriers in some families. Other sites at increased risk of neoplasm formation include the ovary, stomach, small bowel, hepatobiliary system, brain and renal pelvis or ureter.

2. Personal or family history of sporadic CRCs or adenomatous polyps

Patients with a personal history of CRC or adenomatous polyps of the colon are at risk for the future development of colon cancer. The clustering of risk in families may be attributed to an inherited susceptibility, common environmental exposures, or a combination of both. The influence of a more distant family history of CRC on individual risk has not been determined with certainty. Some of the increased risk attributed to family history is due to inheritance of known susceptibility genes, such as mutations in the *APC* gene, *p53* gene, or in MMR genes, particularly *MSH2*, *MLH1*, and *MSH6*.

Importantly, the majority of cases of CRC cannot be attributed to known genetic defects even when associated with a family history of CRC as recognized genetic syndromes account for only a small proportion of all cases of CRC. Additional autosomal dominant genetic defects conferring a high risk of CRC almost certainly is found. However, at least some of the increased risk of CRC associated with a family history is likely attributable to other genetic factors, such as recessive susceptibility genes, autosomal dominant genes with low penetrance, or complex interactions between an individual's genetic makeup and environmental factors.

Despite the importance of family history on the risk of CRC, up to 25% of individuals with a first-degree relative with confirmed CRC do not report having such a family history and even those that do report a history may not be aware of the increased risk associated with this. This has important implications for the assessment of family history as well as patient and family counseling.

3. Inflammatory bowel disease

Patients with long-standing inflammatory bowel disease (IBD) are known to be at an elevated risk of CRC, although it is difficult to precisely estimate the risk. The magnitude of the risk has been studied extensively in ulcerative colitis (UC).

Ulcerativecolitis— There is a well documented association between chronic ulcerative colitis and colonic neoplasia, with the extent, duration, and activity of disease being the primary determinants while for Crohn's disease there are less data. However, there is an association between pancolitis due to Crohn's disease and the risk of colon malignancy. The extent of disease does appear to have a significant influence on CRC risk in UC [38]. Other factors that may modify the risk of CRC in patients with UC include the coexistence of primary sclerosing colangitis (PSC), presence of inflammatory pseudopolyps, and severity of inflammation. For patients with long-standing, extensive UC, colectomy is an effective strategy for the prevention of CRC. Other strategies include endoscopic surveillance for dysplasia and/or the use of chemopreventive agents.

The relationship between Crohn's disease and the development of CRC has been less consistently demonstrated. In studies using data from referral-based practices, the risk of development of CRC appears to be significantly increased in patients with extensive Crohn's colitis. Finally, the risk of CRC in patients with Crohn's disease is elevated, but the exact magnitude of increased risk remains unclear and requires further investigation.

Several additional risk factors have been identified mostly in observational studies. These may include: race/ethnicity and gender, acromegaly, renal transplantation, diabetes mellitus and insulin resistance, use of androgen deprivation therapy, cholecystectomy, alcohol, obesity.

http://dx.doi.org/10.5772/53524

Protectivefactors — A large number of factors have been reported by at least some studies to be associated with a decreased risk of CRC. These *include* regular physical activity, a variety of dietary factors, the regular use of aspirin or nonsteroidal antiinflammatory drugs (NSAIDs), and hormone replacement therapy in postmenopausal women. None of these factors are currently used to stratify CRC screening recommendations.

1. Physical Activity

Over 50 studies have been conducted to evaluate the influence of physical activity on CRC risk. Overall, the literature is relatively consistent with respect to the effect: Greater physical activity (occupational, recreational, or total activity) is associated with a reduced risk of CRC. The effect is relatively small; the estimated increased risk of colon cancer in the sedentary ranges from 1.6 to 2.0. The biological mechanisms that explain the relationship between physical activity and CRC risk are unclear. Increased physical activity leads to changes in insulin sensitivity and IGF levels, and both insulin and IGF are potentially involved with colorectal carcinogenesis. Additional proposed mechanisms include effects of physical activity on prostaglandin synthesis, effects on antitumor immune defenses, and the reduction in percent body fat associated with exercise. The mechanism is almost certainly multifactorial. Nonetheless, for a host of health-related reasons, frequent moderate to vigorous physical activity can be recommended to most patients without hesitation.

2. Fruit and Vegetable Intake

The effect of dietary intake of fruit and vegetables on CRC risk has been evaluated extensively [22]. Fruits and vegetables are a source of antioxidants, including carotenoids and ascorbate. Other bioactive constituents in fruits and vegetables that may protect against carcinogenesis include the indoles and isothiocyanates. The evidence for an association between fruit and vegetable intake and the risk of CRC is inconsistent [23]. Given this, it is unlikely that a large number of cases of CRC can be attributed directly to a lack of intake of fruits or vegetables, or that major additional interventions to increase consumption would lead to a substantial reduction in the incidence of CRC.

3. Aspirin and Nonsteroidal Anti-inflammatory Drugs

There is considerable observational evidence that the use of aspirin or other nonsteroidal anti-inflammatory drugs (NSAIDs) has protective effects at all stages of colorectal carcinogenesis (aberrant crypt foci, adenoma, carcinoma, and death from CRC [14]. The mechanism of antineoplastic action of NSAIDs is incompletely understood, but it is believed that both cyclooxygenase (COX)-dependent and COX-independent pathways may be involved. NSAIDs and aspirin may play an important role in secondary chemoprevention of colorectal adenomas and cancer. Because chemopreventive agents must be used in the general population to substantially reduce the burden of disease, the risks of chemoprophylaxis with aspirin or NSAIDs may outweigh the benefits. Serious GI complications occur in regular users of aspirin and NSAIDs although rare.

4. Hormone Replacement Therapy

Observational studies have demonstrated an association between hormone replacement therapy (HRT) in women and a reduction in both incidence and mortality from CRC. Possible mechanisms for the effect of HRT include a reduction in bile acid secretion (a potential promoter or initiator of CRC), as well as estrogen effects on colonic epithelium, both directly and through alterations in insulin-like growth factor with the use of estrogens. Overall, there appears to be a consistent reduction in the risk of CRC with the use of HRT. However, given the potential adverse effect of HRT, this should not be used as a primary preventive strategy for CRC.

4. Clinical presentation

4.1. Symptoms

Symptoms are common and prominent late in colon cancer when the prognosis is poor but are less common and less obvious early in the disease. Common symptoms include abdominal pain, rectal bleeding, altered bowel habits, and involuntary weight loss [58]. Although colon cancer can present with either diarrhea or constipation, a recent change in bowel habits is much more likely to be from colon cancer than chronically abnormal bowel habits. Less common symptoms include nausea and vomiting, malaise, anorexia, and abdominal distention.

Symptoms depend on cancer location, cancer size, and presence of metastases. Left colonic cancers are more likely than right colon cancers to cause partial or complete intestinal obstruction because the left colonic lumen is narrower and the stool in the left colon tends to be better formed because of reabsorption of water in the proximal colon [59]. Large exophytic cancers are also more likely to obstruct the colonic lumen. Partial obstruction produces constipation, nausea, abdominal distention, and abdominal pain. Partial obstruction occasionally paradoxically produces intermittent diarrhea as stool moves beyond the obstruction.

Distal cancers sometimes cause gross rectal bleeding, but proximal cancers rarely produce this symptom because the blood becomes mixed with stool and chemically degraded during colonic transit. Bleeding from proximal cancers tends to be occult, and the patient may present with iron deficiency anemia without gross rectal bleeding. The anemia may produce weakness, fatigue, dyspnea, or palpitations. Advanced cancer, particularly with metastasis, can cause cancer cachexia, characterized by a symptomatic tetrad of involuntary weight loss, anorexia, muscle weakness, and a feeling of poor health.

4.2. Signs

Just as with symptoms, colon cancer tends not to produce signs until advanced. Anemia from gastrointestinal bleeding may produce pallor. Iron deficiency anemia can cause koilonychia manifested by brittle, longitudinally furrowed, and spooned nails; glossitis manifested by lingual erythema and papillae loss; and cheilitis manifested by scaling or fissuring of the lips. Hypoalbuminemia may clinically manifest as peripheral edema, ascites, or anasarca. Hypoactive or high-pitched bowel sounds suggest gastrointestinal obstruction. A palpable abdominal mass is a rare finding that suggests advanced disease. Rectal examination, including fecal occult blood testing (FOBT), is important in the evaluation of possible colon cancer. Rectal cancer may be palpable by digital rectal examination. Other physical findings, although rare, should be systematically searched for, including peripheral lymphadenopathy, especially a Virchow's node in the left supraclavicular space; hepatomegaly from hepatic metastases; and temporal or intercostal muscle wasting from cancer cachexia. Very rare findings with colon cancer include a Sister Mary Joseph node caused by metastases to a periumbilical node, and a Blumer's shelf caused by perirectal extension of the primary tumor.

4.3. Laboratory abnormalities

Patients with suspected colon cancer should have routine blood tests including a hemogram with platelet count determination, serum electrolytes and glucose determination, evaluation of routine serum biochemical parameters of liver function, and a routine coagulation profile. About half of patients with colon cancer are anemic. Anemia, however, is very common, so that only a small minority of patients with anemia have colon cancer. Iron deficiency anemia of undetermined etiology, however, warrants evaluation for colon cancer, particularly in the elderly [60]. Hypoalbuminemia is uncommon, but not rare, in colon cancer. It usually indicates poor nutritional status from advanced cancer. Routine serum biochemical parameters of liver function are usually within normal limits in patients with colon cancer. Abnormalities, particularly elevation of the alkaline phosphatase level, often indicate hepatic metastases. The serum lactate dehydrogenase level may increase with colon cancer. Diarrhea associated with colon cancer can rarely produce electrolyte derangements or dehydration. Nausea and vomiting from colon cancer can rarely produce metabolic derangements of hypovolemia, hypokalemia, or alkalosis.

The serum carcinoembryonic antigen level is not useful to screen for colon cancer. It is only moderately sensitive. Although patients with very advanced cancer tend to have highly elevated levels, patients with early and highly curable colon cancer tend to have only minimally elevated levels, with considerable overlap with the levels of patients without colon cancer. It is poorly specific. Other colonic diseases or systemic disorders can cause a carcinoembryonic antigen elevation. Preoperative testing is, however, useful to determine cancer prognosis and to provide a baseline for comparison with postoperative levels. An elevated serum level preoperatively is a poor prognostic indicator: the higher the serum level the more likely the cancer is extensive and will recur postoperatively. After apparently complete colon cancer resection the serum level almost always normalizes; failure to normalize postoperatively suggests incomplete resection. A sustained and progressive rise after postoperative normalization strongly suggests cancer recurrence. Patients with this finding require prompt surveillance colonoscopy to exclude colonic recurrence and abdominal imaging to exclude metastases.

4.4. Unusual clinical syndromes caused by colon cancer

Colon cancer can cause acute colonic obstruction, most commonly from exophytic intraluminal growth, and most uncommonly from intussusception or volvulus. Obstruction typically occurs in the sigmoid colon because of the narrow lumen and hard stool in this region. Patients present with abdominal pain, nausea and vomiting, obstipation, abdominal tenderness, abdominal distention, and hypoactive bowel sounds. Colon cancer can rarely perforate acutely through the colonic wall and cause acute generalized peritonitis, and can rarely perforate slowly to form a walled-off inflammatory mass or abscess with localized peritoneal signs [61]. Factors promoting colonic perforation include disruption of mucosal integrity because of transmural malignant extension or colonic ischemia, and increased intraluminal pressure because of colonic obstruction. Presentation with colonic obstruction or perforation indicates a poor prognosis. Colon cancer rarely causes ischemic colitis because of colonic dilatation proximal to malignant obstruction or malignant infiltration of blood vessels. Colon cancer occasionally causes gross rectal bleeding because of cancerous mucosal ulceration.

5. Colorectal cancer (crc) – screening

Colorectal cancer is theoretically a preventable disease and is ideally suited to a population screening programme, as there is a long premalignant phase, during which there is ample opportunity to intervene with a variety of different screening modalities.

Most CRCs are thought to arise from benign adenomatous polyps, a process that takes approximately five to ten years. This long premalignant phase makes the disease ideally suited to a population screening programme.

Early detection and removal of precancerous colon polyps and CRC may reduce both incidence and death rates related of CRC. It is recommended to begin screening at age 50 for asymptomatic persons who are at average risk. High-risk patients should have regular colorectal surveillance [45]. Several screening methods are used to detect CRC lesions. Colonoscopy is the best method and final assessment step for detection of CRC.

The ultimate aim of a screening programme for CRC is to reduce mortality from the disease, which may be achieved in two ways. As five-year survival is closely related to the stage at which the cancer is detected (patients with Dukes' stage A cancer have a greater than 90 per cent five-year survival rate, while those with Dukes' stage D disease have a 7 per cent five-year survival rate), any screening modality that results in early detection of the disease will have a beneficial effect on survival through more effective treatment (figure 5). Additionally, if benign adenomatous polyps are removed, cancer development is prevented, resulting in decreased mortality.

http://dx.doi.org/10.5772/53524

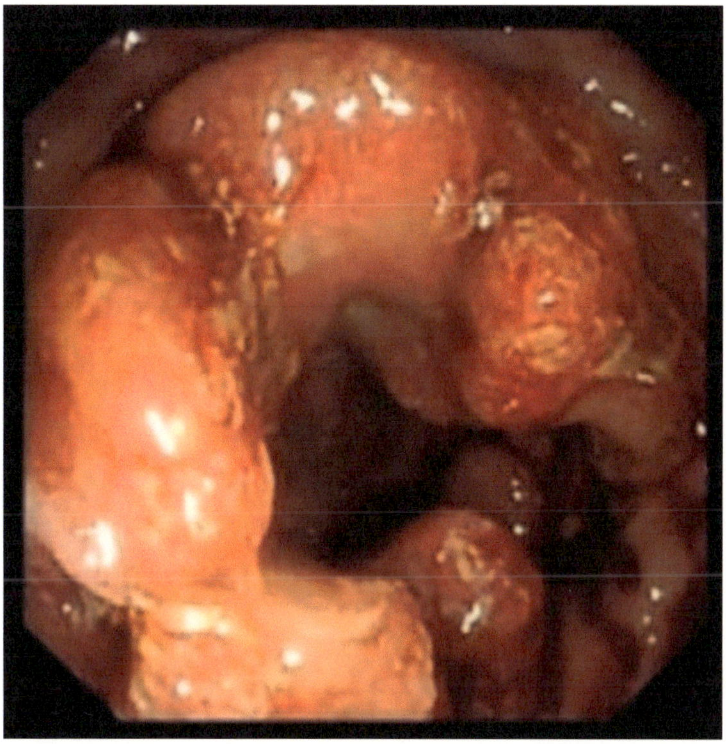

Figure 4. Colorectal cancer

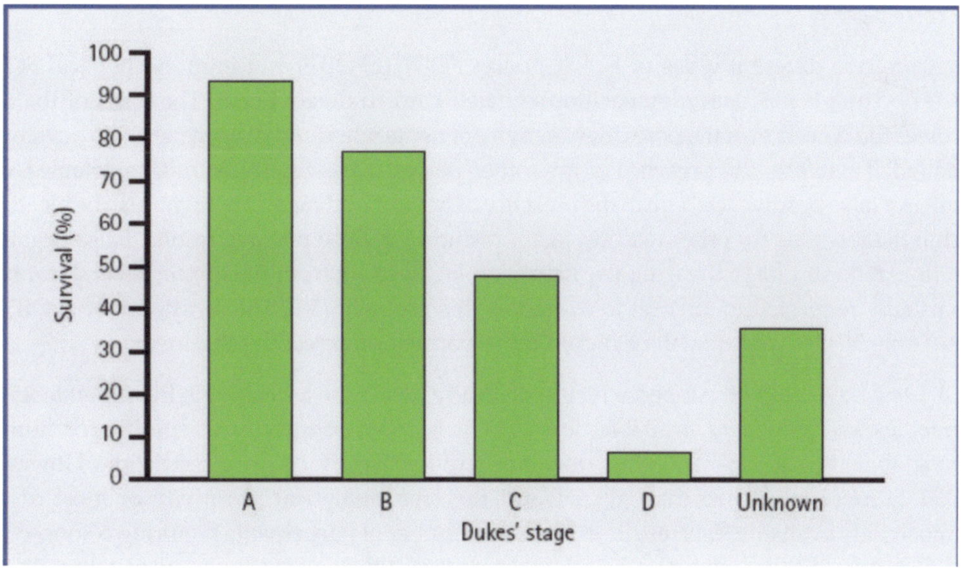

Figure 5. Five-year survival of colorectal cancer for each Dukes' stage at diagnosis

6. Who is at risk of developing colorectal cancer

There is strong tendency that countries with an obviously rising CRC incidence are more "Westernized" in lifestyle, especially in dietary habits, with increased consumption of high fat and protein but less fiber in diet. The change is more evident in urban areas than rural areas of the same country. Most of CRC is sporadic, i.e., caused by the interaction of genetic and environmental factors via the adenomacarcinoma sequence, and cancer may take up to ten years to develop in this way. Adenomas are more common with age, and one in four of the population aged over 50 will develop one or more polyps, with 10% of these polyps progressing to cancer over time.The most common indicator of high risk is a first-degree relative with CRC.

7. Tests for colorectal cancer screening

Tests for CRC include: colonoscopy, flexible sigmoidoscopy (FS), virtual colonoscopy and faecal occult blood testing (FOBt).

7.1. Faecal Occult Blood testing (FOBt)

FOBt has been used widely in CRC screening for several decades. Screening at age 50 for asymptomatic persons who are at average risk with annual and biennial FOBt has been shown in multiple randomized trails to reduce CRC incidence and mortality rates [49].

FOBt can detect occult blood in a small amount of stool sample. It is cheap, non-invasive and easily performed at home. FOBt is based on the propensity of CRC and adenomas to bleed microscopically.

There are two different types of FOBT, guaiac FOBT (gFOBT) and immunochemical FOBT (iFOBT). The gFOBT uses a guaiac-impregnated card to detect heme. The basis of the test involves the detection of the peroxidase activity of heme when a hydrogen peroxide developer is added. Therefore, the presence of any other peroxidases, e.g. from fruit/ vegetables, can result in a false positive test, as can the presence of heme in red meat. There can also be bleeding within the intestine for other reasons, again resulting in false positive results. False negative results can occur due to the irregular nature of the bleeding from the tumor; several samples are usually requested to attempt to overcome this problem [50]. The sensitivity of gFOBT is about only 50% of cancers will be picked up in population screening (figure 6).

iFOBT test have been developed which specifically detect the hemoglobin in human feces by antibodies and is widely available now [51]. It is more sensitive and specific for human hemoglobin than gFOBT and thus does not require dietary or drug restriction. However, iFOBT is more expensive than gFOBT and the high analytical sensitivity of most of the commercially available tests results in a greater number of participants requiring colonoscopy and a greater false positive rate [54]. However, recent developments in quantitative iFOBT may overcome this problem, asthe trigger for investigation can be set at any concentration of fecal hemoglobin. Clinical trials have shown that persons with positive occult-blood tests have

http://dx.doi.org/10.5772/53524

a risk of cancer that is three to four times as high as that among persons with negative tests, and that colonoscopy should be recommended for persons with these positive tests. In a recent study (Quintero et al) it has been shown that both iFOBT and colonoscopy are effective for detecting colorectal cancer but iFOBT is less effective for early detection of premalignant lesions (adenomas) than colonoscopy or sigmoidoscopy [57]. However, comparative studies have shown that iFOBT is more accurate than the gFOBT for the detection of colorectal cancer and advanced adenomas and this new test is now recommended as the first-choice fecal occult blood test in colorectal-cancer screening.

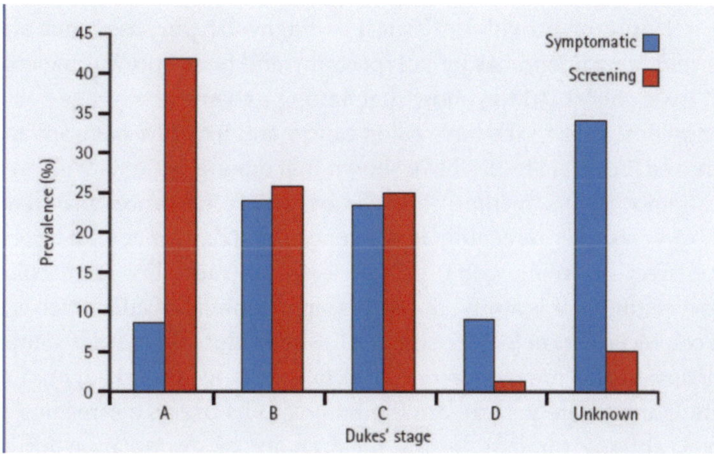

Figure 6. Dukes' stage of colorectal cancers detected by faecal occult blood test screening compared to those diagnosed in patients presenting with symptoms

7.2. Flexible sigmoidoscopy

Flexible sigmoidoscopy has also been used as a screening tool for CRC detection, as half of all cancers are seen in the rectum or sigmoid colon. There have been several studies suggesting benefit from flexible sigmoidoscopy, and their data suggest that flexible sigmoidoscopy would be an effective screening tool. Flexible sigmoidoscopy as an alternative to colonoscopy has the advantage that no oral bowel preparation is required, as the subject uses an enema that can be taken at home.The procedure is quick, requires no sedation and examines the left colon, which is the site of 75 per cent of all colorectal neoplasia. If CO_2 insufflation is used, adenomas can be resected at the initial screening examination. This procedure does not, however, examine the right colon. For many clinicians and patients, colonoscopy is more appealing than flexible sigmoidoscopy because patients can be sedated and undergo a complete colon examination with polypectomy.

7.3. Virtual colonoscopy

Virtual colonoscopy, or computed tomography colonography (CTC), is another modality used to examine the colon. It has been suggested that this examination has fewer complications and increased patient satisfaction when compared to colonoscopy, but with similar sensitivity and specificity for the detection of pathology. There is no requirement for sedation and it has the advantage of detecting extracolonic pathology. It does, however, still require bowel preparation and colonic insufflation with CO_2, the latter still causing discomfort. Furthermore, it is not therapeutic and the lesions detected require endoscopic evaluation and resection.

7.4. Colonoscopy

Colonoscopy is the gold standard investigation for the diagnosis of CRC. It is highly sensitive and specific for detecting both cancers and adenomas of at least 1 cm in diameter and has the added benefit not only of providing tissue for diagnostic purposes, but also affords the opportunity of removing adenomas by polypectomy and hence preventing colorectal cancer (CRC). Several large cohort studies show that among patients at average risk who undergo screening colonoscopy, 0.5 to 1.0% have colon cancer and 5 to 10% have advanced neoplasia that can be removed. Several studies have shown that among patients with an adenoma that is detected and removed at screening colonoscopy, colorectal cancer may develop in 0.3 to 0.9% within 3 to 5 years after screening. In a recent study (Zauber et al) it has been evaluated the long -term effect of colonoscopic polypectomy on mortality from colorectal cancer. According to the results of this study, the endoscopic removal of adenomas ends in reduced mortality from colorectal cancer [56]. To sum up, this procedure is considered the most accurate test for early detection and prevention of colorectal cancer as it markedly reduces the risk of CRC and death. Unfortunately, there are limitations to its use as a screening modality on a population level, although it may be the ideal choice of examination for an individual. Colonoscopy is invasive and time consuming,and requires full bowel preparation; the complication rate, although low, may still be unacceptable within a screening population.

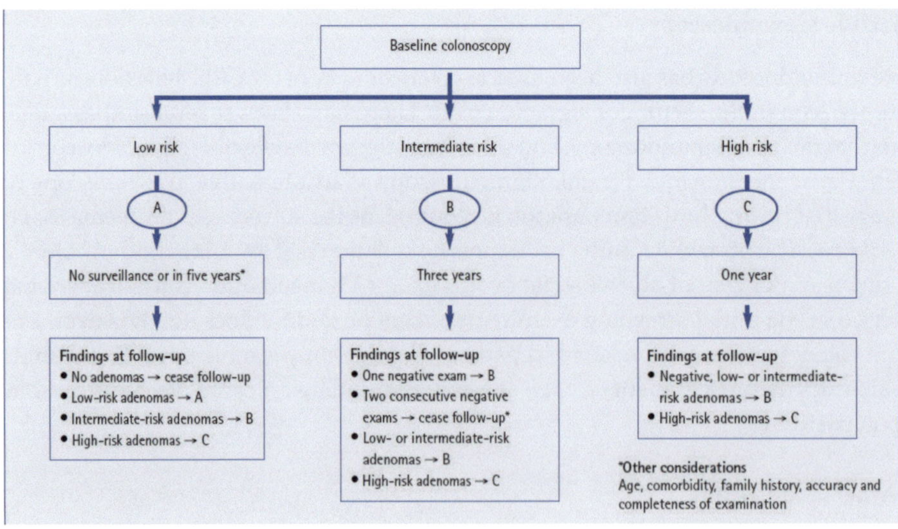

Figure 7. British Society of Gastroenterology guidelines for follow-up of adenoma removal.

http://dx.doi.org/10.5772/53524

8. Conclusions and recommendations

Although there are several methods available for CRC screening, none is optimal. Patients at average risk for CRC should begin screening at age 50 with either annual FOBT, flexible sigmoidoscopy every 5 years or colonoscopy every 10 years. Evidence does not show any strategy as optimal, so clinicians should discuss the advantages and disadvantages of the various screening techniques with patients. Patients with a family history of CRC or adenomas or a personal history of high-risk polyps or inflammatory bowel disease should begin screening earlier (figure 7). Routine screening in persons older than 75 years of age is not recommended. Life expectancy, rather than age alone, should guide decisions about when to stop CRC screening.

Author details

Kouklakis S. Georgios and Asimenia D. Bampali

Medical School Democritus, University of Thrace, Greece

References

[1] Jemal A, Bray F, Center MM, et al. Global cancer statistics. CA Cancer J Clin 2011; 61:69.

[2] Siegel R, Naishadham D, Jemal A. Cancer statistics, 2012. CA Cancer J Clin 2012; 62:10.

[3] Kohler BA, Ward E, McCarthy BJ, et al. Annual report to the nation on the status of cancer, 1975-2007, featuring tumors of the brain and other nervous system. J Natl Cancer Inst 2011; 103:714.

[4] Davis DM, Marcet JE, Frattini JC, et al. Is it time to lower the recommended screening age for colorectal cancer? J Am Coll Surg 2011; 213:352.

[5] Jemal A, Siegel R, Xu J, Ward E. Cancer statistics, 2010. CA Cancer J Clin 2010; 60:277.

[6] Troisi RJ, Freedman AN, Devesa SS. Incidence of colorectal carcinoma in the U.S.: an update of trends by gender, race, age, subsite, and stage, 1975-1994. Cancer 1999; 85:1670.

[7] Jessup JM, McGinnis LS, Steele GD Jr, et al. The National Cancer Data Base.

[8] Colorectal Cancer: Epidemiology, Etiology, and Molecular Basis. Harvey G Moore, Nancy N. Baxter and Jose G. Guillem

[9] Sanoff HK, Sargent DJ, Campbell ME, et al. Five-year data and prognostic factor analysis of oxaliplatin and irinotecan combinations for advanced colorectal cancer: N9741. *J Clin Oncol*. Dec 10 2008;26(35):5721-7.

[10] Chu, E and DeVita VT. Physicians' cancer chemotherapy drug manual. *Jones and Bartlett publishers*. 2008.

[11] Vogelstein B, Fearon ER, Hamilton SR, Kern SE, Preisinger AC, Leppert M, et al. Genetic alterations during colorectal-tumor development. *N Engl J Med*. Sep 1 1988;319(9): 525-32.

[12] Sinicrope FA, Foster NR, Thibodeau SN, et al. DNA mismatch repair status and colon cancer recurrence and survival in clinical trials of 5-fluorouracil-based adjuvant therapy. *J Natl Cancer Inst*. Jun 8 2011;103(11):863-75.

[13] Jemal A, Siegel R, Ward E, et al. Cancer Statistics, 2008. CA Cancer J Clin 2008; 58:71-96; originally published online; DOI: 10.3322/CA2007.0010. Feb 20, 2008

[14] Rothwell PM, Fowkes GR, Belch JF, Ogawa H, Warlow CP, Meade TW. Effect of daily aspirin on long-term risk of death due to cancer: analysis of individual patient data from randomized trials. *Lancet*. Dec 7/2010; Early online publication

[15] Burn J, Gerdes AM, Macrae F, et al. Long-term effect of aspirin on cancer risk in carriers of hereditary colorectal cancer: an analysis from the CAPP2 randomised controlled trial. *Lancet*. Dec 17 2011;378(9809):2081-7.

[16] Baillargeon J, Kuo YF, Lin YL, et al. Effect of mental disorders on diagnosis, treatment, and survival of older adults with colon cancer. *J Am Geriatr Soc*. Jul 2011;59(7):1268-73.

[17] Phipps AI, Baron J, Newcomb PA. Prediagnostic smoking history, alcohol consumption, and colorectal cancer survival: The Seattle Colon Cancer Family Registry. *Cancer*. Nov 1 2011;117(21):4948-57.

[18] Dehal AN, Newton CC, Jacobs EJ, et al. Impact of diabetes mellitus and insulin use on survival after colorectal cancer diagnosis: the Cancer Prevention Study-II Nutrition Cohort. *J Clin Oncol*. Jan 1 2012;30(1):53-9.

[19] Yothers G, Sargent DJ, Wolmark N, et al. Outcomes Among Black Patients With Stage II and III Colon Cancer Receiving Chemotherapy: An Analysis of ACCENT Adjuvant Trials. *J Natl Cancer Inst*. Oct 19 2011;103(20):1498-1506.

[20] Lasser KE, Murillo J, Lisboa S, et al. Colorectal cancer screening among ethnically diverse, low-income patients: a randomized controlled trial. *Arch Intern Med*. May 23 2011;171(10):906-12.

[21] [Best Evidence] Burn J, Bishop DT, Mecklin JP, Macrae F, et al. Effect of aspirin or resistant starch on colorectal neoplasia in the Lynch syndrome. *N Engl J Med*. Dec 11 2008;359(24):2567-78.

[22] Meyerhardt JA, Niedzwiecki D, Hollis D, et al. Association of dietary patterns with cancer recurrence and survival in patients with stage III colon cancer. *JAMA*. Aug 15 2007;298(7):754-64.

[23] Aune D, Chan DS, Lau R, et al. Dietary fibre, whole grains, and risk of colorectal cancer: systematic review and dose-response meta-analysis of prospective studies. *BMJ*. Nov 10 2011;343:d6617.

[24] Pala V, Sieri S, Berrino F, et al. Yogurt consumption and risk of colorectal cancer in the Italian European prospective investigation into cancer and nutrition cohort. *Int J Cancer*. Dec 1 2011;129(11):2712-9.

[25] Yuhara H, Steinmaus C, Cohen SE, Corley DA, Tei Y, Buffler PA. Is diabetes mellitus an independent risk factor for colon cancer and rectal cancer?. *Am J Gastroenterol*. Nov 2011;106(11):1911-21; quiz 1922.

[26] Jacobs ET, Ahnen DJ, Ashbeck EL, Baron JA, Greenberg ER, Lance P, et al. Association between body mass index and colorectal neoplasia at follow-up colonoscopy: a pooling study. *Am J Epidemiol*. Mar 15 2009;169(6):657-66.

[27] Ogino S, Kawasaki T, Kirkner GJ, Ohnishi M, Fuchs CS. 18q loss of heterozygosity in microsatellite stable colorectal cancer is correlated with CpG island methylator phenotype-negative (CIMP-0) and inversely with CIMP-low and CIMP-high. *BMC Cancer*. May 2 2007;7:72.

[28] [Best Evidence] Quasar Collaborative Group, Gray R, Barnwell J, et al. Adjuvant chemotherapy versus observation in patients with colorectal cancer: a randomised study. *Lancet*. Dec 15 2007;370(9604):2020-9.

[29] Saltz LB, Kelsen DP. Adjuvant treatment of colorectal cancer. *Annu Rev Med*. 1997;48:191-202.

[30] Ribic CM, Sargent DJ, Moore MJ, et al. Tumor microsatellite-instability status as a predictor of benefit from fluorouracil-based adjuvant chemotherapy for colon cancer. *N Engl J Med*. Jul 17 2003;349(3):247-57.

[31] Mlecnik B, Tosolini M, Kirilovsky A, Berger A, Bindea G, Meatchi T, et al. Histopathologic-based prognostic factors of colorectal cancers are associated with the state of the local immune reaction. *J Clin Oncol*. Feb 20 2011;29(6):610-8.

[32] [Best Evidence] Gunderson LL, Jessup JM, Sargent DJ, Greene FL, Stewart AK. Revised TN categorization for colon cancer based on national survival outcomes data. *J Clin Oncol*. Jan 10 2010;28(2):264-71.

[33] Tournigand C, Andre T, Achille E, et al. FOLFIRI followed by FOLFOX6 or the reverse sequence in advanced colorectal cancer: a randomized GERCOR study. *J Clin Oncol*. Jan 15 2004;22(2):229-37.

[34] [Best Evidence] Arkenau HT, Arnold D, Cassidy J, Diaz-Rubio E, Douillard JY, Hochster H, et al. Efficacy of oxaliplatin plus capecitabine or infusional fluorouracil/leucovorin in patients with metastatic colorectal cancer: a pooled analysis of randomized trials. *J Clin Oncol*. Dec 20 2008;26(36):5910-7.

[35] Meat and cancer. *Meat Sci*. 2010;84(2):308-13.

[36] Case-control study on beneficial effect of regular consumption of apples on colorectal cancer risk in apopulation with relatively low intake of fruits and vegetables. Eur J Cancer Prev. 2010;19(1):42-7.

[37] Lifestyle, occupational, and reproductive factors and risk of colorectal cancer. *Dis Colon Rectum*.2010;53(5):830-7.

[38] Colorectal cancer and inflammatory bowel disease: epidemiology, risk factors, mechanisms of carcinogenesisand prevention strategies. *Anticancer Res*. 2009;29(7):2727-37.

[39] Ferlay J, Shin HR, Bray F, Forman D, Mathers C, Parkin DM. GLOBOCAN 2008, Cancer Incidence and Mortality Worldwide: IARC CancerBase No. 10 Lyon, France: International Agency for Research on Cancer; 2010. Available from: http://globocan.iarc.fr

[40] Miladinov-Mikov M. Epidemiologija raka debelog creva i rektuma. In: Gudurić B, Breberina M, Jovanović D, editors. Rak debelog creva u Vojvodini. Monografija. Novi Sad: Vojvođanska akademija nauka i umetnosti, Institut za onkologiju Vojvodine; 2009. p. 9-25.

[41] Registar za maligne neoplazme Vojvodine, Institut za onkologiju Vojvodine, nepublikovani podaci

[42] Miladinov-Mikov M, Lukic N, Petrovic T. Epidemiological characteristics of colorectal cancer in Vojvodina. In: Riboli E, Lambert R, editors. Nutrition and Lifestyle: Opportunities for Cancer Prevention. International Agency for Research on Cancer. Lyon: IARC Sci Publ; 2002;156:547-8.

[43] Ferlay J, Parkin DM, Steliarova-Foucher E. Estimates of cancer incidence and mortality in Europe in 2008. *Eur J Cancer*. 2010;46(4):765-81.

[44] Rachet B, et al. Population-based cancer survival trends in England and Wales up to 2007: an assessment of the NHS cancer plan for England. *The Lancet Oncology*. 2009.

[45] 45.Chien-Kuo Liu *Division of Colorectal Surgery, Mackay Memorial Hospital,Taipei, Taiwan*

[46] 46. Mandel JS, Bond JH, Church TR, et al. Reducing mortality from colorectal cancer by screening for fecal occult blood. Minnesota Colon Cancer ControlStudy. N Engl J Med 328: 1365-71, 1993.

[47] Bureau of National Health Insurance, Department of Health, R.O.C. (Taiwan). Cancer mortality in Taiwan, 2009.

[48] Levin B, Lieberman DA, McFarland B, et al. Screening and surveillance for early detection of colorectal cancer and adenomatous polyps, 2008:a joint guideline from the American Cancer Society, the US Multi-Society Task Force on Colorectal Cancer, and the American College of Radiology. Gastroenterology 134: 1570-95, 2008.

[49] Levin B, Brooks D, Smith R, et al. Emerging technologies in screening for colorectal cancer:CT colonography, immunochemical fecal occult blood tests and stool screening using molecular markers. CA Cancer J Clin 53: 44-55, 2003.

[50] Hardcastle JD, Chamberlain JO, Robinson MH, et al. Randomized controlled trial of fecal-occult blood screening for colorectal cancer. Lancet 348: 1472-7, 1996.

[51] Smith A, Young GP, Cole SR, et al. Comparison of a brush-sampling fecal immunochemical test for hemoglobin with a sensitive guaiac-based fecal occult blood test in detection of colorectal neoplasia. Cancer 107: 2152-9, 2006.

[52] Fraser CG, Mathew CM, Mowat NA, et al. Evaluation of a card collection-based fecal immunochemical test in screening for colorectal cancer using two-tier reflex approach. Gut 56: 1415-8, 2007.

[53] Imperiale TF. Quantitative immunochemical fecal occult blood tests: is it time to go back to the future? Ann Intern Med 146: 309-11, 2007.

[54] Mandel JS, Bond JH, Church TR, et al. Reducing mortality from colorectal cancer by screening for fecal occult blood. Minnesota Colon Cancer Control Study. N Engl J Med 328: 1365-71, 1993. [Erratum, N Engl J Med 1993;329:672.]

[55] Kronborg O, Fenger C, Olsen J, et al. Randomised study of screening for colorectal cancer with faecal-occult-blood test. Lancet 348: 1467-71, 1996.

[56] Colonoscopic Polypectomy and Long-Term Prevention of Colorectal-Cancer Deaths Ann G. Zauber, Ph.D., Sidney J. Winawer, M.D., Michael J. O'Brien, M.D., M.P.H., Iris Lansdorp-Vogelaar, Ph.D., Marjolein van Ballegooijen, M.D., Ph.D., Benjamin F. Hankey, Sc.D., Weiji Shi, M.S., John H. Bond, M.D., Melvin Schapiro, M.D., Joel F. Panish, M.D., Edward T. Stewart, M.D., and Jerome D. Waye, M.D. N Engl J Med 2012; 366:687-696 February 23, 2012

[57] Colonoscopy versus Fecal Immunochemical Testing in Colorectal-Cancer Screening Enrique Quintero, M.D., Ph.D., Antoni Castells, M.D., Ph.D., Luis Bujanda, M.D., Ph.D., Joaquín Cubiella, M.D., Ph.D., Dolores Salas, M.D., Ángel Lanas, M.D., Ph.D., Montserrat Andreu, M.D., Ph.D., Fernando Carballo, M.D., Ph.D., Juan Diego Morillas, M.D., Ph.D., Cristina Hernández, B.Sc., Rodrigo Jover, M.D., Ph.D., Isabel Montalvo, M.D., Ph.D., Juan Arenas, M.D., Ph.D., Eva Laredo, R.N., Vicent Hernández, M.D., Ph.D., Felipe Iglesias, R.N., Estela Cid, R.N., Raquel Zubizarreta, M.D., Teresa Sala, M.D., Marta Ponce, M.D., Mercedes Andrés, M.D., Gloria Teruel, M.D., Antonio Peris, M.D., María-Pilar Roncales, R.N., Mónica Polo-Tomás, M.D., Ph.D., Xavier Bessa, M.D., Ph.D., Olga Ferrer-Armengou, R.N., Jaume Grau, M.D., Anna Serradesanferm, R.N., Akiko Ono, M.D., José Cruzado, M.D., Francisco Pérez-Riquelme, M.D., Inmaculada Alonso-Abreu, M.D., Mariola de la Vega-Prieto, M.D., Juana Maria Reyes-Melian, M.D., Guillermo Cacho, M.D., José Díaz-Tasende, M.D., Alberto Herreros-de-Tejada, M.D., Carmen Poves, M.D., Cecilio Santander, M.D., and Andrés González-Navarro, M.D. for the COLONPREV Study Investigators N Engl J Med 2012; 366:697-706February 23, 2012

[58] Bond JH. Polyp guidelines: diagnosis, treatment, and surveillance for patients with colorectal polyps. Practice Parameters Committee of the American College of Gastroenterology. Am J Gastroenterol 2000;95:3053–63.

[59] Smith R, Cokkinides V, Eyre H. American Cancer Society guidelines for the early detectionof cancer. CA Cancer J Clin 2003;53:27–43.

[60] Smith RA, von Eschenbach AC, Wender R, Levin B, Byers T, Rothenberger D, et al.American Cancer Society guidelines for the early detection of cancer: update of early detection guidelines for prostate, colorectal, and endometrial cancers. Also: update 2001 –testing for early lung cancer detection. CA Cancer J Clin 2001;51:38–75.

[61] Winawer SJ, Fletcher RH, Miller L, Godlee F, Stolar MH, Mulrow CD, et al. Colorectal cancer screening: clinical guidelines and rationale. Gastroenterology 1997;112:594-642.

Chapter 2

Issues in Screening and Surveillance Colonoscopy

Anjali Mone, Robert Mocharla, Allison Avery and
Fritz Francois

Additional information is available at the end of the chapter

http://dx.doi.org/10.5772/53111

1. Introduction

Colorectal cancer (CRC) is a major cause of morbidity and mortality throughout the world. However timely screening and treatment can dramatically impact outcomes. The association with well-defined precancerous lesions and long asymptomatic period provides the opportunity for effective screening and early treatment of CRC. The current options for CRC screening are strongly anchored in evidence demonstrating utility in reducing morbidity and mortality. This chapter will review the epidemiology of CRC, risk stratification, strategies for screening, as well as factors that threaten achieving health equity through appropriate screening programs.

2. Epidemiologic trends in colorectal cancer

Worldwide CRC is the third most common cancer and fourth most common cause of death. Interestingly this disease affects men and women almost equally (Haggar and Boushey, 2009). In the United States CRC is the third most commonly diagnosed cancer and constitutes 10% of new cancers in men and women (Society, 2011). In 2011, there were approximately 141,120 new cases and it is estimated that 143,460 Americans will be diagnosed with colorectal cancer in 2012 (NIH, 2009). Furthermore it is estimated up to 30% of new cases are found in the general population without known risk factors for this disease (Imperiale et al., 2000). Although there are still approximately one million new cases of CRC diagnosed each year, incidence has been steadily declining over the past 15 years (Bresalier, 2009; Ferlay et al., 2010; Kohler et al., 2011). In the United States mortality from CRC has also declined with a 7% decrease in men and 12% decrease in women between 1980 and 1990 (Jemal et al., 2008). Since 1990 decreases in CRC incidence and mortality have been even more substantial, and is largely attributable to improvements in screening rates (Lieberman, 2010), especially the growing use of colonoscopy procedures (Edwards et al., 2010). Nevertheless, important trends remain in the worldwide epidemiology of CRC.

2.1. Geographic variations in CRC epidemiology

There is significant diversity in colorectal cancer incidence worldwide. Surprisingly industrialized nations have a remarkably greater occurrence of CRC accounting for 63% of all cases. In fact CRC incidence rates range from more than 40 per 100,000 people in the United States, Australia, New Zealand, and Western Europe to less than 5 per 100,000 in Africa and parts of Asia. It is notable that the US is the only country with significantly declining CRC incidence rates for both genders, and this is most likely a reflection of better screening practices and early prevention (Jemal et al., 2011).

While there is substantial disparity in CRC occurrence globally, CRC incidence has been increasing in places previously reporting low rates. For example the number of new CRC diagnoses has been rising in a number of Asian countries that recently transitioned from low-income to high-income economies. Individuals residing in China, Japan, India, Singapore, and Eastern European countries were previously reported to have the lowest rates of CRC. Countries with the highest incidence rates include Australia, New Zealand, Canada, the United States, and parts of Europe, however incidence has started stabilizing and even declining in these regions (Haggar and Boushey, 2009; Jemal et al., 2010).

Interestingly CRC incidence seems to have a close association with location. In fact studies show that migrants rapidly acquire the risk patterns for CRC associated with their new surroundings. For example the incidence rates in Japanese immigrants have been found to significantly increase after moving to the United States. Geographic influence is also evident in a study done in Israel where male Jews of Western descent were found to have a higher likelihood of developing CRC than those born in Africa or Asia. Furthermore environment may be responsible for variations within ethnic groups. This is demonstrated by higher rates of CRC among American Indians living in Alaska than those residing in the Southwest. Incidence rates among black males were found to range from 46.4 cases per 100,000 individuals in Arizona to 82.4 per 100,000 in Kentucky. In white men rates range from 44.4 per 100,000 in Utah to 68.7 per 100,000 in North Dakota (The Centers for Disease Control and Prevention [CDC], 2011).

The importance of location can also be seen by differences in CRC incidence within specific genders. CRC mortality rates for men are lower in Western states excluding Nevada, and higher in Southern and Midwestern states. These differences in CRC rates may be attributable to regional variations in risk factors including diet and lifestyle as well as access to screening and treatment. In fact one study found that up to 43% of colorectal cancers are preventable through diet and lifestyle modifications (Perera P.S., 2012).

2.2. Racial and ethnic variations

There is substantial evidence demonstrating racial disparities in CRC risk particularly for black men. In the USA this group has been found to have 20% higher incidence rate and 45% higher mortality rate from colorectal cancer compared to whites (Jemal et al., 2008; Wallace and Suzuki, 2012). There are also significant differences in life expectancy among blacks compared to whites. While there was a 39% reduction in mortality rate for white men between 1960-2005, during the same period there was a dramatic 28% increase in mortality for black men (Soneji et al., 2010). Of note incidence rates among other racial groups including Hispanics, Asian Americans, and American Indians are lower than those among whites. The factors that underlie these differences have not been fully elucidated but most likely encompass both modifiable factors (e.g. smoking, socioeconomic status, body mass index, and cultural beliefs) as well as non-modifiable factors (e.g. race/ethnicity, gender, and genetic predisposition). These findings do suggest there is a need for appropriate risk stratification for CRC and for more aggressive screening in high-risk populations, particularly among blacks in the United States. Such an approach has been recommended by both the American College of Gastroenterology as well as the American Society for Gastrointestinal Endoscopy with the suggestion to start screening blacks at the age of 45 (Cash et al., 2010; Rex et al., 2009).

2.3. The gender gap

According to SEER 2012 statistics, the overall prevalence of colorectal cancer does not vary substantially between the genders. The lifetime risk of being diagnosed with CRC is similar for men 5.7% and women 5.2%. The lifetime risk of dying from CRC is also similar; 2.3% and 2.1% for men and women respectively (NIH, 2009). Even though annually the new diagnoses of CRC have roughly been equal in men (187,973) and women (185,983), men have higher age-adjusted CRC incidence rates (Abotchie et al., 2012). Women seem have a delay of approximately 7-8 years in the development of advanced polyps (Jaroslaw Regula, 2012; Lieberman et al., 2005). Additionally age adjusted mortality rates can be up to 35-40% higher in men compared to women (CDC, 2011). Gender related disparities are not completely understood but may be attributable to variations in hormonal exposure (Chlebowski et al., 2004). These biological differences related to sex raise the issue of whether men and women should be screened differently for CRC. However current screening guidelines have not been modified based on gender (Levin et al., 2008).

2.4. Modifiers of the epidemiologic trends

Despite some overall gains, several factors remain that impact the epidemiology of CRC. Advancements in elucidating CRC pathogenesis allow for explanations of the above epidemiologic trends and have the potential for more efficient screening and treatment. It is estimated that up to 70% of CRC cases occur sporadically in individuals with no identifiable risks (Hardy et al., 2000). Factors that predispose individuals to a higher risk for developing CRC include any personal or family history of CRC or adenomatous polyps, inflammatory bowel disease (IBD), and inherited genetic syndromes such as familial adenomatous polyposis (FAP), hereditary nonpolyposis colorectal cancer (HNPCC). Guidelines recommend earlier and more aggressive screening for this high-risk population.

As evidenced by the presence of both modifiable and non-modifiable risk factors, the pathogenesis of CRC seems to be influenced by a combination of genetics and the environment. Indeed the disease results from the progressive accumulation of both genetic as well as epigenetic changes in the colonic epithelium. Currently genetic tests are available that identify patients with inherited mutations associated with FAP and HNPCC. While this technology is promising, only 2-6% of CRC cases are attributable to common inherited mutations, suggesting other variables are playing a role in the development of this disease (Winawer et al., 2003).

Some of the environmental influences that have been investigated include the role of Streptococcus Bovis. Although infections are recognized as a major preventable cause in cancer, an infectious etiology has not been identified in cases of sporadic CRC, strongly suggesting that more factors are involved in the development of this disease (Boleij and Tjalsma, 2012). Similar to many other cancers, an important common thread in the pathogenesis of CRC is the presence of chronic inflammation that is thought to increase the probability of mutagenic events that lead to the production of oxidative species and damage DNA causing genomic instability (Zauber et al., 2008). This is demonstrated by patients with inherited genetic mutations who are found on colonoscopic examination to have chronic inflammatory changes that precede tumor development (Terzic et al., 2010). This can also be seen in patients colonized with S. Bovis who are found to have inflammatory changes in the bowel wall (Terzic et al., 2010). Further support for an inflammatory basis is found in recent studies showing aspirin and non-steroidal, anti-inflammatory drugs greatly reduce the risk of CRC (Rothwell et al., 2012).

2.5. Impact of screening on the epidemiology of CRC

Numerous studies show favorable CRC outcomes if the cancer is identified and treated at an early stage. In fact the 5-year survival rate is greater than 90% if CRC is identified at an early stage. However if the cancer extends beyond the colon, 5-year survival is less than 10% (Collett et al., 1999). Continuing advances in CRC therapies hold the promise of adequate treatment for advanced stages of the disease. A recent study in Nature suggests the possibility of helping patients with advanced stage CRC with targeted drugs. This study suggests that there are a finite number of genetic pathways in CRC that can be therapeutically targeted. Although these findings are promising much work is still needed before there will be a cure for CRC (Muzny et al., 2012).

Given the limited effective treatment for advanced CRC, prevention through early detection is paramount. CRC is a model disease for routine population screening since it is prevalent, has a long asymptomatic period, and precancerous lesions can be identified and treated (Pezzoli et al., 2007). Compared to other cancers where the primary goal is early detection of neoplasia, CRC can actually be prevented with detection and removal of cancer precursor lesions (Inadomi et al., 2012). It is estimated that 30% of people over the age of 50 with no history of CRC risk factors harbor adenomatous polyps (Alberti et al., 2012; Pezzoli et al., 2007), and the incidence of these polyps increases with age. Early adenoma resection is asso-

http://dx.doi.org/10.5772/53111

ciated with considerable reductions in CRC (Rex et al., 2009; Winawer et al., 1993b), and has now been demonstrated to have mortality benefit (Zauber et al., 2012).

Although it is difficult to identify precisely which adenomas will undergo neoplastic transformation, there are certain pathologic features that can help predict their level of risk: increased size ≥10 mm, increased number of 3 or more adenomas, villous histology, and high-grade dysplasia (Alberti et al., 2012; Lieberman et al., 2012). Most adenomas undergo a similar progression to invasive cancer termed the adenoma-carcinoma sequence (Levin et al., 2008; Sano et al., 2009). Given that these cancer precursors are often asymptomatic, there is compelling evidence to support early screening for healthy individuals. In fact the average-risk individuals compose 70-75% of the CRC population (Lieberman, 2010). In response to mounting evidence suggesting that screening of average-risk individuals allows for early cancer detection and prevention, CRC guidelines from several organizations were updated in 2008 (USPSTF, 2008).

2.6. CRC prevention tests

Colonoscopy allows for the direct visualization of the entire colon and for the potential to remove lesions that are identified. Results from the National Polyp Study confirm that colonoscopy and adenoma removal is associated with decreased rates of developing colon cancer in the future (Winawer S.J., 2006) and reduces mortality (Zauber et al., 2012). The finding that mortality is reduced by polypectomy is of major significance because it suggests that colonoscopy can identify a subset of adenomas which can potentially become aggressive cancers and provides further evidence that colonoscopy is in fact the best screening option because of its added benefit of decreased mortality, particularly in individuals at increased risk. In patients with no lesions detected during a screening colonoscopic examination, the interval for follow-up surveillance can be extended to 10 years compared to 5 years for sigmoidoscopy (which visualizes only the left side of the colon) along with FOBT every 3 years. The known draw backs to colonoscopy include the need for bowel prep, sedation that may be associated with cardiopulmonary risks, higher cost compared to other methods, association with greater risk of bleeding and perforation, and a miss rate of up to 5% for malignant colon lesions.

While colonoscopy remains the gold standard for CRC prevention, economic constraints and patient attitudes may prevent screening with this technique. In an effort to improve participation alternative tests have been endorsed. There are a range of screening methods that are categorized into two major groups, prevention and detection. Prevention tests detect cancer as well as pre-cancerous polyps, and are generally structural exams such as the colonoscopy, flexible sigmoidoscopy, CT colonography, and double-contrast barium enema. Detection tests are only able to identify CRC lesions and consist of fecal tests including the fecal immunochemical test (FIT), fecal occult blood testing (FOBT), and Fecal DNA testing (Rex et al., 2009).

Flexible Sigmoidoscopy remains an acceptable alternative to colonoscopy for colorectal cancer screening (Levin et al., 2008; USPSTF, 2008; Winawer et al., 2003; Winawer et al., 1997). Although both screening techniques are similar, sigmoidoscopy requires more frequent screenings at 5–year intervals and the benefits are confined to the distal colon only. In addition the USPSTF recommends screening with FOBT every 3 years (USPSTF, 2008). Prior studies have demonstrated a significant mortality benefit for the section of the colon examined (Wilkins and Reynolds, 2008). A recent study in the NEJM confirmed this data showing that flexible sigmoidoscopy decreases CRC incidence and mortality (Schoen et al., 2012). The advantages of sigmoidoscopy include lower cost, lower risk profile, and need for less bowel preparation compared to colonoscopy. However a major setback for this alternative is that polyp visualization is limited to the distal colon. Studies have shown that up to 30% of patients with distal colon cancer also have synchronous proximal lesions that will be missed by sigmoidoscopy (Francois et al., 2006; Imperiale et al., 2000; Lieberman et al., 2000). As such individuals with polyps in the distal colon should undergo follow up with colonoscopy given the increased prevalence of synchronous right-sided lesions. Screening only 50% of colon will preclude detection of the lesions in the portion of the colon not within reach of the sigmoidoscope. This test would also not be an appropriate screening tool for women, patients over the age of 60, patients with HIV, and African Americans who have a higher likelihood of harboring proximal polyps (Bini et al., 2006; Lieberman et al., 2000; Lieberman et al., 2005; Schoenfeld et al., 2005).

Double contrast Barium enema allows for visualization of the entire colon and must be completed every 5 years. Its high polyp miss rate (as high as 23%), lack of therapeutic intervention (another procedure is needed to remove detected polyps), and concerns regarding radiation exposure, have limited its use (Toma et al., 2008; Wilkins and Reynolds, 2008).

CT colonography is able to provide information about the entire colon and has been proposed as a possible screening option for patients who decline conventional colonoscopy. This test is less invasive compared to conventional colonoscopy, is associated with decreased risk of perforation and does not require sedation (Lieberman, 2010). Not only are detection rates far superior to the barium enema, but CT colonography (CTC) has comparable sensitivity to colonoscopy for polyps 10mm or greater in size (Johnson et al., 2008). However relative to other options, this modality is costly, and has poor sensitivity for polyps less than 7mm (Lieberman, 2010). Due to insufficient evidence for performance metrics this test is currently not supported by established guidelines. The United States Preventive Services Task Force expresses additional concern about the impact and extra costs related to following-up extra-colonic findings (USPSTF, 2008). In fact an estimated 27% to 69% of tests performed uncover abnormal extra-colonic findings (Lieberman, 2010). More studies are needed to assess this procedure's benefits and risks, particularly to determine whether this method may be missing significant lesions.

Capsule Endoscopy provides direct visualization of the colonic mucosa via an ingestible capsule with video cameras at both ends that wireless transmits images to a receiver. Given that bowel motility significantly affects results, this test is not performed regularly and is not supported by current guidelines.

http://dx.doi.org/10.5772/53111

2.7. CRC detection tests

Fecal occult blood testing (FOBT) is an annual stool test that detects cancer at an early stage. The USPSTF now specifically recommends the high-sensitivity guaiac-based testing (Hemoccult Sensa) over the standard guaiac-based testing (Hemoccult II) (USPSTF, 2008). Based on the premise that colon cancer intermittently bleeds, the FOBT tests for blood by detecting the peroxidase activity of heme (Lieberman, 2010). Not only is the test economical and convenient, patients with a positive test result have an almost 4 fold increased likelihood having cancer (Winawer et al., 2003). In fact studies have found FOBT reduces mortality by approximately 33% over a 10-year period (Lieberman, 2010). Another study reported approximately 20% reduction in mortality when FOBT was compared to controls over an 18-year period (Lieberman, 2010). Supporters of the FOBT question whether invasive measures such as the colonoscopy are harmful given that computer simulated modeling shows similar life-years gained in both tests (Zauber et al., 2008). Furthermore advocates assert that FOBT has the greatest potential for impact at the population level because it is directed at healthy people (Harvard Medical School, 2012). Additionally asymptomatic people may be more willing to participate in a less invasive and generally less inconvenient test.

While a case can be made that FOBT has some quantifiable mortality benefits, evidence suggests that colonoscopy is still the superior screening option. FOBT has many disadvantages. One major drawback of this modality is the high false positive rate because the test is not specific for human blood. In fact the test will not be accurate if patients consume red meat or any other peroxidase containing substances. Additionally three-stool sample are required on separate days (Lieberman, 2010). Single sample FOBT is estimated to miss 95% of CRC (Wilkins and Reynolds, 2008). Furthermore the test must be repeated annually to be effective. In addition to these drawbacks, this test only detects potentially high-risk individuals which means that abnormal test results require subsequent follow up with colonoscopy. Compliance with all of the aforementioned recommendations is unknown making the effectiveness of the test uncertain. In fact one survey found that up to 30% of doctors recommended inappropriate forms of follow up rendering the FOBT not useful (Nadel et al., 2005). Despite these drawbacks the FOBT sampling test is still preferable to the no screening option.

Fecal immunochemical testing (FIT) is a newer test that is easier to use and specific for humans. This means that the FIT is less susceptible to interference by diet or drugs. This modality uses antibodies to detect human blood components such as hemoglobin and albumin in stool samples (School, 2012). This alternative is appealing because it is less invasive than colonoscopy but potentially more accurate than the FOBT. Studies show over 50% sensitivity for cancer after using as small an amount as one stool sample (Lieberman, 2010). FIT may be superior to the FOBT given that one study showed higher participation in the FIT group. Participation is key for fecal tests making the previously mentioned study clinically relevant. However no randomized trials have shown that FIT decreases mortality (Wilkins and Reynolds, 2008).

Given that participation may be negatively impacted by hesitation to undergo colonoscopy screening, a recent study investigated whether FIT can serve as a valid screening alternative and no significant differences were found between FIT and colonoscopy in terms of participation (Quintero et al., 2012). Furthermore colonoscopy still detected substantially higher numbers of cancerous polyps. It is difficult from this study to declare that FIT testing is non-inferior because of colonoscopy's mortality benefit.

Fecal DNA testing detects a finite number of gene mutations in stool samples associated with colon neoplasia (Alberti et al., 2012). One large prospective trial found stool DNA testing to have greater sensitivity for cancer than standard FOBT (Imperiale et al., 2004). Furthermore patients were found to prefer fecal DNA testing to both FOBT and colonoscopy (Wilkins and Reynolds, 2008). However this option is not recommended by current guidelines because of insufficient evidence. Also there have been other studies comparing stool DNA testing to FOBT that suggest this fecal DNA testing does not measure up in terms of cost or efficacy (Lansdorp-Vogelaar et al., 2010).

2.8. Which screening test should be done?

Each of the aforementioned screening options has strengths and setbacks, however patient adherence to CRC screening remains more critical than the specific method chosen (Vijan et al., 2001). Simply put, the best test is the one that the patient accepts and complies with. Despite mounting evidence that screening is life saving, screening rates remain surprisingly low for this preventable cancer. In fact awareness of the importance of CRC screening has only recently started to approach that of other cancers. Statistics indicate only 24% of Americans have completed the FOBT within the past few years and only 57.1% have ever had a sigmoidoscopy or colonoscopy (Wilkins and Reynolds, 2008). Data from the NHIS, a national survey of the general population, shows that only 58.3% of the US population met recommendations for CRC screening in 2010 (Shapiro et al., 2012). This is increased from 54.5% in 2008. Although there has been progress in the use of CRC testing, 40-50% of individuals over the age of 50 still are not receiving routine screening for colorectal cancer.

It is apparent from these suboptimal screening rates that there is a demand for novel screening strategies that are not only effective but also economical and non-invasive. Continued research in this field is ongoing and in a fascinating study published in *Gut*, Citarda et al (Citarda et al., 2001) took steps towards attempting to find this desired formula. Their study is evidence of the increasing knowledge about the molecular properties of cancer. Based on the theory that a specific cancer smell exists, they found that a trained labrador retriever could detect the presence of colorectal cancer with 91% sensitivity and 99% specificity in breath samples and 97% sensitivity and 99% specificity in watery stool samples. Surprisingly the study dog's ability to detect cancer was not confounded by benign colorectal disease, inflammatory bowel disease, or smoking. Even though the routine use of canines for cancer screening is not practical, this study suggests there is potential for future screening tests based on cancer-specific chemical compounds.

2.9. Cost effectiveness of CRC screening

CRC screening has been found to reduce mortality and to be cost-effective. The challenge remains to make screening affordable and available to individuals who will experience the

http://dx.doi.org/10.5772/53111

greatest benefit. Several models have been proposed to estimate the costs of various screening programs. The 2005 Institute of Medicine comprehensive summary of CRC screening effectiveness concluded that all of the screening options are relatively comparable in terms of life-years gained as well as cost when compared with a no-screening option. FOBT was the least costly option, however most modalities are estimated to cost <$40,000 per life-year saved (Lieberman, 2010; Pignone et al., 2002). However it is difficult to rely on these models alone as they may not be entirely accurate and are not able to account for other factors such as patient compliance. In general cost benefit analysis studies suggest that CRC screening is overall a cost-effective measure and it is estimated that routine screening can save more than 18,800 lives per year (Maciosek et al., 2006; Wilkins and Reynolds, 2008).

2.10. Surveillance guidelines

Currently the United States Multi-Society Task Force (MSTF) on CRC supports a 10-year interval between subsequent screening colonoscopies for average risk patients. Case-control and observational studies indicate that the mortality benefit from colonoscopy lasts at least 10 years. However patients who are found to have adenomas on baseline colonoscopy are at increased risk of developing future adenomas and cancerous lesions (Martinez et al., 2009). Certain higher-risk patients can develop cancer as soon as 3-5 years after a colonoscopy. These are termed interval cancers. These patients require a shorter interval between subsequent follow up because this has been shown to reduce colorectal cancer incidence by as much as 66% (Citarda et al., 2001; Winawer et al., 1993a). Guidelines from the GI consortium panel advocate repeat colonoscopy 5 years after removal of a low-risk polyp and after 3 years if the polyp has higher risk features. The selection of a 3-year screening interval for subsequent follow-up is based on evidence that shows detection of advanced lesions is not improved at 1 year versus 3 years (Winawer et al., 1993b). Further research is still needed to determine whether a single negative follow up colonoscopy is sufficient (Lieberman et al., 2012).

The use of risk stratification to determine the optimal screening interval is important because physicians that refer patients for surveillance at intervals shorter than recommended may be exposing patients to unnecessary risks and costs (Lieberman, 2010). In fact a recent study revealed underuse of colonoscopies in high-risk patients and overuse in low risk patients. By ineffective allocation of resources high-risk patients are placed at increased risk for developing cancer. Furthermore optimization of screening is important in light of low screening rates for a preventable cancer. Customized screening recommendations based on risk allows for more streamlined and effective screening leaving resources that can be devoted to colon cancer education targeting the challenging subset of the population at high risk with poor adherence. Ultimately screening program success depends not only on quality but patient participation (Lieberman et al., 2012). In addition to risk stratification, the MSTF on CRC believes that high-quality baseline examination is key for effective surveillance. Interval cancers have been found to occur more frequently in patients with negative baseline exams. There is evidence to suggest that important lesions are often missed at baseline colonoscopy and it is estimated that up to 17% of 10 mm lesions are missed. This variability in adenoma detection rates may be attributable to biologic differences in missed adenomas or disparities in endoscopist proficiency.

3. When to start screening?

As with any effective screening technique, the most important issue is always *when* to start offering the test. Although the lifetime risk of CRC is estimated to be 6%, we now understand that the chance of developing the disease increases with age. In the United States the annual incidence of CRC in people of ages 50 to 54 was found to be approximately double that found in individuals ages 45 to 49 (Imperiale et al., 2000). A successful screening test, if used on 100% of the population has the potential to save many more lives than if the test is used on only a portion of the population. However given limited medical resources, strategic optimization is necessary for maximum impact. Current recommendations support initiation of screening at age 50 for average risk men and women with earlier screening recommended for high-risk populations (Levin et al., 2008; Rex et al., 2009; USPSTF, 2008; Winawer et al., 2003). In addition to identifying optimal timing for initiation, the goals of screening have shifted to focus on cancer prevention rather than simply cancer detection (Winawer et al., 2003). As a result recent guidelines from the American College of Gastroenterology (ACG) and USPSTF now endorse colonoscopy as the preferred modality for screening (Rex et al., 2009; USPSTF, 2008).

Screening guidelines must be tailored to maximize benefit while minimizing cost to both the individual and society as a whole (Rembold, 1998). The term "number needed to screen" is defined as the amount of people needed to be screened over a timed duration to prevent one death or adverse event. Many studies have looked at the cost-effectiveness of colon cancer screening with the three most common methods (i.e. fecal occult blood annually, sigmoidoscopy every 5 years, colonoscopy every 10 years - all beginning at age 50 and stopping at age 85). Current estimates range from $6,000 – $11,900 spent for every year of life gained (Maciosek et al., 2006; Telford et al., 2010). In contrast, studies on the cost effectiveness of screening mammography estimate roughly $58,000 spent for every one year of life gained (Stout et al.). Many experts suggest that a screening policy should result in expenditure of $50,000 or less per year of life gained. Thus, it is clear that colon cancer screening makes sense medically and financially. The question of when colon cancer screening should begin and end remains, and is a complex one. While colon cancer is typically a disease of the middle age to elderly, there are many groups of high-risk patients that need screening much earlier than current guidelines. The remainder of this section will attempt to elucidate screening strategies in low-risk, average-risk, and high-risk groups.

It is important to emphasize that colon cancer is a diverse entity with many paths leading to a common endpoint, carcinoma. The adenoma-carcinoma sequence can encompass a multitude of genetic mutations that lead to the eventual progression to cancer (i.e. mismatch repair genes, tumor suppressor genes, base excision repair genes, micro-satellite genes). No single mutation results in adenocarcinoma, but as mutations compile, a carcinoma eventual-

http://dx.doi.org/10.5772/53111

ly develops. For the majority of colon cancers, there is a significant amount of time between development of an adenoma and its progression to a malignant lesion. The time interval for progression is often determined by type of adenoma found. Current studies estimate that the dwelling time for a tubular adenoma is roughly 26 years, 9 years for tubulovillous adenoma, and 4 years for a villous adenoma (with an overall annual transition rate of 2.2%) (Chen et al.). It is this significant window period of detection time that allows screening for colon cancer to be so incredibly effective, and thus important to optimize timing and frequency of screening. While these concepts hold true for the majority of colon cancers, not all cancers are created equal. Certain high-risk groups progress to cancer much more rapidly than the above data suggests, and these groups will be detailed ahead.

3.1. Distribution of colorectal cancer types

The vast majority (70-75%) of colorectal cancers develop in sporadic (nonhereditary) fashion and no risk factors are identified in the individuals. The next most common form (15-20%) occurs in those with a family history of colon cancer (excluding known cancer syndromes). Hereditary Non-polyposis colorectal cancer (i.e. Lynch Syndrome) makes up roughly 3-8%. Familial Adenomatous Polyposis 1%, and Colitis Associated Cancer (i.e. Inflammatory Bowel Disease) also 1% (Winawer et al.). Keeping these figures in mind, colon cancer screening has the largest absolute impact on average-risk individuals. As such, the next section will focus on screening recommendations for the average-risk group.

3.2. Approach to average-risk individuals

As mentioned before, colon cancer is a disease of the middle age to elderly. According to a review by the National Cancer Institute conducted from 2005-2009, the median age at time of diagnosis of a colorectal cancer is 69. Thus, if we extrapolate from the data provided previously (~2% annual transformation from adenoma to carcinoma), we can see that it makes sense to exclude the younger population from screening tests. In fact, the most recent USPSTF recommendations support the initiation of colon cancer screening in average-risk individuals at age 50 (Grade A Recommendation) (USPSTF). These recommendations were made based in part on the results of two microsimulation models (MISCAN and SimCRC models) that incorporated current data on colon cancer incidence and adenoma progression, and simulated the natural history of colon cancer in a large population. The models then estimated the life-years gained if screening colonoscopy was performed vs. no screening at all. Further data analysis detailed age to begin screening, age to stop screening, and time intervals between screening. The models concluded that the optimal age to initiate screening is 50 (when compared to ages 40 and 60). Of note, one simulation showed better outcomes when screening was initiated at age 40, however the alternate simulation did not corroborate the data. The Task Force concluded, "Because the evidence for both adenoma prevalence at age 40 and the duration of the adenoma-carcinoma sequence is weak, we restricted further analysis to start ages of 50 and 60." This led to the recommendation of initiating screening at age 50. Regarding interval time period between colonoscopy, the authors reviewed data on 5-year, 10-year, and 20-year intervals. They concluded, as could be expected, shorter intervals resulted in more life-years gained (their primary endpoint). However, when comparing 5-year to 10-year, there was only a modest increase in life years gained when compared to the corresponding increase in colonoscopies performed. 20-year intervals resulted in significantly less life-years gained, so was not considered optimal. While these authors agree with the recommendations by the USPSTF for average-risk individuals, it is important that practitioners further tailor their screening strategies based on several additional factors. As mentioned, 75% of colon cancers occur in average-risk individuals, thus representing a large absolute number of persons. As such, there is much variability and associated risks among the average-risk population.

Factors that increase the risk for colorectal cancer or are protective have been identified. While these factors have not been incorporated into the USPSTF Guidelines, knowledge about their existence and influence on overall risk may be helpful in directing clinicians toward screening colonoscopy practices. Additionally, and some may argue more importantly, clinicians must take into account a patient's expected adherence to their colonoscopy recommendations. Will the patient have regular and predictable access to a skilled gastroenterologist? Will they be willing to comply with frequent colonoscopy should their risk factors or findings require it? A new concept known as once in a lifetime screening with colonoscopy is being proposed as an effective technique in some groups. Knowledge of risk factors can be especially helpful in these cases, in which a clinician can strongly encourage adherence to recommendations based on each individual's risk factors. Additionally, it is important to note that the following discussion applies only to individuals classified as average-risk, and excludes those with a family history, diagnosed genetic condition, and Inflammatory Bowel Disease. These groups will be discussed separately.

3.3. Modifiable CRC risk factors

To date, several modifiable risk factors have been clearly linked with the development of colorectal carcinoma. Starting from the 10,000-foot view, many of the risk factors can be collectively grouped under the heading of total energy balance (i.e. caloric intake vs. caloric expenditure). Numerous studies have shown a clear link between Body Mass Index and resultant risk of colon cancer. For example, investigators looked at the lifetime incidence of colon cancer among the Framingham Cohort in Massachusetts, and divided the group by age group to a 30-54 year old group and a 55-79 year old group. They then looked at the overall incidence of colon cancer among the groups, and related the information to average Body Mass Index. In the 55-79 year old group, they separated the cohort into BMI >30 and BMI <30 groups. They noticed a significant 2.4 fold increased risk for the development of colon cancer for those with a BMI >30 (95% CI: 1.5-3.9) (Moore et al., 2004). Interestingly, the same study also analyzed the results with relation to waist size measurement. As BMI can be notoriously misleading, especially among males, the authors pursued this alternate measure for further support. They concluded that central adiposity (defined as a waist size >39 inches), was associated with a two-fold increase in risk for colon cancer. They further noted that the risk increased linearly with increases in waist size. This data has been replicated among many other studies, in both men and women. A large study by the Nurses' Health

Study Research Group concluded similarly that increasing BMI is associated with increased risk of colon cancer, and particularly noted a higher risk among women with an increased waist-to-hip ratio (Martinez et al., 1997). It is now widely accepted that obesity, and particularly central obesity, is an independent risk factor for the development of colon cancer. Several theories have been proposed as to why exactly this clear association exists. For now, the most supported theory proposes that insulin resistance (along with hyperinsulinemia and increased Insulin-like Growth Factor-1) plays a large role in this relationship. In fact, a recent meta-analysis has concluded that Diabetes Mellitus is itself an independent risk factor for colon cancer. Even after controlling for physical activity, smoking, and obesity, the authors found an increase in relative risk among those with Diabetes Mellitus of 1.43 and 1.35 in men and women, respectively (both statistically significant) (Yuhara et al., 2011). Pathophysiologically, both insulin and IGF-1 are involved in cell proliferation and regulation of apoptosis and it is enough to recognize that states with elevated levels of both hormones have been clearly linked to increased risk for colon cancer. Additionally, multiple studies have looked at the effect of physical activity and its influence on colon cancer. These studies and their respective meta-analyses have shown clearly an inverse relationship between physical activity and colon cancer. Among data taken from the group exhibiting the highest level of exercise, one study showed a 50% reduction in lifetime colon cancer risk (Colditz et al., 1997). Thus, an important conclusion can be reached based on the data reviewed as well as others: obese, sedentary individuals are at higher risk for colon cancer. While the USPSTF guidelines do not currently reflect this information for screening recommendations, clinicians most certainly can make use of it to provide patient-centered care. Patients should be counseled regarding overall health and the potential for primary prevention of colon cancer via improved dieting and exercise habits.

The next most common modifiable risk factors a clinician is likely to encounter is tobacco and/or alcohol use, both clearly linked with colon cancer. Multitudes of studies have been undertaken in the last two decades examining the potential link between cigarette smoking and colorectal cancer. A meta-analysis from 2009 conducted by Liang et al examined 36 such studies (Liang et al., 2009). The results of the analysis showed a clear association between age of initiation of tobacco use, amount smoked per day, and total duration of tobacco use. Data showed a relative-risk of 1.38 for an increase in 40-cigarretes per day, 1.20 for an increase of 40 years total duration, and 1.51 for an increase of 60-pack years. Interestingly, they also noted a predilection for rectal cancer over colon cancer when analyzing incidence of site-specific carcinoma. Next, studies emerging over the last decade have begun to note increases in risk for colorectal cancer even in light to moderate alcohol use. A pooled analysis of 8 cohort studies involving nearly 490,000 men and women was published in the Annals of Internal Medicine in 2004. Data showed, when compared with non-drinkers, a relative-risk of 1.41 (CI 1.16-1.72) in individuals who consumed 45g of daily alcohol (roughly three drinks) (Cho et al., 2004). There was no statistically significant correlation among daily consumption of 30-44g/daily. More recently, a meta-analysis from 2011 from the Annals of Oncology examined 27 cohort studies and 34 case-control studies (Fedirko et al., 2011). They also concluded a strong association between alcohol consumption and colorectal cancer risk. The association was strongest among heavy drinkers, relative-risk 1.82 if >100g/day. Surprisingly, they even found a statistically significant increase in relative-risk to 1.07 for individuals drinking one alcoholic beverage per day (10g/day), which throws into question the current recommendations of the USDA (two drinks or less daily for men, one drink or less daily for women). Interestingly, even stronger associations were noted in studies examined the Asian population (specifically Japanese men). Clearly, there is a link between both tobacco and alcohol use and risk of colorectal cancer. Over the next few years, additional studies and meta-analyses will likely emerge further elucidating just which populations are at risk and what usage levels are most harmful. For now, clinicians should clearly state that tobacco use and even light daily alcohol ingestion increases their likelihood of developing colorectal cancer. As the current data suggests only a modest increase in relative-risk, this information may be more pertinent among individuals with additional risk factors. Clinicians should certainly take a patient's tobacco and alcohol use into account when determining how frequent they will advise screening colonoscopies.

3.4. Protective measures against CRC

Just as risk factors have been identified, there are also several clear factors that are protective against colon cancer. Physical activity was discussed earlier, thus will not be repeated here, but suffice it to mention again that it is highly protective against colon cancer. Moreover, the medical community already advocates daily exercise for a multitude of other health benefits, and the fact that it also protects against colon cancer would not alter a clinician's management of colonoscopy screening. However, several studies have clearly shown a protective relationship between common pharmaceuticals and colon cancer. Both Aspirin and Non-steroidal anti-inflammatory drugs have been shown to decrease the incidence of colon cancer. Studies from as early as the 1980s began to show a relationship between anti-inflammatory medications and colon cancer. Initial studies performed on patients with Rheumatoid Arthritis, as they were often on chronic NSAID therapy, were the first to show this relationship in the 1980s. Further studies conducted in patients on long-term aspirin therapy showed similar results. The exact mechanism by which anti-inflammatory medications provide this protective benefit currently remains unknown. Several hypotheses exist which primarily center on COX-1 and COX-2 inhibition, as they are known to promote inflammation, tumorigenesis, and angiogenesis. In a study published in the Lancet in 2007 by Flossman et al, British researchers pooled data from two large Aspirin trials in the UK (British Doctors Aspirin Trial, UK-TIA Aspirin Trial) (Flossmann and Rothwell, 2007). Among patients with complete compliance for 5 years or more of aspirin therapy, they found a statistically significant relative-risk of 0.26 (CI 0.12-0.56). The effect was less substantial among non-compliant patients, but nevertheless protective (RR 0.37). It is important to note in this study, as in many other studies, the protective benefit was most clearly seen after a latency period of at least 10 years. Moreover, study data pooled from trials related to cardiovascular protection often have used differing doses of aspirin (or NSAIDs). At this time, no clear dose, duration of therapy or type of NSAID has shown to be of greatest benefit in primary colorectal cancer chemoprevention. As such, the USPSTF has not recommended NSAIDS as a primary preventive measure for colorectal cancer. As more and more studies specifically geared and powered toward colorectal carcinoma prevention (as opposed to data analysis of

http://dx.doi.org/10.5772/53111

trials geared toward cardiovascular effects), it can likely be expected that clearer relationships between NSAID type, dosing, and duration will be elucidated. As it is not officially recommended by the USPSTF, clinicians are not currently advocating for NSAID use as primary prevention. However, a large portion of those at greatest risk for developing colorectal cancer (i.e. middle-age to elderly) are already on Aspirin for its cardiovascular benefits. Thus, clinicians can take this fact into account when assessing an individual's colorectal cancer risk. Again, there is no current recommendation to decrease screening intervals in patients on Aspirin therapy, however, when taken collectively with other risk factors, clinicians may further tailor how aggressive they wish to be with screening.

Another common protective measure a clinician may encounter regards the use of postmenopausal hormonal therapy. Again, as early as the 1980s, studies emerged showing an unexpected link between hormonal therapy and colorectal cancers. As in many other associations, the exact mechanism by which estrogen/progestin can inhibit cancer development is unknown. However, speculations on its pathophysiology are under active investigation. Researchers hypothesize that hormonal therapy can alter levels of bile acids, Insulin-Like Growth Factor-1, and IGF Binding Protein-3. Moreover, estrogen receptors have been found on colonic epithelial cells, and it is unclear if this may also provide a route of protection. Nevertheless, numerous studies (one of which will be described below) have shown the inverse relationship between hormonal therapy and colon cancer risk. In a prospective study of nearly 57,000 women (taken from the Breast Cancer Detection Demonstration Project) published in 2009, Johnson et al looked at hormonal therapy (including estrogen alone, combination with progestin, and duration of therapy) and its relation to colon cancer incidence (Johnson et al., 2009). Results are astoundingly clear that hormonal therapy is protective against colon cancer. The results were as follows: ever users of unopposed estrogen RR 0.83 (95% CI, 0.70-0.99), current users unopposed estrogen >10 years RR 0.74 (95% CI, 0.56-0.96). The results among estrogen + progestin users showed an even stronger relationship: estrogen + progestin RR 0.78 (95% CI, 0.6-1.02), estrogen + sequential progestin RR 0.64 (95% CI, 0.43-0.95), and strongest effect with 2-5yr use of estrogen + sequential progestin RR 0.52 (95% CI, 0.32-0.87). Similar studies conducted by the WHI (Women's Health Initiative) have shown similar results for estrogen + progestin therapy, but not estrogen therapy alone. Interestingly, they also noted that although the frequency of cancer was less in the hormonal group, the cancers were detected at later stages (increased lymph node involvement and metastatic disease) (Chlebowski et al., 2004). So, as before, we have clear evidence of a protective measure against colon cancer. Unfortunately, the same WHI trial showed an increase in myocardial infarction, stroke, dementia, pulmonary emboli, and breast cancer among hormonal therapy users. As such, there have been no widespread recommendations for primary prevention of colorectal cancer by means of hormonal therapy. However, clinicians may encounter women who are on hormonal therapy. While estrogen therapy alone may not have clear benefits, estrogen + progestin therapy has repeatedly shown to be of benefit in prevention of colorectal cancer. In fact, based on the results of the first-mentioned study, risk was decreased by a staggering 25-46%. Taking this information into account, assuming no additional risk factors exist, and clinician may be able to tailor their screening colonoscopy frequency toward a less aggressive and frequent approach.

A clinician may also encounter questions from a patient regarding diet recommendations. While a healthy, balanced diet high in non-processed, low animal fat calories is always recommended, there has been non conclusive data regarding diet and its relation to colorectal cancer. As such, the decision on when to initiate and how often to perform screening colonoscopies should not be influenced by a patient's diet. It is possible that more clear relationships will be clarified in the future, but for now, data displaying strong associations does not exist.

The next question that must be answered is what role should gender and race/ethnicity of a patient play in a clinician's screening colonoscopy recommendations? According to the most recent data from the Center for Disease Control (CDC) males have a higher incidence of colorectal cancer vs females (52.7 vs. 39.7/100,000) (Prevention). The highest incidence is found in African American males (62/100,000), followed by Caucasian males (51.5/100,000). Hispanics, Asians, and Native American/Alaskan Native groups all had a lower incidence than the comparative African-American and Caucasian groups in both the male and female categories. When comparing death rates from colorectal cancer by race, again males have an overall higher rate vs. females (20.2 vs 14.1/100,000).(NIH, 2009) African-American males displayed the highest rate at 29.8/100,000, and African-American Females the next highest rate at 19.8/100,000. The remainder of the groups showed death rates below the average of respective male and female groups analyzed. Compiling the above data, it is evident that African-Americans are most affected by colorectal cancer in comparison to other race/ethnicities. In fact, a study examining 5-year survival rates among Caucasians vs. African-Americans (among all stages of colorectal cancer) revealed a staggering difference of 64% vs. 52% (Ries). Initially, arguments were made postulating that perhaps the African-American community rate of screening colonoscopy was much lower, thus accounting for the higher incidence and mortality rate. According to the CDC data on screening rates, Caucasians are most screened at 66.2% and African-Americans are next most screened at 62.9% (Rim S.H., 2011). The lowest screening rate is found in the Hispanic population at 51.2%. While African-Americans have a higher mortality rate from colorectal cancer, it is clear that it is not solely due to inadequate screening, as African-Americans have much higher screening rates than Hispanics, yet also a much higher mortality rate. A study examining this finding concluded that African-Americans are more likely to be diagnosed at an earlier age and present at later stages of disease, as compared to Caucasians, however this data has not been consistently replicated (Chien et al., 2005). Another study postulated that socioeconomic status and access to medical care may be partially involved in this mortality discrepancy (Wudel et al., 2002). This study found that African-Americans are more likely to be treated at city hospital vs university hospitals (which are associated with better outcomes). However, when comparing survival data even among Caucasians and African-Americans at each type of hospital, African-Americans fared worse. Another study has pointed to type of care offered (i.e. adjuvant chemotherapy and radiation) as a potential factor (Govindarajan et al., 2003). This study found that African-Americans are treated less with both chemotherapy and radiation therapy vs. Caucasian patients. It is still unclear why exactly African-Americans are more often diagnosed and more often killed by colorectal cancer. Regardless of the reason, it is clear that there is a difference that needs to be addressed. It seems that while the reasons are being elucidated, more aggressive screening among African-Americans needs to be established. Data may eventually and conclusively show that colorectal cancer appears earlier and is more aggressive in African-Americans. In the meantime, these authors would argue for earlier age at initiation of screening and more frequent screening intervals.

Finally, in the average-risk population, the issue of access to colonoscopy need always remain in the back of a clinician's mind. Many patients may not have access due to socioeconomic or geographic barriers, or simply they may choose not to undergo screening based on underlying psychological barriers or misconceptions regarding colon cancer and/or colonoscopy. As mentioned previously, many organizations are working toward colon cancer and screening awareness, however clinicians must keep public unawareness as part of their screening practice. If a patient presents at age 45 and there is concern for eventual adherence to the screening guidelines at age 50, he/she should be screened at age 45.

3.5. Risk associated with family history of CRC

As mentioned previously, the next largest group of the population diagnosed with colon cancer involves those with a family history (excluding individuals with a known colorectal cancer syndrome). This group makes up ~15-20% of all diagnoses. Currently, there are multiple efforts and studies looking into what exactly confers this higher risk among individuals with a positive family history of colon cancer. At this time, it remains unclear what genetic and/or environmental factors are involved in the pathogenesis, however, it is abundantly clear that patients with 1st degree relatives diagnosed with colon cancer, are at a significantly higher risk of developing colon cancer themselves. In fact, in one of the seminal studies published on the topic from the New England Journal Of Medicine, individuals with one 1st-degree relative with colon cancer were found to have a 1.7 fold increase in their own risk for colon cancer (Rex et al., 2009). This risk increased further as the number of diseased 1st-degree relatives increased as well. Further, they found that the increased risk was irrespective of location of diagnosed tumor in the relative (i.e. proximal vs. distal site of malignancy). As such, the American College of Gastroenterology revised its guidelines regarding individuals with a positive family history. If an individual has a 1st degree relative that was diagnosed with colon cancer before the age of 60 (or 2 or more relatives with colon cancer or advanced adenomas irrespective of age at diagnosis), they are considered to have a positive family history. If a patient is identified as having a positive family history, they should then begin colonoscopy screening at age 40 (or 10 years before the youngest age of diagnosis), and they should have an interval follow-up colonoscopy every 5 years. According to these recommendations, 2nd-degree relatives or relatives diagnosed >60 years of age are not considered as a conferring a positive family history.

3.6. Polyposis syndromes

While the exact genetic predisposition for the majority of colon cancer remains unknown, there are several well-known (and identifiable) cancer syndromes that a clinician must take into account when making colon cancer screening advice. The most common of these is Familial Adenomatous Polyposis. It affects roughly 1 in 5,000-7,000 individuals and confers a 100% risk of eventual colorectal cancer, with the average age at diagnosis 40 (Bussey et al.,

1978). These individuals should begin screening colonoscopy in adolescence (usually started 10-12 years old), and this should be repeated annually. Ultimately these patients should receive prophylactic colectomy. Another such polyposis includes Attenuated Adenomatous Polyposis. As opposed to FAP (which involves hundreds to thousands of polyps diffusely spread throughout the colon), AAP is an oligopolyposis and typically involves <100 polyps. These polyps are more often right-sided and with a flat morphology. Patient's typically begin to have polyps appear in the 4th-5th decade of life and an average age of diagnosis of cancer at age 55 (Knudsen et al., 2003). Roughly 69% of patients with APP will eventually develop colon cancer. These patients should begin screening colonoscopy at age 25 and this should be repeated annually. Less common genetic polyposes a clinician may encounter involve: MUTYH-Associated Polyposis, Peutz-Jeghers Syndrome, and Juvenile Polyposis Syndrome. MUTYH-Associated Polyposis is an autosomal recessive cancer syndrome (heterozygotes with one affected allele are at increased risk, but homozygotes show the largest increase in risk). Variations in phenotype have been described, from hundreds to thousands of polyps distributed throughout the colon. Lifetime prevalence of colon cancer is reported at 80% (Jenkins et al., 2006). These individuals should begin annual screening at age 18-20. Clinicians may also encounter Peutz-Jeghers Syndrome, which is an autosomal dominant disorder characterized by numerous hamartomatous polyps throughout the colon. These individuals carry a 39% lifetime risk of colon cancer and should have colonoscopy screening every 2-3 years beginning in their late teen years (McGarrity and Amos, 2006). Finally, pediatric clinicians may encounter Juvenile Polyposis, which is an autosomal dominant condition characterized by numerous polyps throughout the gastrointestinal tract. These individuals are often brought to the attention of a physician following an intestinal obstruction or gastrointestinal bleed as a consequence of the numerous polyps. These patients carry a 10-38% lifetime colon cancer risk and should be screened annually beginning at age 15 (Howe et al., 1998; Jass et al., 1988).

3.7. Non-polyposis syndromes

The most common hereditary colon cancer syndrome is Lynch Syndrome, or Hereditary Non-Polyposis Colorectal Cancer. This too is an autosomal dominant condition, which is characterized by numerous, proximal adenomas. Affected individuals carry a 48-68% risk of colon cancer by age 60, with the majority being diagnosed between age 40-50 (Mecklin et al., 2007). Even more importantly, adenomas associated with HNPCC are typically more aggressive and advance to carcinoma quicker than would be otherwise expected. As such, these individuals should begin screening at age 20, and this should be repeated every 1-3 years.

3.8. CRC risk associated with Inflammatory Bowel Disease

Nearly every clinician is sure to encounter a patient afflicted with Inflammatory Bowel Disease (IBD). As such, it is important to recognize that these patients carry an increased risk for colon cancer, and they cannot be treated as average-risk individuals. The entity is referred to as Colitis-Associated Cancer, or CAC, and the resultant risk of eventual colon cancer is related to the severity of disease (in both Ulcerative Colitis, and Crohn's Disease). The cumulative risk of colon cancer among patients with ulcerative colitis (U.C.) is thought to be roughly 2% after 10-years of disease, and up to 18% after 30-years of disease (Eaden et al., 2001). Although Crohn's Disease (C.D.) classically involves the small intestine, it can also involve the large bowel, which confers an increased risk of colon cancer as well. Crohn's patients with large intestinal involvement carry an 8.3% risk of colon cancer after 30 years of disease (Canavan et al., 2006). Currently, the recommendation is to begin screening both U.C. and C.D. patients 8-10 years post-diagnosis, and institute 1-2 year screening intervals.

4. When to stop screening?

As touched on previously, equally important to the initiation of an effective screening program involves the optimal age to finish the screening process. The question could be posed: "Why stop screening at all if it is an effective means to prevent morbidity and mortality from colon cancer?" However several factors should be considered including the fact that colonoscopy is not entirely without risk. The known complications associated with colonoscopy (e.g. bleeding, perforation, infection, diverticulitis), occur particularly in the elderly population. Furthermore, and especially true with regard to colorectal cancer screening, there exists a potentially long latency period from adenoma to carcinoma which may take years and even decades in some individuals. Elderly patients with an adenoma seen on screening may, and oftentimes do, perish as a result of other disease processes. Finally, limited resources must also be taken into account. Each and every colonoscopy takes a concerted effort from a skilled colonoscopist and their support staff, and the required financial means on the part of the patient and/or government. As such it is necessary to establish evidence-based guidelines on when patients can safely stop colon cancer screening. The following section will delve further into this topic and the current recommendations for age at which to stop screening.

4.1. Complications from screening colonoscopy

In general, colonoscopy is a relatively safe, well-tolerated procedure by patients. The majority of patients will never experience any complications, even if undergoing multiple colonoscopies throughout their lifetime. There are, however, significant and life-threatening complications that can occur. Although rare, given the enormous number of colonoscopies performed annually, it is important to be cognizant of the associated complications. In 2010, an analysis was released tracking complications rates among 18 large studies and involving over 685,000 colonoscopies (Ko and Dominitz, 2010). The most common complication seen was lower gastrointestinal bleeding, at roughly 0.1-0.6%. Fortunately, the far majority of these were not mortal bleeds. However, as most colonoscopies are undertaken in the outpatient setting, gastrointestinal hemorrhage can develop into a life-threatening event very quickly in a non-monitored setting. Next most common, bowel perforation posed a risk of less than 0.3% (Ko and Dominitz, 2010). These most often occur following barotrauma or mechanical trauma to the bowel wall. Again, although exceedingly rare, a perforated bowel has the potential to be lethal. A perforation can be clinically evident immediately after the incident occurs, however, small perforations in the bowel can lead to an insidious course that can ultimately result in severe peritonitis and rapid clinical decompensation. Diverticulitis is also a well-established complication of colonoscopy, with a rate estimated at 0.04-0.08% (Ko and Dominitz, 2010). There also exists the known entity of post-polypectomy electrocoagulation syndrome (or post-polypectomy syndrome). Following electrocautery of the bowel wall, there is risk for a partial or transmural burn of the bowel wall. In cases of a transmural burn, patients experience symptoms of clinical peritonitis. This rarely proceeds to actual peritonitis (radiography does not visualize actual perforated bowel with free air in the peritoneum), and these patients can be managed via supportive care and antibiotics. However, resultant hospitalization and treatment is not without its own associated risks and costs, so this cannot be taken lightly either. The incidence of post-polypectomy electrocoagulation syndrome appears to be roughly 0.003%-0.01% (Ko and Dominitz, 2010). Infection as a result of colonoscopy is exceedingly rare, and can most times be attributed to poor infection control procedures involving equipment. Although the risk of transient bacteremia is postulated to be higher, the actual risk of an infection transmission purely as a result of colonoscopy is estimated at roughly 1 per 1.8 million procedures, with Pseudomonas and Salmonella species being the most commonly identified (Spach et al., 1993). Other case-reportable complications have included splenic rupture, acute appendicitis, and subcutaneous emphysema (Hirata et al., 1996; Humphreys et al., 1984; Kamath et al., 2009). Overall mortality from colonoscopy remains controversial due to complicated comorbidities among those in studies tracking colonoscopy-related mortality. Estimates range from 0%-0.09% (Ko and Dominitz, 2010). Less serious complications include nausea, vomiting, diarrhea and bloating. Fortunately, these are usually self-limited within several days following the colonoscopy. As evidenced above, colonoscopy does have rare but serious complications. However, it is important to note that complications are also related to the type of procedure performed (screening colonoscopy or polypectomy) and the age of those undergoing the procedure.

In assessing the risk of complications from colonoscopies it is important to consider the type of intervention to be employed during the procedure and the baseline characteristics of the patient. Many studies have analyzed data pertaining to complications particularly associated with different age groups. For example, a retrospective cohort study from 1994-2009 examined these risks among over 43,000 patients ages 40-85 (Rutter et al., 2012). They pooled hemorrhage, perforation, and diverticulitis as serious adverse events. They found an event rate of 4.7/1000 screening colonoscopies and 6.8/1000 for follow-up colonoscopies. Interestingly, there were significant differences between age groups. Among ages 40-49 there was a serious event rate of 4.2/1000, ages 50-64 3.7/1000, ages 65-74 7.9/1000, and for ages 75-84 13.3/1000. Thus the rate of complications clearly increases with age. They also noted an increase in events following polypectomy vs no intervention, however this proves less clinically relevant, as a clinician would certainly not forgo polypectomy based on this fact alone. With the above data, and other studies like it (Gatto et al., 2003), it becomes evident that beyond a certain age, colonoscopies may be causing more harm than good.

4.2. Timing of progression from adenoma to carcinoma

As mentioned previously, the progression from adenoma to carcinoma may take years and even decades. Some adenomas may never make the entire progression. The adenoma may never acquire all the necessary genetic mutations, or simply, an individual may not live long enough for the adenoma to significantly progress. As such, detecting an asymptomatic polyp in an elderly individual may have no significance whatsoever. In fact, while the risk of colonoscopy complications poses a real threat, the adenoma may prove to have no bearing on a patient's health. Currently, the most recent CDC data estimates that the average life expectancy in the United States is 78.7 years (76.2 for males and 81.1 for females) (Centers for disease control and prevention, 2012). This brings into question the utility of screening elderly age individuals. At what age will a screening colonoscopy likely provide no benefit to the average-risk elderly patient?

The following discussion pertains to those at average-risk as identified previously in the chapter. Individuals with predisposing factors (family history, genetic syndromes, inflammatory disease) are not included in this grouping, and should continue with regularly scheduled colonoscopies as defined previously. Many of the adenomas identified in these high-risk groups have demonstrated a more rapid rate of progression to carcinoma, and thus, they continue to need aggressive screening measures throughout their lifetime.

The incidence of colon cancer rises sharply with advancing age. Many studies have examined this relationship over the past decades, and conclusive evidence supports this claim. In fact, the rate of colon cancer among those over 65 years of age is 254.2/100,000 persons, while the risk is substantially lower among those under 65, at 18.1/100,000 persons (NIH, 2009). Clearly, the elderly are at highest risk for developing colon cancer. Likewise, the elderly are also highest at risk for complications of colonoscopy. Extrapolating from the data previously provided, the complication rate amongst individuals 75-84 is 1330/100,000 people. Therefore, there would be roughly 5 times as many serious complications from colonoscopy as there would be actual diagnoses of cancer in the age group 75-84. Further, studies have been conducted looking at the chances of actually dying from colon cancer if diagnosed late in life. Among those at age 75 (and in the middle quartile of expected life remaining), they have a 1.9% chance of actually dying from colon cancer (Walter and Covinsky, 2001). By age 85, this risk decreases to 1.6%. Among elderly patients with multiple co-morbidities, the chance of dying from colon cancer falls to 0.85%. For comparison, a 50-year old male in the middle quartile of life expectancy has a 2.3% and female a 2.2% chance of eventually dying from colon cancer. While the incidence of colon cancer increases with age, it appears the mortality from the disease actually declines (if the cancer develops at the later age). These elderly patients succumb to an illness other than colon cancer. Additionally, studies have likewise examined the actual amount of life gained due to screening colonoscopy among different age groups. Here too there is a clear association with age. Among asymptomatic individuals undergoing screening colonoscopy, younger age groups experience a much larger benefit in terms of life gained. Among 50-54 year olds undergoing asymptomatic screening, there is roughly 0.84 years of life years gained (Lin et al., 2006). However, among individuals 80 years and above, only 0.13 additional years of life are gained. Thus, there is roughly a 6-fold difference in the actual effect of colon cancer screening between the two groups. Although younger patients have a much lower chance of developing colon cancer, they experience the lowest complication rate and benefit from the largest amount of life years gained if diagnosed and treated.

4.3. The resource allocation factor

It is also equally important to consider allocation of valuable resources when debating whether or not to forego colon cancer screening in the elderly. Colonoscopies, while cost-effective, are expensive. Those uninsured may have to pay thousands of dollars for the procedure, and those insured may have to pay copays, deductibles, etc. Moreover, the cost to society is enormous. Considering there are currently 74,008,000 Americans age 55 and above, there are millions of colonoscopies completed annually (Wagner et al., 1970). If there are no established recommendations on when it is appropriate to stop colonoscopy screening, millions of dollars will be spent for a procedure that may have minimal impact on the health of those screened. Moreover, funding that could go toward more cost-effective treatments or screening programs would be needlessly diverted. Fortunately, the Affordable Care Act (ACA) recently instated a policy in which Medicare and Medicaid "shall not impose any cost sharing requirements for evidence-based items or services that have in effect a rating of 'A' or 'B' in the current recommendations of the United States Preventive Services Task Force." Therefore, the cost of a colonoscopy to the individual may be minimized, however the cost to society will only grow. It is important to take into account the number of providers who can safely and effectively offer colonoscopy screening as well. Studies have demonstrated that colonoscopies performed by Gastroenterologists vs. non-Gastroenterologists are both more cost-effective and more beneficial to the patient (i.e. trained endoscopists are better at detection) (Hassan et al., 2012). In fact, the American Cancer Society estimates a savings of roughly $200,000,000 per year if all colonoscopies were performed by Gastroenterologists (currently both Gastroenterologists and non-Gastroenterologists are able to perform colonoscopy). Unfortunately, the number of gastroenterologists available to provide screening colonoscopies remains limited. Currently, there are roughly 10,400 practicing Gastroenterologists in the United States. As screening compliance increases (and the absolute number of individuals meeting the indication for screening increases as well), there will be a severe shortage of practicing Gastroenterologists. As mentioned previously, as of now, there is a 58.3% compliance rate to colon cancer screening. As this number increases, the limited supply of Gastroenterologists will ultimately be overwhelmed. Even those who meet indications for screening may be unable to obtain a colonoscopy in a timely manner. In effect, every colonoscopy performed on an elderly patient may mean one less colonoscopy for a young, healthy individual. Simply put, there must be established guidelines followed by all practitioners to ensure that screening colonoscopies are performed in the most cost-effective and life-preserving manner. Therefore, it is of paramount importance to take resource allocation into account when advising patients on whether to proceed with colonoscopy or not.

http://dx.doi.org/10.5772/53111

4.4. Evidence based approach to ending screening

The USPSTF currently recommends that colon cancer screening via colonoscopy be terminated at age 75 (USPSTF, 2008). This recommendation is based upon a Decision Analysis published in 2008. Again, using two simulation models, the authors examined the average life-years gained and the number of colonoscopies that would be required based upon the age at which colonoscopy screening was stopped (and assuming a 10-year interval screening method in average-risk individuals). The authors primarily tested ceasing colonoscopy at age 75 vs 85. In essence, they found that by stopping screening at age 75, they decreased the number of life-years gained by only 2-5/1000 people. However, the number of colonoscopies needed decreased by 348-398/1000 people. The ranges given signify the results from both simulation models. While some may argue that adding 2-5 life-years per 1000 people should take paramount importance, this unfortunately cannot be the case given the limited resources as discussed above. Until resources are infinite, it is necessary to funnel finances and medical staff toward the population that will most benefit from screening. Distributing the additional 348-398 colonoscopies to a younger population will result in more life-years gained, lives saved, and far fewer complications. Therefore, for the time being, it seems that ceasing colonoscopy screening at age 75 is both responsible and in the best interest of society.

4.5. Surveillance after late stage cancer diagnosis

Lastly, it is important to recognize that not all colonoscopies will be performed for strictly screening purposes. Ultimately, the goal of colonoscopy is early diagnosis and curative treatment by either polypectomy or bowel resection. However, as colon cancer is unfortunately still such a large cause of mortality in the United States and the screening rate is not 100%, many individuals will still be diagnosed with late-stage and unresectable colon cancer. This then poses the question, what is the utility in surveillance colonoscopy in these individuals?

To date, limited data exists concerning this topic. The primary treatment for patients with diagnosed Stage IV inoperable colon cancer is palliative chemotherapy. Occasionally, chemotherapy may be able to shrink the tumor(s) to an operable state, but this is more often not the case among late-stage diagnoses due to multiple metastases. Studies have analyzed prognostic indicators among patients with inoperable disease and found that performance status, ASA-class, CEA level, metastatic load, extent of primary tumor, and chemotherapy were the only independent variables affecting prognosis in these patients (Stelzner et al., 2005). While the initial diagnostic colonoscopy can provide valuable tissue data and information regarding depth of invasion, at this time surveillance colonoscopy does not appear to play a role in the management beyond initial diagnosis. Given that there is no clear benefit to surveillance colonoscopy after diagnosis of inoperable colon cancer and there are a multitude of risks associated with the procedure, surveillance colonoscopy is not indicated in these patients.

5. Factors that impact effective screening

Colonoscopy is an accurate and effective screening technique that is endorsed by many societies including the American Cancer Society, U.S. Multi-society Task Force, American College of Radiology, and American College of Gastroenterology (ACG) (Levin et al., 2008; Rex et al., 2009; USPSTF, 2008). While it may seem that screening for CRC is a well-established and accepted standard of care, screening rates for CRC have only recently started to approach that of other cancers. Increasing interest in the issue of best practice for CRC screening is attributable to updates to screening guidelines as a result of recent studies indicating significant mortality benefits. In addition to changes in the actual screening guidelines, the goal of screening has shifted to focus on cancer prevention by removing polyps rather than simply cancer detection (USPSTF, 2008). Important factors exist that impact the effectiveness of available screening modalities for CRC, and these originate from physicians, patients, as well as from society. While current recommendations support initiation of screening at age 50 for all average risk men and women, earlier initiation is advocated for those at higher risk including African American men and women. Knowledge about these guidelines can impact screening practice. Consideration must also be given to the modality of CRC screening. The ACG recommends colonoscopy as the preferred mode of screening, and the gold standard given it diagnostic and therapeutic potential (Rex et al., 2009). Studies demonstrate that most physicians overwhelmingly prefer colonoscopy as the test of choice (Guerra et al., 2007). In fact, 70% of PCPs strongly believe colonoscopy is the best available colorectal cancer-screening test. Furthermore, a large proportion of physicians are concerned over lawsuits if they do not offer screening colonoscopies. The fear of facing a lawsuit over colonoscopy complications can be outweighed by the fear of being sued if the procedure is not offered at all (McGregor et al., 2010; Varela et al., 2010). While CRC screening saves lives, the use of colonoscopy and other available options, remains suboptimal. Pinpointing the reasons why people are not getting screened, either by choice or by circumstance, is essential in order to increase screening outcomes and compliance. There are unquestionably many barriers to effective healthcare delivery in the US, let alone being able to appropriately screen for CRC (Hoffman et al., 2011). Barriers can be sorted into a few main categories: physician, patient, societal related factors. This section will touch on some of these obstacles.

5.1. The role of the physician in CRC screening

Physician recommendations play a crucial role in the decision to get screened for CRC (Zapka et al., 2011). A mere discussion of CRC screening at the time of an office visit may be sufficient and motivate patients to complete CRC screening. Given the prominence of the physician factor it is important to consider elements that impact physician recommendation of colonoscopy to their patients. Collegial norms, patient preferences, and published evidence including guidelines from the ACS and USPSF have been identified as important elements. Physicians in the US favor endoscopy and often fail to adequately present alternatives such as stool testing. One study found that 50% of the patients surveyed did not receive the test they requested, and most underwent a colonoscopy instead (Hawley et al., 2012). However, since all screening tests have some benefit, even if they are not on par with

http://dx.doi.org/10.5772/53111

colonoscopy, physicians need to be sensitive and attuned to patient preferences. Techniques other than colonoscopy may be more suitable for specific patients, given their individual circumstances. For example, a recent study published in *Cancer* found that wealthy patients frequently opt for colonoscopy while lower socioeconomic groups tended to choose at home stool testing over endoscopy (Bandi et al., 2012). Patient preference varies by ethnicity as well, with African Americans less likely to choose endoscopy than Caucasians (Dimou et al., 2009). From their trial data, Inadomi and colleagues (Inadomi et al., 2012) predict that if colonoscopy were the only option offered, fewer patients would be screened. It is evident that the choice of screening test should take into consideration not only the physician's, but also the patient's perspective because some form of screening still remains superior to no screening at all. Considering the evidence above, physicians should recommend one best option to their patients using evidence-based medicine and taking into account patient specific factors. CRC screening guidelines are complicated and offering multiple options still requires shared decision making in practice (Zapka et al., 2011).

Although Medicare coverage has lessened these concerns, many physicians reported that health insurance remains very influential for screening recommendations (White et al., 2012). Of note, individuals of lower socioeconomic classes have expressed concerns that they experience a lack of screening offers from doctors. This is supported by physicians who admit they do not recommend colonoscopy, if patients do not have insurance or ready access. Another interesting difference in physician screening recommendation was the age of the physician, with younger physicians recommending the test more. Although this is merely speculation, younger physicians may be more comfortable ordering this newer test (Zapka et al., 2011).

In practice, physicians often fail to mention CRC screening because of limited time, competing issues, and forgetfulness. At times the many pressing issues that need to be addressed, preclude the lengthy discussion about available cancer screening tests. Additionally, many patients only go to a clinic to address urgent issues. These clinics are often overbooked and the main focus is to stabilize the acute problem. Some patients lack health insurance or are unwilling to wait for appointments (Guerra et al., 2007). At best, some physicians may recommend a follow up health maintenance visit. In addition, one national survey suggested that the primary care physicians may not adequately discuss all test options available with average risk patients because they are under the assumption that this will be addressed in more depth by specialists. Screening rates suffer from lack of coordination between specialists and PCPs (Doubeni et al., 2010). Physician forgetfulness and unfamiliarity with guidelines is a preventable obstacle to screening (White et al., 2012). The screening and surveillance recommendations differ significantly for a subset of CRC patients with hereditary syndromes. There is a marked lack of knowledge about screening guidelines for high-risk populations based on family history and also ethnicity. Primary care physician recommendations are often inconsistent with published guidelines. Among those most intimate with guidelines, the gastroenterologists, only a fraction recommended genetic counseling, which is also a part of appropriate screening (White et al., 2012).

Studies have suggested that physicians may not be fully aware of patient's attitudes and values towards screening. Physicians underestimated test discomfort and did not recognize the importance of helping patients make informed decisions for screening. In addition, several studies have shown that PCPs recommendations are affected by their demography including age, sex and ethnicity. For example, non-Caucasian physicians are less likely to recommend cancer screening compared to Caucasian doctors. Hispanic physicians in the US were found to be less likely to recommend CRC screening. In a study in Australia, general practitioners of Middle Eastern ethnicity estimated CRC incidence to be lower in immigrants compared to patients born in Australia, which may have resulted in lower recommendations of CRC screening for immigrants (Koo et al., 2012). Thus in general, primary care physicians need greater awareness about CRC rates and screening.

While patients cite physician recommendation as the number one motivator for screening, other factors might impact compliance. Research demonstrates that providing excessive choices can be overwhelming subsequently leading to confusion and indecision. Selection of one preferred alternative may help simplify the discussion about screening (Inadomi et al., 2012). Studies that target physician recommendations have been shown to be more effective than those that focus only on the patient (Guerra et al., 2007). In contrast, others argue that options are needed because every CRC screening modality has its own strengths and limitations. Additionally, there does not seem to be a clear consensus among patients about preferred methods. Thus, an important question arises: would patients be more willing to participate in screening, if they are given the opportunity to choose? Engaging patients in the decision-making process can improve satisfaction by taking into account each patient's unique needs. A patient-centered approach improves screening compliance (Inadomi et al., 2012).

5.2. Patient-based factors in CRC screening

At the center of the discussion related to screening is the patient's participation in completing the process. While low participation rates in screening related to infrequent or lack of follow-up is a difficult barrier to overcome, other factors are also important. It is notable that most of the data about reasons for screening non-compliance comes from direct physician report (Hoffman et al., 2011). Physicians reported offering screening to all of their high risk and most of their average risk patients, and most were surprised at the low adherence rates. Through their interactions with patients, physicians believed barriers to screening were fear of the test, embarrassment, lack of insurance, and lack of knowledge about cancer and screening. Interestingly, when patients were asked the same questions, they did not feel that discomfort or embarrassment kept them from undergoing the procedure. Patients reported lack of physician recommendation as one of the main factors for not getting tested, along with lack of symptoms that might suggest a colon neoplasm (Jones et al., 2010). Of course these studies are limited in terms of the particular patient population sampled and may not be applicable to all patients; however, it is important to note that patients place great importance on the conversation with primary care providers about CRC screening (Fenton et al., 2011). Furthermore, this is directly linked to patient's knowledge about CRC and screening. Misconceptions continue to prevail as barriers to CRC screening, indicating a continued need for brief, direct encouragement from providers to educate patients about screening, particularly in the absence of symptoms or family history of CRC. Physicians can have great impact on CRC screening, particularly with lifesaving colonoscopy, which is greatly underutilized in the US.

In a questionnaire investigating the patient barriers to CRC screening, hesitation about screening was highest among never-screened respondents, intermediate among ever-screened respondents who were overdue for testing, and lowest among the people adherent with guidelines suggesting that different obstacles exist within each target group. The only difference between those groups of patients is *prior screening status*. These results also demonstrate that people who have undergone screening are less fearful of the test itself, this could be attributed to the fact that they have first hand experience instead of false information or misconceptions. Patients who are more educated are likely to be aware of the risks and benefits of CRC screening (Winterich et al., 2011).

5.2.1. *Patient attitudes, beliefs, and knowledge of CRC*

Low compliance for CRC screening by patients can be attributed to several factors including lack of insurance, cost, lack of knowledge of cancer and screening, not seeing a need for testing, embarrassment, lack of symptoms or health problems, fear of perceived pain, and anxiety of testing. This is in addition to failure by recommendation from a physician (Jones et al., 2010). Studies have suggested that many patients dread getting ready for and having the test and also worry about the test results. Additional research has found that the participants did not understand the purpose of screening for cancer, were not able to distinguish between screening tests from any other tests and did not realize that screening is performed when a person feels well (Shokar et al., 2005).

Lack of knowledge is a major barrier to screening, particularly for immigrants, ethnic minorities, and underserved populations because of challenges in effective communication, as will be discussed later. Studies looking into lack of knowledge about colon cancer screening identified many other knowledge gaps including low health literacy. Some individuals did not have a basic understanding of human anatomy and were not able to identify the location of the colon nor its purpose. A subset of these individuals did not believe colon cancer existed. Furthermore, a surprising amount of educated individuals could not accurately describe the colon's function, confusing it with the rectum and anus (Francois et al., 2009; Winterich et al., 2011).

Those that had some fundamental knowledge of colon anatomy lacked an adequate understanding about the causes and risk factors of colon cancer. Many individuals without symptoms or family history do not feel concerned about this disease. Some are under the impression that causes of colon cancer center around food and thought that bowel cleansing was a good way to maintain or re-establish health. Others cited that they did not get screened because they did not smoke, drink, eat unhealthy foods, or participate in anal sex, all of which they perceived to be high-risk behaviors (Francois et al., 2009).

In addition to poor understanding about colon cancer, many misperceptions about colonoscopy itself were identified. One study captured the reasons some people did not like colonoscopy including that the preparation was "inconvenient", "uncomfortable", and involved a "compromising position". Men of all races and levels of educational attainment shared the male specific gender barrier that they were turned off by the invasive nature of the colonoscopy. While males and females have similar screening rates, men expressed more initial hesitation about screening because of the fear that it threatens their masculinity. Men who associated their masculinity with these exams experienced them more negatively (Winterich et al., 2011). Interestingly, Winterich et al. (Winterich et al., 2011) found that as education increased, men's negative views of colonoscopy also seemed to increase. Most individuals of a low-educational attainment generally described the colonoscopy as a "good" test because of the culturally dominant view that medical care is important (Winterich et al., 2011).

5.2.2. Racial and ethnic disparities in CRC screening

As mentioned earlier, screening rates differ based on race and ethnic groups. The National Health Interview Survey reported that racial disparities seen with CRC screening are related to socioeconomic status, however, racial disparities persist despite coverage for CRC screening in a Medicare population (Wilkins et al., 2012). Compared to whites, blacks and Hispanics are less likely to be screened. Overall rates of CRC screening are estimated to be 50% and it is even lower for minorities. Screening rates vary even within a racial or ethnic group, e.g among Asians, Koreans and Vietnamese have lower rates of screening; among whites, those living in Appalachia have lower screening rates. Minority populations and low socioeconomic status are considered to be factors resulting in low CRC screening rates (Linsky et al., 2011). Research studies also suggest that immigrants may experience unique barriers such as language and cultural differences with their health care providers which can lead to poorer communication about the importance of screening (Goel et al., 2003).

5.2.3. The language divide

Patients who do not speak English are less likely to be screened (Linsky et al., 2011). According to the 2005-2007 American Community Survey, minorities comprise 26% of the population, and nearly 20% of Americans speak a language other than English at home. By 2050, minorities could make up about half of the US population, with a similar increase in individuals speaking a language other than English at home. Spanish speaking Hispanics are 43% less likely to receive CRC screening. Communication problems when discussing cancer screening are also documented with Vietnamese Americans (Linsky et al., 2011). Additionally, for Creole speaking Haitian Americans the language barrier may also be a factor in communicating with physicians (Francois et al., 2009). While patient-physician language discordance presents a barrier, it is possible to address it through initiatives such as translation services so that disparities in screening rates can be reduced.

5.2.4. Cultural chasms

Cultural beliefs can result in lower screening rates, for example, Italian- Australians, Macedonian-Australians and Greek- Australians were found to believe that nothing can be done to treat 'malignant' cancers and that in fact, treatment of cancers may hasten death (Severino et al., 2009). They also believe that consumption of 'unnaturally' grown foods, eating foods sprayed with pesticides or experiencing strong emotions may cause cancer. Studies with African Americans have indicated that the lack of CRC knowledge, lack of physician recommendation, and a distrust of the health care system and providers impede screening; as well as a fatalistic belief (beliefs that screening and treatments are 'futile' since it is in "God's hands") which has also been reported as a barrier for CRC screening (James et al., 2002). A subset of individuals connected colon cancer with "someone putting a curse on you" (Francois et al., 2009). Studies in Latino population suggest that fatalistic attitudes and fear of cancer are barriers to cancer screening and misconceptions about the causes of cancer as well as perceived discomfort and embarrassment (Walsh et al., 2004).

Among other factors, family recommendations and cultural norms weighed heavily on perceptions about cancer and colonoscopy. For example, studies with Mexican and Hispanic communities have cited the need for strategies to distribute the information without causing any stigma or embarrassment. Privacy is highly valued in Mexican culture and thus individualized educational sessions are a good approach. On the other hand, Hispanic communities prefer group educational workshops. Emphasis on family and being healthy to provide for the family was effective, as well as convincing women within families of the importance of screening. Latinos also tend to see doctors only when sick and combine traditional and home healing with physician prescribed medications. Religion and spirituality seem to impact the willingness to accept CRC screening, as does low income and less education (Getrich et al., 2012).

In a study of Haitian immigrants, preventive care was not emphasized by the community. Haitians make one of the largest immigrant groups in US and have the lowest percentage of insurance coverage. Instead of having a primary physician they seem to rely on emergency rooms and do not see a doctor unless there is something wrong, there is not an operating concept valuing 'check ups'. Undocumented persons, seek help only in an emergency situation and instead rely on home remedies. These individuals expressed that they simply did not want to know if there was something wrong with them, because finding one problem might lead to other ones (Francois et al., 2009).

5.2.5. Health literacy and educational outreach in CRC screening

Efforts to empower patients to become involved in their own care have proven to be effective. Health literacy campaigns in New York City have improved CRC screening rates. Community education is required to promote screening and public education campaigns are shown to be effective. For example Mr. Polyp ads, a public service announcement from the American Cancer Society, led many to ask their doctors about colonoscopies (Guerra et al., 2007). Population based interventions aimed at increasing the demand for screening include, reminders and incentives, mass and small media, group and one-on-one education. Bilingual verbal communication and 'word of mouth' are also potentially very effective modalities. Blumenthal et al. (Blumenthal et al., 2010) tested three interventions intended to increase the rate of CRC screening among African Americans. They concluded that group education doubled screening rates and reduced out of pocket expenses. Furthermore, differences in attitudes and perceived barriers among ethnic and minority population may need culturally tailored interventions. Focus groups with Hispanics identified fear of finding cancer and fear of embarrassment from the examination, as screening obstacles. With this information, Varela et al. (Varela et al., 2010) developed targeted educational materials to promote colonoscopies among Hispanics. Similar educational materials could tap into faith-based programs like the successful Witness Project for breast cancer.

5.2.6. Patient navigators and customized CRC screening

As previously mentioned, ethnic and cultural differences can pose a great barrier to effective cancer screening. Patient advocates who help coordinate care provide an option for tackling screening disparities. Termed patient navigators, these individuals are laypersons from the community who help patients navigate the intricacies of the health care system (Lasser et al., 2011). They can better address the unique needs of a patient and are responsible for almost anything such as helping patients get insurance, finding transportation to doctors' appointments, healthcare education, and emotional support. For example, patients that require interpreters are found to be less compliant with screening recommendations. Providing patients with a healthcare ambassador who speaks their preferred language has proven to be a simple yet extremely powerful intervention. In a randomized controlled trial, recently published in the Archives of Internal Medicine, researchers found quantifiable benefits from assigning black and non-English speaking patients with a healthcare navigator. These patients had a greater likelihood of being screened by FOBT than control subjects (33.6% vs 20.0%; P<.001) and were also more likely to undergo colonoscopy (26.4% vs 13.0%; P,.001). Moreover, these patients had more adenomas detected (8.1% vs 3.9%; P<.06) and more cases of CRC prevented (Lasser et al., 2011). This study highlights the importance of a multidisciplinary approach to medicine. The impact of patient navigators, especially on urban and racial minorities, is demonstrated by numerous studies (Chen et al., 2008; Lasser et al., 2011; Lasser et al., 2009; Ma et al., 2009; Myers et al., 2008; Nash et al., 2006). A recent study found patient navigators to be effective for Creole or Portuguese speaking patients. This model can be observed in practice in Boston where Partners in Health routinely trains paramedical personnel to assist in providing customized care for patients with HIV and TB in Haiti and Rwanda.

The benefit of a team approach to healthcare is further evidenced by studies demonstrating that the use of nurse practitioners and physicians assistants further streamlines healthcare delivery and improves screening compliance. Moreover, telephone counseling and printed materials can help improve follow up and overall quality of life in colorectal cancer survivors. Clouston et al. (Clouston et al., 2012) performed a study to evaluate use of a website and telephones on CRC screening rates and concluded that both increased compliance significantly. However, a strong and trusting family physician-patient relationship must be maintained; otherwise, patients will experience a fundamental disconnect in the patient-physician relationship that may discourage screening. The team-based approach does not look to replace the physician, but can enhance patient-physician discourse.

Customized programs targeted to specific individuals may help improve patient participation rates. Tailored screening guidelines have been advocated for certain groups based on noted prevalence and anatomic location of colonic lesions in these populations. For example, women are known to have an increased risk of right-sided polyps and cancer (Chu et al., 2011), while African Americans tend to develop colorectal cancer at an earlier age (Agrawal et al., 2005). The recommendation for tailored screening guidelines as suggested by the ACG have the potential to help address existing disparities in CRC but must be balanced by ease of implementation as well as healthcare financing concerns.

5.3. Public policies, outreach, and CRC screening

Although screening rates for CRC remain suboptimal, there has been an overall upward trend. Endorsement from various recommending organizations helped promote awareness of CRC screening in the medical community. Supported by population-based studies, gastroenterology organizations have promoted screening with colonoscopy as the best screening test. The healthcare policy to support CRC screening through Medicare reimbursement was impactful in developing further acceptance. Medicare's decision to support screening colonoscopy had a significant impact on the popularity of this modality as other payers followed suit. With insurance companies willing to pay, doctors were more inclined to recommend screening and free to choose their preferred modality, colonoscopy. In fact, gastroenterologists report they are now performing many more colonoscopies than before. Some spend 50% to 80% of their time performing this one procedure, a dramatic increase from before (Ransohoff, 2005).

Public perception and support has greatly impacted the implementation of screening, especially colonoscopy. All of the aforementioned factors are geared at gaining strong popular support, a necessary ingredient for any widespread screening practice. For example, prostate cancer screening became widely practiced on the basis of popular support, even without evidence of mortality reduction. Arguably the most influential aspect of colon cancer and screening awareness was the increasing presence of colonoscopy in the media. Famous people affected by colon cancer include Ronald Reagan, Audrey Hepburn, and Daryl Strawberry to name a few. Public interest in colonoscopy reached a turning point in March of 2000, the first colon cancer awareness month. This initiative was spearheaded by news icon Katie Couric, who advocated for CRC screening on the national stage by televising her own colonoscopy after her husband's death (Cram et al., 2003). Similar appearances of colonoscopy in the media impacted CRC screening practices in the United States. Most recently, Dr. Oz underwent a colonoscopy on his eponymous television show. An editorial featured in the New York Times entitled "Going the distance-the case for true colorectal-cancer screening" garnered further support for colonoscopies stating that sigmoidoscopy, that only screens part of the colon, is comparable to mammography for only one breast. Numerous editorials and front page articles have featured colonoscopies (Ransohoff, 2005). For example a newspaper ad made the assertion, "your golden years deserve the gold standard of colon cancer screening" (American College of Gastroenterology [ACG], 2012). Additional marketing on the web has helped improve awareness among the public who increasingly use the web for health information (Cohen and Adams, 2011).

5.3.1. Healthcare access

For patients to consider screening, it is important that to have insurance coverage, access to healthcare or both. Only 24% of uninsured Americans, who do not have a usual source of health care and are eligible, participate in CRC screening (Shapiro et al., 2012). Patients with higher incomes are likely to have health insurance and tend to have a consistent source of care. A recent systemic review reported that lower socioeconomic status was correlated with a higher incidence and mortality rate (Wilkins et al., 2012). Subramanian et al. (Subramanian et al., 2010) argue that when budgets are tight, options other than colonoscopies are better for screening, basing this on the premise that some form of screening is better than no screening at all. This study asserts that state and federal agencies have screening programs for the uninsured and underinsured that may not be able to support colonoscopy in their limited budget. However efficacy of the guaiac based fecal blood test depends on 100% compliance. This is often not practical and the study's authors admit that colonoscopy is still a better screening test if annual testing is not feasible.

In addition to financial access, geographic access can pose a problem for individuals in rural areas. In New York City and other urban centers, most hospitals and many private practices will offer colonoscopy; however, this is not the case in every part of the country. Several studies have found lower screening rates in rural versus nonrural areas (Wilkins et al., 2012). Geographic distance is a factor and individuals are less likely to be screened if the nearest colonoscopy-offering center is over an hour away. The rural countries in the study by Wilkins et al. (Wilkins et al., 2012) had higher poverty rates, lower educational level, limited access to doctors, and less insurance coverage.

5.3.2. National programs

The benefits of a team approach to healthcare is further evidenced by national programs that help promote patient awareness and education about CRC screening. Health policy initiatives need to underscore the importance of screening programs to improve quality of cancer screening. Cancer registries may be of use to identify and monitor the incidence, stage of cancer and screening rate across regions. A CRC screening registry similar to Breast Cancer Surveillance Consortium could be established to monitor rates of screening, overuse, quality and complications. An ideal monitoring system should be able to estimate rates of screening regardless of patient's insurance status and demographic characteristics, assess use, appropriateness and outcomes. Efforts should be made to support expansion, analysis and collaboration of existing data sources and databases such as Clinical Outcome Research Initiative (CORI) endoscopy data base, the Cancer Research Network (CRN) and the Computed Tomography Colonography Registry.

http://dx.doi.org/10.5772/53111

5.3.3. Communication via current technologies

The use of systems strategies can improve physician delivery of healthcare. Systems strategies employ patient and physician screening reminders, performance reports of screening rates, and electronic medical records (Yabroff et al., 2011). Given time constraints, remembering to perform all routine screenings for every patient is difficult. The increasing use of electronic medical records (EMR) has helped physicians overcome this obstacle. Pop-up reminders can help minimize forgetfulness, as well as the added pressure of remembering individualized guidelines. These electronic prompts have the additional advantage of flexibility, which allows for screening to account for the patient's personal and family history. In one retrospective survey, the physicians that utilized this technology, which automatically provided appointments for CRC screening at a certain age, had the highest screening rates (Fenton et al., 2011).

In addition to physician prompts, organized screening programs make use of patient reminders to improve screening compliance. These programs reach out to all members of the population due for CRC screening via mailed reminders (Levin et al., 2011). In addition to outreach mailings, the Task Force on Community Preventive Services of the Centers for Disease Control and Prevention recommend performance reports for doctors. Monetary incentive from insurance companies for completing age-appropriate screening is effective. Additionally, better reimbursements are needed to encourage spending time on preventive medicine (Guerra et al., 2007). Brouwers (Brouwers et al., 2011) conducted a systemic review that included 66 randomized controlled studies and a cluster of randomized controlled trials. They concluded that client reminders, small media and provider audit and feedback appear to increase screening rates significantly. Despite evidence that systems strategies are effective, relatively few physicians report using a comprehensive plan to promote cancer screening (Yabroff et al., 2011).

5.3.4. Health insurance coverage for colonoscopy

Ensuring health insurance coverage and usual source of care will most likely increase use among those who have never been screened. Following Medicare's example, private insurance coverage of CRC screening will be a step towards resolving the cost issue for physicians and patients. Asking patients to pay thousands of out of pocket expenses to undergo a colonoscopy, will not help increase the rates of this life saving procedure. In a step to increase testing accessibility and affordability, the Affordable Care Act will ask insurers to cover screening colonoscopies. This will include not only colonoscopy, but the use of anesthesia (e.g. propofol) as opposed to conscious sedation (e.g., midazolam, fentanyl). Providing increased options for sedation is likely to remove the patient barrier related to discomfort and make it more likely that individuals will comply with colonoscopy as a life-saving screening modality (Liu et al., 2012).

6. Conclusion

This chapter has summarized the current body of knowledge related to colorectal cancer screening and surveillance recommendations in the context of addressing risk stratification, when to start and stop screening, as well as factors that impact screening rates. Overall, screening, detection, and removal of precancerous lesions allow for the prevention of CRC. It is notable that although strong evidence now exists for the mortality benefits of CRC screening, significant disparities remain in the disease thus giving rise to opportunities to address physician, patient, as well as societal factors that can improve screening rates.

Acknowledgements

We thank the Office of Diversity Affairs at the New York University School of Medicine for its support.

Author details

Anjali Mone, Robert Mocharla, Allison Avery and Fritz Francois

New York University Langone Medical Center, USA

References

[1] Abotchie, P.N., Vernon, S.W., and Du, X.L. (2012). Gender differences in colorectal cancer incidence in the United States, 1975-2006. J Womens Health (Larchmt) 21, 393-400.

[2] American College of Gastroenterology. 2012. Your golden years deserve the gold standard of colon cancer screening. Retrieved from s3.gi.org/patients/ccrk/crcad2.pdf.

[3] Agrawal, S., Bhupinderjit, A., Bhutani, M.S., Boardman, L., Nguyen, C., Romero, Y., Srinivasan, R., and Figueroa-Moseley, C. (2005). Colorectal cancer in African Americans. Am J Gastroenterol 100, 515-523; discussion 514.

[4] Alberti, L.R., De Lima, D.C., De Lacerda Rodrigues, K.C., Taranto, M.P., Goncalves, S.H., and Petroianu, A. (2012). The impact of colonoscopy for colorectal cancer screening. Surg Endosc.

[5] Bandi, P., Cokkinides, V., Smith, R.A., and Jemal, A. (2012). Trends in colorectal cancer screening with home-based fecal occult blood tests in adults ages 50 to 64 years, 2000 to 2008. Cancer.

[6] Bini, E.J., Park, J., and Francois, F. (2006). Use of flexible sigmoidoscopy to screen for colorectal cancer in HIV-infected patients 50 years of age and older. Arch Intern Med 166, 1626-1631.

[7] Blumenthal, D.S., Smith, S.A., Majett, C.D., and Alema-Mensah, E. (2010). A trial of 3 interventions to promote colorectal cancer screening in African Americans. Cancer 116, 922-929.

[8] Boleij, A., and Tjalsma, H. (2012). Gut bacteria in health and disease: a survey on the interface between intestinal microbiology and colorectal cancer. Biological reviews of the Cambridge Philosophical Society 87, 701-730.

[9] Bresalier, R.S. (2009). Early detection of and screening for colorectal neoplasia. Gut and liver 3, 69-80.

[10] Brouwers, M.C., De Vito, C., Bahirathan, L., Carol, A., Carroll, J.C., Cotterchio, M., Dobbins, M., Lent, B., Levitt, C., Lewis, N., et al. (2011). What implementation interventions increase cancer screening rates? a systematic review. Implementation science : IS 6, 111.

[11] Bussey, H.J., Veale, A.M., and Morson, B.C. (1978). Genetics of gastrointestinal polyposis. Gastroenterology 74, 1325-1330.

[12] Canavan, C., Abrams, K.R., and Mayberry, J. (2006). Meta-analysis: colorectal and small bowel cancer risk in patients with Crohn's disease. Aliment Pharmacol Ther 23, 1097-1104.

[13] Cash, B.D., Banerjee, S., Anderson, M.A., Ben-Menachem, T., Decker, G.A., Fanelli, R.D., Fukami, N., Ikenberry, S.O., Jain, R., Jue, T.L., et al. (2010). Ethnic issues in endoscopy. Gastrointest Endosc 71, 1108-1112.

[14] Chen, C.D., Yen, M.F., Wang, W.M., Wong, J.M., and Chen, T.H. (2003). A case-cohort study for the disease natural history of adenoma-carcinoma and de novo carcinoma and surveillance of colon and rectum after polypectomy: implication for efficacy of colonoscopy. Br J Cancer 88, 1866-1873.

[15] Chen, L.A., Santos, S., Jandorf, L., Christie, J., Castillo, A., Winkel, G., and Itzkowitz, S. (2008). A program to enhance completion of screening colonoscopy among urban minorities. Clin Gastroenterol Hepatol 6, 443-450.

[16] Chien, C., Morimoto, L.M., Tom, J., and Li, C.I. (2005). Differences in colorectal carcinoma stage and survival by race and ethnicity. Cancer 104, 629-639.

[17] Chlebowski, R.T., Wactawski-Wende, J., Ritenbaugh, C., Hubbell, F.A., Ascensao, J., Rodabough, R.J., Rosenberg, C.A., Taylor, V.M., Harris, R., Chen, C., et al. (2004). Estrogen plus progestin and colorectal cancer in postmenopausal women. N Engl J Med 350, 991-1004.

[18] Cho, E., Smith-Warner, S.A., Ritz, J., van den Brandt, P.A., Colditz, G.A., Folsom, A.R., Freudenheim, J.L., Giovannucci, E., Goldbohm, R.A., Graham, S., et al. (2004).

Alcohol intake and colorectal cancer: a pooled analysis of 8 cohort studies. Ann Intern Med 140, 603-613.

[19] Chu, L.L., Weinstein, S., and Yee, J. (2011). Colorectal cancer screening in women: an underutilized lifesaver. AJR American journal of roentgenology 196, 303-310.

[20] Citarda, F., Tomaselli, G., Capocaccia, R., Barcherini, S., and Crespi, M. (2001). Efficacy in standard clinical practice of colonoscopic polypectomy in reducing colorectal cancer incidence. Gut 48, 812-815.

[21] Clouston, K.M., Katz, A., Martens, P.J., Sisler, J., Turner, D., Lobchuk, M., and McClement, S. (2012). Does access to a colorectal cancer screening website and/or a nurse-managed telephone help line provided to patients by their family physician increase fecal occult blood test uptake?: A pragmatic cluster randomized controlled trial study protocol. BMC Cancer 12, 182.

[22] Cohen, R.A., Adams P.F. Use of the Internet for Health Information: United States, 2009. NCHS data brief, no 66. Hyattsville, MD: National Center for Health Statistics. 2011.

[23] Colditz, G.A., Cannuscio, C.C., and Frazier, A.L. (1997). Physical activity and reduced risk of colon cancer: implications for prevention. Cancer Causes Control 8, 649-667.

[24] Collett, J.A., Platell, C., Fletcher, D.R., Aquilia, S., and Olynyk, J.K. (1999). Distal colonic neoplasms predict proximal neoplasia in average-risk, asymptomatic subjects. J Gastroenterol Hepatol 14, 67-71.

[25] Cram, P., Fendrick, A.M., Inadomi, J., Cowen, M.E., Carpenter, D., and Vijan, S. (2003). The impact of a celebrity promotional campaign on the use of colon cancer screening: the Katie Couric effect. Arch Intern Med 163, 1601-1605.

[26] Dimou, A., Syrigos, K.N., and Saif, M.W. (2009). Disparities in colorectal cancer in African-Americans vs Whites: before and after diagnosis. World J Gastroenterol 15, 3734-3743.

[27] Doubeni, C.A., Laiyemo, A.O., Young, A.C., Klabunde, C.N., Reed, G., Field, T.S., and Fletcher, R.H. (2010). Primary care, economic barriers to health care, and use of colorectal cancer screening tests among Medicare enrollees over time. Annals of family medicine 8, 299-307.

[28] Eaden, J.A., Abrams, K.R., and Mayberry, J.F. (2001). The risk of colorectal cancer in ulcerative colitis: a meta-analysis. Gut 48, 526-535.

[29] Edwards, B.K., Ward, E., Kohler, B.A., Eheman, C., Zauber, A.G., Anderson, R.N., Jemal, A., Schymura, M.J., Lansdorp-Vogelaar, I., Seeff, L.C., et al. (2010). Annual report to the nation on the status of cancer, 1975-2006, featuring colorectal cancer trends and impact of interventions (risk factors, screening, and treatment) to reduce future rates. Cancer 116, 544-573.

[30] Fedirko, V., Tramacere, I., Bagnardi, V., Rota, M., Scotti, L., Islami, F., Negri, E., Straif, K., Romieu, I., La Vecchia, C., et al. (2011). Alcohol drinking and colorectal cancer risk: an overall and dose-response meta-analysis of published studies. Annals of oncology : official journal of the European Society for Medical Oncology / ESMO 22, 1958-1972.

[31] Fenton, J.J., Jerant, A.F., von Friederichs-Fitzwater, M.M., Tancredi, D.J., and Franks, P. (2011). Physician counseling for colorectal cancer screening: impact on patient attitudes, beliefs, and behavior. J Am Board Fam Med 24, 673-681.

[32] Ferlay, J., Shin, H.R., Bray, F., Forman, D., Mathers, C., and Parkin, D.M. (2010). Estimates of worldwide burden of cancer in 2008: GLOBOCAN 2008. Int J Cancer 127, 2893-2917.

[33] Flossmann, E., and Rothwell, P.M. (2007). Effect of aspirin on long-term risk of colorectal cancer: consistent evidence from randomised and observational studies. Lancet 369, 1603-1613.

[34] Francois, F., Elysee, G., Shah, S., and Gany, F. (2009). Colon cancer knowledge and attitudes in an immigrant Haitian community. J Immigr Minor Health 11, 319-325.

[35] Francois, F., Park, J., and Bini, E.J. (2006). Colon pathology detected after a positive screening flexible sigmoidoscopy: a prospective study in an ethnically diverse cohort. Am J Gastroenterol 101, 823-830.

[36] Gatto, N.M., Frucht, H., Sundararajan, V., Jacobson, J.S., Grann, V.R., and Neugut, A.I. (2003). Risk of perforation after colonoscopy and sigmoidoscopy: a population-based study. J Natl Cancer Inst 95, 230-236.

[37] Getrich, C.M., Sussman, A.L., Helitzer, D.L., Hoffman, R.M., Warner, T.D., Sanchez, V., Solares, A., and Rhyne, R.L. (2012). Expressions of machismo in colorectal cancer screening among New Mexico Hispanic subpopulations. Qualitative health research 22, 546-559.

[38] Goel, M.S., Wee, C.C., McCarthy, E.P., Davis, R.B., Ngo-Metzger, Q., and Phillips, R.S. (2003). Racial and ethnic disparities in cancer screening: the importance of foreign birth as a barrier to care. J Gen Intern Med 18, 1028-1035.

[39] Govindarajan, R., Shah, R.V., Erkman, L.G., and Hutchins, L.F. (2003). Racial differences in the outcome of patients with colorectal carcinoma. Cancer 97, 493-498.

[40] Guerra, C.E., Schwartz, J.S., Armstrong, K., Brown, J.S., Halbert, C.H., and Shea, J.A. (2007). Barriers of and facilitators to physician recommendation of colorectal cancer screening. J Gen Intern Med 22, 1681-1688.

[41] Haggar, F.A., and Boushey, R.P. (2009). Colorectal cancer epidemiology: incidence, mortality, survival, and risk factors. Clinics in colon and rectal surgery 22, 191-197.

[42] Hardy, R.G., Meltzer, S.J., and Jankowski, J.A. (2000). ABC of colorectal cancer. Molecular basis for risk factors. BMJ 321, 886-889.

[43] Hassan, C., Rex, D.K., Zullo, A., and Cooper, G.S. (2012). Loss of efficacy and cost-effectiveness when screening colonoscopy is performed by nongastroenterologists. Cancer.

[44] Hawley, S.T., McQueen, A., Bartholomew, L.K., Greisinger, A.J., Coan, S.P., Myers, R., and Vernon, S.W. (2012). Preferences for colorectal cancer screening tests and screening test use in a large multispecialty primary care practice. Cancer 118, 2726-2734.

[45] Hirata, K., Noguchi, J., Yoshikawa, I., Tabaru, A., Nagata, N., Murata, I., and Itoh, H. (1996). Acute appendicitis immediately after colonoscopy. Am J Gastroenterol 91, 2239-2240.

[46] Hoffman, R.M., Espey, D., and Rhyne, R.L. (2011). A public-health perspective on screening colonoscopy. Expert review of anticancer therapy 11, 561-569.

[47] Howe, J.R., Mitros, F.A., and Summers, R.W. (1998). The risk of gastrointestinal carcinoma in familial juvenile polyposis. Ann Surg Oncol 5, 751-756.

[48] Humphreys, F., Hewetson, K.A., and Dellipiani, A.W. (1984). Massive subcutaneous emphysema following colonoscopy. Endoscopy 16, 160-161.

[49] Imperiale, T.F., Ransohoff, D.F., Itzkowitz, S.H., Turnbull, B.A., and Ross, M.E. (2004). Fecal DNA versus fecal occult blood for colorectal-cancer screening in an average-risk population. N Engl J Med 351, 2704-2714.

[50] Imperiale, T.F., Wagner, D.R., Lin, C.Y., Larkin, G.N., Rogge, J.D., and Ransohoff, D.F. (2000). Risk of advanced proximal neoplasms in asymptomatic adults according to the distal colorectal findings. N Engl J Med 343, 169-174.

[51] Inadomi, J.M., Vijan, S., Janz, N.K., Fagerlin, A., Thomas, J.P., Lin, Y.V., Munoz, R., Lau, C., Somsouk, M., El-Nachef, N., et al. (2012). Adherence to colorectal cancer screening: a randomized clinical trial of competing strategies. Arch Intern Med 172, 575-582.

[52] James, A.S., Campbell, M.K., and Hudson, M.A. (2002). Perceived barriers and benefits to colon cancer screening among African Americans in North Carolina: how does perception relate to screening behavior? Cancer Epidemiol Biomarkers Prev 11, 529-534.

[53] Jaroslaw Regula, A.C., Michal F. Kaminski (2012). Should There Be Gender Differences in the Guidelines for Colorectal Cancer Screening? Curr Colorectal Cancer Rep 8, 32-35.

[54] Jass, J.R., Williams, C.B., Bussey, H.J., and Morson, B.C. (1988). Juvenile polyposis--a precancerous condition. Histopathology 13, 619-630.

[55] Jemal, A., Bray, F., Center, M.M., Ferlay, J., Ward, E., and Forman, D. (2011). Global cancer statistics. CA: a cancer journal for clinicians 61, 69-90.

[56] Jemal, A., Center, M.M., DeSantis, C., and Ward, E.M. (2010). Global patterns of cancer incidence and mortality rates and trends. Cancer Epidemiol Biomarkers Prev 19, 1893-1907.

[57] Jemal, A., Siegel, R., Ward, E., Hao, Y., Xu, J., Murray, T., and Thun, M.J. (2008). Cancer statistics, 2008. CA Cancer J Clin 58, 71-96.

[58] Jenkins, M.A., Croitoru, M.E., Monga, N., Cleary, S.P., Cotterchio, M., Hopper, J.L., and Gallinger, S. (2006). Risk of colorectal cancer in monoallelic and biallelic carriers of MYH mutations: a population-based case-family study. Cancer Epidemiol Biomarkers Prev 15, 312-314.

[59] Johnson, C.D., Chen, M.H., Toledano, A.Y., Heiken, J.P., Dachman, A., Kuo, M.D., Menias, C.O., Siewert, B., Cheema, J.I., Obregon, R.G., et al. (2008). Accuracy of CT colonography for detection of large adenomas and cancers. N Engl J Med 359, 1207-1217.

[60] Johnson, J.R., Lacey, J.V., Jr., Lazovich, D., Geller, M.A., Schairer, C., Schatzkin, A., and Flood, A. (2009). Menopausal hormone therapy and risk of colorectal cancer. Cancer Epidemiol Biomarkers Prev 18, 196-203.

[61] Jones, R.M., Woolf, S.H., Cunningham, T.D., Johnson, R.E., Krist, A.H., Rothemich, S.F., and Vernon, S.W. (2010). The relative importance of patient-reported barriers to colorectal cancer screening. Am J Prev Med 38, 499-507.

[62] Kamath, A.S., Iqbal, C.W., Sarr, M.G., Cullinane, D.C., Zietlow, S.P., Farley, D.R., and Sawyer, M.D. (2009). Colonoscopic splenic injuries: incidence and management. J Gastrointest Surg 13, 2136-2140.

[63] Knudsen, A.L., Bisgaard, M.L., and Bulow, S. (2003). Attenuated familial adenomatous polyposis (AFAP). A review of the literature. Familial cancer 2, 43-55.

[64] Ko, C.W., and Dominitz, J.A. (2010). Complications of colonoscopy: magnitude and management. Gastrointest Endosc Clin N Am 20, 659-671.

[65] Kohler, B.A., Ward, E., McCarthy, B.J., Schymura, M.J., Ries, L.A., Eheman, C., Jemal, A., Anderson, R.N., Ajani, U.A., and Edwards, B.K. (2011). Annual report to the nation on the status of cancer, 1975-2007, featuring tumors of the brain and other nervous system. J Natl Cancer Inst 103, 714-736.

[66] Koo, J.H., You, M.Y., Liu, K., Athureliya, M.D., Tang, C.W., Redmond, D.M., Connor, S.J., and Leong, R.W. (2012). Colorectal cancer screening practise is influenced by ethnicity of medical practitioner and patient. J Gastroenterol Hepatol 27, 390-396.

[67] Lansdorp-Vogelaar, I., Kuntz, K.M., Knudsen, A.B., Wilschut, J.A., Zauber, A.G., and van Ballegooijen, M. (2010). Stool DNA testing to screen for colorectal cancer in the Medicare population: a cost-effectiveness analysis. Ann Intern Med 153, 368-377.

[68] Lasser, K.E., Murillo, J., Lisboa, S., Casimir, A.N., Valley-Shah, L., Emmons, K.M., Fletcher, R.H., and Ayanian, J.Z. (2011). Colorectal cancer screening among ethnically

diverse, low-income patients: a randomized controlled trial. Arch Intern Med 171, 906-912.

[69] Lasser, K.E., Murillo, J., Medlin, E., Lisboa, S., Valley-Shah, L., Fletcher, R.H., Emmons, K.M., and Ayanian, J.Z. (2009). A multilevel intervention to promote colorectal cancer screening among community health center patients: results of a pilot study. BMC family practice 10, 37.

[70] Levin, B., Lieberman, D.A., McFarland, B., Andrews, K.S., Brooks, D., Bond, J., Dash, C., Giardiello, F.M., Glick, S., Johnson, D., et al. (2008). Screening and surveillance for the early detection of colorectal cancer and adenomatous polyps, 2008: a joint guideline from the American Cancer Society, the US Multi-Society Task Force on Colorectal Cancer, and the American College of Radiology. Gastroenterology 134, 1570-1595.

[71] Levin, T.R., Jamieson, L., Burley, D.A., Reyes, J., Oehrli, M., and Caldwell, C. (2011). Organized colorectal cancer screening in integrated health care systems. Epidemiologic reviews 33, 101-110.

[72] Liang, P.S., Chen, T.Y., and Giovannucci, E. (2009). Cigarette smoking and colorectal cancer incidence and mortality: systematic review and meta-analysis. Int J Cancer 124, 2406-2415.

[73] Lieberman, D. (2010). Progress and challenges in colorectal cancer screening and surveillance. Gastroenterology 138, 2115-2126.

[74] Lieberman, D.A., De Garmo, P.L., Fleischer, D.E., Eisen, G.M., and Helfand, M. (2000). Patterns of endoscopy use in the United States. Gastroenterology 118, 619-624.

[75] Lieberman, D.A., Holub, J., Eisen, G., Kraemer, D., and Morris, C.D. (2005). Prevalence of polyps greater than 9 mm in a consortium of diverse clinical practice settings in the United States. Clin Gastroenterol Hepatol 3, 798-805.

[76] Lieberman, D.A., Rex, D.K., Winawer, S.J., Giardiello, F.M., Johnson, D.A., and Levin, T.R. (2012). Guidelines for Colonoscopy Surveillance After Screening and Polypectomy: A Consensus Update by the US Multi-Society Task Force on Colorectal Cancer. Gastroenterology.

[77] Lin, O.S., Kozarek, R.A., Schembre, D.B., Ayub, K., Gluck, M., Drennan, F., Soon, M.S., and Rabeneck, L. (2006). Screening colonoscopy in very elderly patients: prevalence of neoplasia and estimated impact on life expectancy. JAMA 295, 2357-2365.

[78] Linsky, A., McIntosh, N., Cabral, H., and Kazis, L.E. (2011). Patient-provider language concordance and colorectal cancer screening. J Gen Intern Med 26, 142-147.

[79] Liu, H., Waxman, D.A., Main, R., and Mattke, S. (2012). Utilization of anesthesia services during outpatient endoscopies and colonoscopies and associated spending in 2003-2009. JAMA 307, 1178-1184.

[80] Ma, G.X., Shive, S., Tan, Y., Gao, W., Rhee, J., Park, M., Kim, J., and Toubbeh, J.I. (2009). Community-based colorectal cancer intervention in underserved Korean Americans. Cancer epidemiology 33, 381-386.

[81] Maciosek, M.V., Solberg, L.I., Coffield, A.B., Edwards, N.M., and Goodman, M.J. (2006). Colorectal cancer screening: health impact and cost effectiveness. Am J Prev Med 31, 80-89.

[82] Martinez, M.E., Baron, J.A., Lieberman, D.A., Schatzkin, A., Lanza, E., Winawer, S.J., Zauber, A.G., Jiang, R., Ahnen, D.J., Bond, J.H., et al. (2009). A pooled analysis of advanced colorectal neoplasia diagnoses after colonoscopic polypectomy. Gastroenterology 136, 832-841.

[83] Martinez, M.E., Giovannucci, E., Spiegelman, D., Hunter, D.J., Willett, W.C., and Colditz, G.A. (1997). Leisure-time physical activity, body size, and colon cancer in women. Nurses' Health Study Research Group. J Natl Cancer Inst 89, 948-955.

[84] McGarrity, T.J., and Amos, C. (2006). Peutz-Jeghers syndrome: clinicopathology and molecular alterations. Cellular and molecular life sciences : CMLS 63, 2135-2144.

[85] McGregor, S., Hilsden, R., and Yang, H. (2010). Physician barriers to population-based, fecal occult blood test-based colorectal cancer screening programs for average-risk patients. Canadian journal of gastroenterology = Journal canadien de gastroenterologie 24, 359-364.

[86] Mecklin, J.P., Aarnio, M., Laara, E., Kairaluoma, M.V., Pylvanainen, K., Peltomaki, P., Aaltonen, L.A., and Jarvinen, H.J. (2007). Development of colorectal tumors in colonoscopic surveillance in Lynch syndrome. Gastroenterology 133, 1093-1098.

[87] Moore, L.L., Bradlee, M.L., Singer, M.R., Splansky, G.L., Proctor, M.H., Ellison, R.C., and Kreger, B.E. (2004). BMI and waist circumference as predictors of lifetime colon cancer risk in Framingham Study adults. Int J Obes Relat Metab Disord 28, 559-567.

[88] Muzny, D. (2012). Comprehensive molecular characterization of human colon and rectal cancer. Nature 487, 330-337.

[89] Myers, R.E., Hyslop, T., Sifri, R., Bittner-Fagan, H., Katurakes, N.C., Cocroft, J., Dicarlo, M., and Wolf, T. (2008). Tailored navigation in colorectal cancer screening. Med Care 46, S123-131.

[90] Nadel, M.R., Shapiro, J.A., Klabunde, C.N., Seeff, L.C., Uhler, R., Smith, R.A., and Ransohoff, D.F. (2005). A national survey of primary care physicians' methods for screening for fecal occult blood. Ann Intern Med 142, 86-94.

[91] Nash, D., Azeez, S., Vlahov, D., and Schori, M. (2006). Evaluation of an intervention to increase screening colonoscopy in an urban public hospital setting. Journal of urban health : bulletin of the New York Academy of Medicine 83, 231-243.

[92] NIH (2009). Surveillance Epidemiology and End results. US National Institutes of Health. Cancer Facts 2006 (online). .

[93] Pezzoli, A., Matarese, V., Rubini, M., Simoni, M., Caravelli, G.C., Stockbrugger, R., Cifala, V., Boccia, S., Feo, C., Simone, L., et al. (2007). Colorectal cancer screening: results of a 5-year program in asymptomatic subjects at increased risk. Dig Liver Dis 39, 33-39.

[94] Pignone, M., Saha, S., Hoerger, T., and Mandelblatt, J. (2002). Cost-effectiveness analyses of colorectal cancer screening: a systematic review for the U.S. Preventive Services Task Force. Ann Intern Med 137, 96-104.

[95] Prescilla S. Perera, R.L.T.a.M.J.W. (2012). Recent Evidence for Colorectal Cancer Prevention Through Healthy Food, Nutrition, and Physical Activity: Implications for Recommendations. Current Nutrition Reports 1, 44-54.

[96] Prevention, C.f.D.C.a. Colorectal (Colon) Cancer Incidence Rates. In CDC Features, Data & Statistics by Date (Atlanta, GA).

[97] Center for disease control and prevention. 2011. Data & Statistics. Retrieved from http://www.cdc.gov/features/dsColorectalCancer/

[98] Center for disease control and prevention. 2012. Life Expectancy. Retrieved from http://www.cdc.gov/nchs/fastats/lifexpec.htm

[99] Ransohoff, D.F. (2005). Colon cancer screening in 2005: status and challenges. Gastroenterology 128, 1685-1695.

[100] Rembold, C.M. (1998). Number needed to screen: development of a statistic for disease screening. BMJ 317, 307-312.

[101] Rex, D.K., Johnson, D.A., Anderson, J.C., Schoenfeld, P.S., Burke, C.A., and Inadomi, J.M. (2009). American College of Gastroenterology guidelines for colorectal cancer screening 2009 [corrected]. The American journal of gastroenterology 104, 739-750.

[102] Ries, L.A., Kosary C.L., Hankley B.F., Miller B.A., Edwards B.K., editors SEER cancer statistics review, 1973-1995. Bethesda (MD): National Cancer Institue; 1998.

[103] Rim S.H., J.D.A., Steele C.B., Thompson T.D., Seeff L.C. (2011). Colorectal Cancer Screening-United States, 2002, 2004, 2006, and 2008. In Morbidity and Mortality Weekly Report (MMWR).

[104] Rothwell, P.M., Price, J.F., Fowkes, F.G., Zanchetti, A., Roncaglioni, M.C., Tognoni, G., Lee, R., Belch, J.F., Wilson, M., Mehta, Z., et al. (2012). Short-term effects of daily aspirin on cancer incidence, mortality, and non-vascular death: analysis of the time course of risks and benefits in 51 randomised controlled trials. Lancet 379, 1602-1612.

[105] Rutter, C.M., Johnson, E., Miglioretti, D.L., Mandelson, M.T., Inadomi, J., and Buist, D.S. (2012). Adverse events after screening and follow-up colonoscopy. Cancer Causes Control 23, 289-296.

[106] Sano, Y., Ikematsu, H., Fu, K.I., Emura, F., Katagiri, A., Horimatsu, T., Kaneko, K., Soetikno, R., and Yoshida, S. (2009). Meshed capillary vessels by use of narrow-band

imaging for differential diagnosis of small colorectal polyps. Gastrointest Endosc 69, 278-283.

[107] Schoen, R.E., Pinsky, P.F., Weissfeld, J.L., Yokochi, L.A., Church, T., Laiyemo, A.O., Bresalier, R., Andriole, G.L., Buys, S.S., Crawford, E.D., et al. (2012). Colorectal-cancer incidence and mortality with screening flexible sigmoidoscopy. N Engl J Med 366, 2345-2357.

[108] Schoenfeld, P., Cash, B., Flood, A., Dobhan, R., Eastone, J., Coyle, W., Kikendall, J.W., Kim, H.M., Weiss, D.G., Emory, T., et al. (2005). Colonoscopic screening of average-risk women for colorectal neoplasia. N Engl J Med 352, 2061-2068.

[109] School, H.M. (2012). Does colonoscopy save lives? A recent study suggests it might, but it isn't the last word. Harvard Health Letter.

[110] Does colonoscopy save lives? A recent study suggest it might, but it isn't the last word. Harvard health letter/from Harvard Medical School 2012; 37:3.

[111] Shapiro, J.A., Klabunde, C.N., Thompson, T.D., Nadel, M.R., Seeff, L.C., and White, A. (2012). Patterns of Colorectal Cancer Test Use, Including CT Colonography, in the 2010 National Health Interview Survey. Cancer Epidemiol Biomarkers Prev 21, 895-904.

[112] Shokar, N.K., Vernon, S.W., and Weller, S.C. (2005). Cancer and colorectal cancer: knowledge, beliefs, and screening preferences of a diverse patient population. Family medicine 37, 341-347.

[113] Society, A.C. (2011). Colorectal Cancer Facts & Figures 2011-2013. Atlanta: American Cancer Society.

[114] Soneji, S., Iyer, S.S., Armstrong, K., and Asch, D.A. (2010). Racial disparities in stage-specific colorectal cancer mortality: 1960-2005. Am J Public Health 100, 1912-1916.

[115] Spach, D.H., Silverstein, F.E., and Stamm, W.E. (1993). Transmission of infection by gastrointestinal endoscopy and bronchoscopy. Ann Intern Med 118, 117-128.

[116] Stelzner, S., Hellmich, G., Koch, R., and Ludwig, K. (2005). Factors predicting survival in stage IV colorectal carcinoma patients after palliative treatment: a multivariate analysis. Journal of surgical oncology 89, 211-217.

[117] Stout, N.K., Rosenberg, M.A., Trentham-Dietz, A., Smith, M.A., Robinson, S.M., and Fryback, D.G. (2006). Retrospective cost-effectiveness analysis of screening mammography. J Natl Cancer Inst 98, 774-782.

[118] Subramanian, S., Bobashev, G., and Morris, R.J. (2010). When budgets are tight, there are better options than colonoscopies for colorectal cancer screening. Health Aff (Millwood) 29, 1734-1740.

[119] Telford, J.J., Levy, A.R., Sambrook, J.C., Zou, D., and Enns, R.A. (2010). The cost-effectiveness of screening for colorectal cancer. CMAJ : Canadian Medical Association journal = journal de l'Association medicale canadienne 182, 1307-1313.

[120] Terzic, J., Grivennikov, S., Karin, E., and Karin, M. (2010). Inflammation and colon cancer. Gastroenterology 138, 2101-2114 e2105.

[121] Toma, J., Paszat, L.F., Gunraj, N., and Rabeneck, L. (2008). Rates of new or missed colorectal cancer after barium enema and their risk factors: a population-based study. Am J Gastroenterol 103, 3142-3148.

[122] USPSTF (2008). Screening for colorectal cancer: U.S. Preventive Services Task Force recommendation statement. Ann Intern Med 149, 627-637.

[123] Varela, A., Jandorf, L., and Duhamel, K. (2010). Understanding factors related to Colorectal Cancer (CRC) screening among urban Hispanics: use of focus group methodology. Journal of cancer education : the official journal of the American Association for Cancer Education 25, 70-75.

[124] Vijan, S., Hwang, E.W., Hofer, T.P., and Hayward, R.A. (2001). Which colon cancer screening test? A comparison of costs, effectiveness, and compliance. Am J Med 111, 593-601.

[125] Wagner, M., Kiselow, M.C., Keats, W.L., and Jan, M.L. (1970). Varices of the colon. Arch Surg 100, 718-720.

[126] Wallace, P.M., and Suzuki, R. (2012). Regional, Racial, and Gender Differences in Colorectal Cancer Screening in Middle-aged African-Americans and Whites. Journal of cancer education : the official journal of the American Association for Cancer Education.

[127] Walsh, J.M., Kaplan, C.P., Nguyen, B., Gildengorin, G., McPhee, S.J., and Perez-Stable, E.J. (2004). Barriers to colorectal cancer screening in Latino and Vietnamese Americans. Compared with non-Latino white Americans. J Gen Intern Med 19, 156-166.

[128] Walter, L.C., and Covinsky, K.E. (2001). Cancer screening in elderly patients: a framework for individualized decision making. JAMA 285, 2750-2756.

[129] White, P.M., Sahu, M., Poles, M.A., and Francois, F. (2012). Colorectal cancer screening of high-risk populations: A national survey of physicians. BMC research notes 5, 64.

[130] Wilkins, T., Gillies, R.A., Harbuck, S., Garren, J., Looney, S.W., and Schade, R.R. (2012). Racial disparities and barriers to colorectal cancer screening in rural areas. J Am Board Fam Med 25, 308-317.

[131] Wilkins, T., and Reynolds, P.L. (2008). Colorectal cancer: a summary of the evidence for screening and prevention. American family physician 78, 1385-1392.

[132] Winawer, S., Fletcher, R., Rex, D., Bond, J., Burt, R., Ferrucci, J., Ganiats, T., Levin, T., Woolf, S., Johnson, D., et al. (2003). Colorectal cancer screening and surveillance: clinical guidelines and rationale-Update based on new evidence. Gastroenterology 124, 544-560.

[133] Winawer, S.J. (2006). The achievements, impact, and future of the National Polyp Study. Gastrointest Endosc 64, 975-978.

[134] Winawer, S.J., Fletcher, R.H., Miller, L., Godlee, F., Stolar, M.H., Mulrow, C.D., Woolf, S.H., Glick, S.N., Ganiats, T.G., Bond, J.H., et al. (1997). Colorectal cancer screening: clinical guidelines and rationale. Gastroenterology 112, 594-642.

[135] Winawer, S.J., Zauber, A.G., Ho, M.N., O'Brien, M.J., Gottlieb, L.S., Sternberg, S.S., Waye, J.D., Schapiro, M., Bond, J.H., Panish, J.F., et al. (1993a). Prevention of colorectal cancer by colonoscopic polypectomy. The National Polyp Study Workgroup. N Engl J Med 329, 1977-1981.

[136] Winawer, S.J., Zauber, A.G., O'Brien, M.J., Ho, M.N., Gottlieb, L., Sternberg, S.S., Waye, J.D., Bond, J., Schapiro, M., Stewart, E.T., et al. (1993b). Randomized comparison of surveillance intervals after colonoscopic removal of newly diagnosed adenomatous polyps. The National Polyp Study Workgroup. N Engl J Med 328, 901-906.

[137] Winterich, J.A., Quandt, S.A., Grzywacz, J.G., Clark, P., Dignan, M., Stewart, J.H., and Arcury, T.A. (2011). Men's knowledge and beliefs about colorectal cancer and 3 screenings: education, race, and screening status. American journal of health behavior 35, 525-534.

[138] Wudel, L.J., Jr., Chapman, W.C., Shyr, Y., Davidson, M., Jeyakumar, A., Rogers, S.O., Jr., Allos, T., and Stain, S.C. (2002). Disparate outcomes in patients with colorectal cancer: effect of race on long-term survival. Arch Surg 137, 550-554; discussion 554-556.

[139] Yabroff, K.R., Zapka, J., Klabunde, C.N., Yuan, G., Buckman, D.W., Haggstrom, D., Clauser, S.B., Miller, J., and Taplin, S.H. (2011). Systems strategies to support cancer screening in U.S. primary care practice. Cancer Epidemiol Biomarkers Prev 20, 2471-2479.

[140] Yuhara, H., Steinmaus, C., Cohen, S.E., Corley, D.A., Tei, Y., and Buffler, P.A. (2011). Is diabetes mellitus an independent risk factor for colon cancer and rectal cancer? Am J Gastroenterol 106, 1911-1921; quiz 1922.

[141] Zapka, J.M., Klabunde, C.N., Arora, N.K., Yuan, G., Smith, J.L., and Kobrin, S.C. (2011). Physicians' colorectal cancer screening discussion and recommendation patterns. Cancer Epidemiol Biomarkers Prev 20, 509-521.

[142] Zauber, A.G., Lansdorp-Vogelaar, I., Knudsen, A.B., Wilschut, J., van Ballegooijen, M., and Kuntz, K.M. (2008). Evaluating test strategies for colorectal cancer screening: a decision analysis for the U.S. Preventive Services Task Force. Ann Intern Med 149, 659-669.

[143] Zauber, A.G., Winawer, S.J., O'Brien, M.J., Lansdorp-Vogelaar, I., van Ballegooijen, M., Hankey, B.F., Shi, W., Bond, J.H., Schapiro, M., Panish, J.F., et al. (2012). Colonoscopic polypectomy and long-term prevention of colorectal-cancer deaths. N Engl J Med 366, 687-696.

Chapter 3

The Future of Colonoscopy: The Use of Data Envelopment Analysis (DEA) for Colorectal Cancer Screening — Italian Experience

Alberto Vannelli, Michel Zanardo, Valerio Basilico,
Baldovino Griffa, Fabrizio Rossi,
Massimo Buongiorno, Luigi Battaglia,
Vincenzo Pruiti, Sara De Dosso and Giulio Capriata

Additional information is available at the end of the chapter

http://dx.doi.org/10.5772/52310

1. Introduction

René Descartes (1596-1650) in the published Discourse on Method, wrote: "...And because the actions of life often brook no delay, it is certainly very true that, when it is not in our power to determine the truest opinions, we ought to follow the most probable ones, and even when we see no difference in probability among this group of truths or that one, nevertheless, we have to decide on some for ourselves and then to consider them, not as something doubtful with regard to the practical matter at hand, but as manifestly true and very certain, because the reason which made us choose them has these qualities". [1] Colonoscopy (COL) issues this doubt.

Everybody known the effect of COL on colorectal cancer (CRC) until 2009, when an observational case–control study did not identify a reasonable explanation for COL: much less effective in preventing death from colorectal cancer (CRC) of the right colon compared with the left colon [2]. Moreover to prevent one cancer death, 1,250 colonoscopies need to be performed, but perforation of the colon occurs at a rate of about 1 in 1000 procedures [3].

Since polyps often take 10 to 15 years to transform into cancer, in someone at average risk of colorectal cancer, guidelines recommend 10 years after a normal screening COL before the next COL. [4,5]. By removing premalignant adenomas and detecting early cancer, COL should lower colorectal cancer mortality. Although gastroenterologists strongly believe that

COL lowers colorectal cancer mortality, evidence in support of this belief is indirect. Robert S. Sandler in 2010 wrote: "The mortality from colorectal cancer has actually been decreasing steadily since 1980, long before widespread use of COL or any other screening, and before use of effective adjuvant therapy for cancer" [6].

However the high cost of biological therapy for advanced CRC, and the high risk of CRC in low-income population are likely to affect the cost-effectiveness of COL in the future [7,8].

In Italy CRC rank third for incidence among male (second among female) and second among the most frequent causes of tumour death for both men and women [9]. The current trend of the incidence shows a slow-down among male patients and stabilization among women. Mortality seems to be in decrease in particular in the population under 50 years old. In Southern Italy and in the Italian islands the incidence is lower (like mortality), but its trend is less favourable than in central-northern Italy. In the Southern Italy trends on the increase are reported both among men and women. The success of Colorectal cancer screening (CCS) is the success of COL. However there are critical points: complications of COL programmes; low coverage; low compliance; overload on endoscopy facilities. Faecal occult blood screening (FOBT) for CRC in men and women aged 50 to 74 is the Italian and European Union recommendation [10]. CCS is widely accepted as a public health policy in Italy [11]. On the contrary few regions have adopted widespread CCS programmes, although some are inching their way to that goal [12]. The reason, is the burden that extensive CCS places on COL services [13]. Behind every CCS test, no matter what kind, is the potential need for a COL, who can detect and remove adenomas, and detect asymptomatic cancers [14-19].

The social and economical impact of CRC is such, to warrant the decisions of the Italian government to implement the screening as a form of prevention. According to the Italian government agreements, on September 30th 2010, the Italian Regions should have implemented the Plan of National Prevention and transformed it into Plan of Regional Prevention: April 24th 2010 agreement between Government, Regions and Autonomous Provinces of Trento and Bolzano: "… the regions are committed to implement by September 30, 2010, the Regional Plan of Prevention to carry out the interventions established by the National Plan of Prevention …" [20].

Two authorities coordinate activities and research projects for both general and specific, population. The Italian Network of Cancer Registries (AIRTUM), and the National Centre for Disease Prevention and Control (Ccm) [21,22].

AIRTUM, called AIRT until 2006, was born in 1997, in 2005, AIRTUM created a centralized database where data from Cancer Registries are stored and, after checked for quality and completeness, used for collaborative studies on cancer epidemiology in Italy [14]. Cancer registration in Italy began in the 1970s with a steady increase in experiences and coverage of an increasing proportion of the Italian resident population. The density of registries is greater in northern Italy, especially in the North-east, compared with Central and Southern Italy (Figure 1).

http://dx.doi.org/10.5772/52310

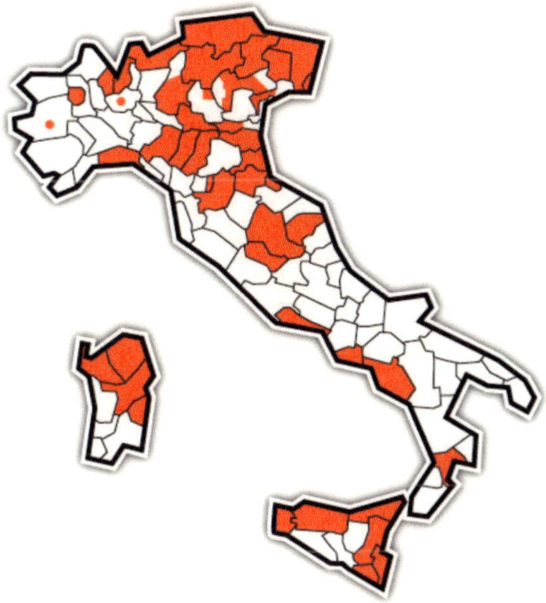

Figure 1. Italian Network of Cancer Registries: red actived, white not yet actived.

On the other hand, especially in the South of Italy, cancer registration has remarkably expanded in recent years with several new registries, which provide a more detailed and descriptive dataset of the oncologic illnesses in this area of Italy. Figure 1 shows the proportion of the resident population covered by cancer registries according to region and geographic macroareas (Northwest, Northeast, Centre, and South). Regional coverage varies from 0% in several southern regions (Puglia, Basilicata, Abruzzi, Molise), as well as Val d'Aosta, to 100% (e.g., Umbria, Friuli Venetia Giulia, Trento, and Bolzano). Nevertheless, Southern Italy reported an increase in cancer reporting. Today more than a third of the Italian population lives in an area with an active cancer registry. This proportion differs between areas (37% in the Northwest, 68% in the Northeast, 26% in the Centre, and 18% in South). Overall, AIRTUM Registries involve more than 19.000.000 subjects, or 34% of the entire Italian resident population. The importance of AIRTUM, is supported by the growing number of accredited registries contributing to the centralized dataset, thus improving representation at the national level. Furthermore, the presence of historic registries, operating since the 1980s, has helped calculate 20-year incidence trends, and stable, robust prevalence estimates. Ccm is to liaise between the Ministry of health on the one side, and regional governments on the other as regards surveillance, prevention and promptly responding to emergencies [23-25]. Over the years, Ccm has acquired a specific identity, which makes it unique within the framework of Italian public health; its main features are: analyze health hazards implementation in prevention secondary and tertiary prevention. The Centre is a bridge between the world of research and health facilities on the one hand, and the best practices and entities being developed on the other, by activating institutional partnerships and professional collaborations: its aim is to build an Italian prevention network. The goal of Ccm is to optimise the national prevention Plan checking surveillance plans and active prevention with the Regions.(Figure 2).

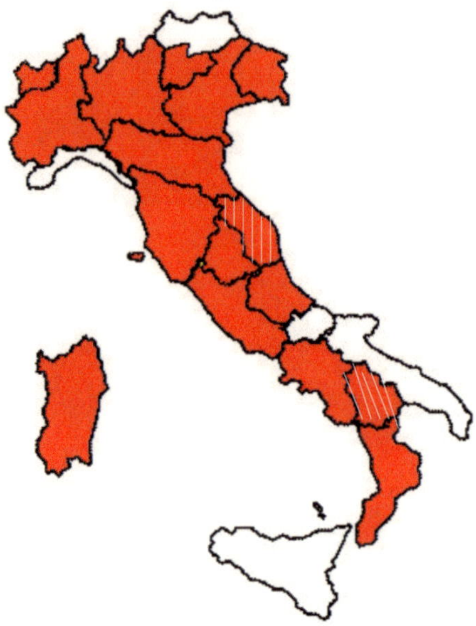

Figure 2. Regional colorectal cancer screening: red actived, white not yet actived, red and white partial actived.

The cooperation with these two authorities introduced design standards and evaluation criteria, as part of an active collaboration relationship between AIRTUM, CCM and the partners with which it has agreements, both in the design and monitoring phase of programmes and projects of CCS.

At the present days, no studies are ongoing to define the cause-effect relationship between costs, CCS programme, and COL.

In this paper we show how both the choice of specific constraints on output weights (CCS programme) can affect the measurement of COL efficiency using the "Data Envelopment Analysis" (DEA).

In their originating study, Charnes, Cooper, and Rhodes on 1978, described DEA as a "mathematical programming model applied to observational data [that] provides a new way of obtaining empirical estimates of relations - such as the production functions and/or efficient production possibility surfaces – that are cornerstones of modern economics" [27].

DEA is a relatively new "data oriented" approach for evaluating the performance of a set of peer entities called Decision Making Units (DMUs) which convert multiple inputs into multiple outputs.

DEA is applied by the management control to evaluate the relative efficiency of human resources, the results are related to the cost of diagnostic procedures, standardized by the case-mix, and both scatter plot and cluster analysis are produced to find out related area of performance and to plan a strategy for the continuous quality improvement. The objective of this study therefore, is to propose one model of study of the costs in the strategy of CCS supporting the benefits of COL using DEA model.

2. Materials and methods

The absence in the literature of previous experience or analogous models can makes difficult to create a logistic model. At the present days, there are many studies to define the cause-effect relationship between costs, and CCS programme, or between costs and COL. The objective of this study is to propose one model of study of the costs in the strategy of CCS supporting the benefits of COL using DEA model. Since the incidence of colorectal cancer shows a geographical variability, we considered the epidemiological data in the light of the different Italian cancer records, which are often referred to provincial or regional results and we compared them with the screening tests available in each Region.

In the first part of the paper, we calculated the global population in Italy and the number of current colorectal cancer cases using the historical archive of ISTAT (Italian National Institute of Statistics). The ISTAT produces and distributes information that describes the social, economic and environmental conditions of the Country, and the changes taking place within it, in strict compliance with legal provisions on confidentiality. As the main producer of national statistics, it provides data and releases information to European statistical authorities and international organizations. We then evaluated the economical impact considering every single available regional result obtained from the archives of Age.Na.S. (Italian Agencies for Regional Health Care Services), AIRTUM, and CCM, and comparing them with the available Italian data obtained from the Italian Ministry of Health and the statistical registers of INAIL (Italian institute for insurance against industrial accident) and INPS (Italian Institute of social insurance). The Age.Na.S. is a public agency founded in 1993. In the Italian healthcare service the Agency plays as a technical body supporting the Ministry of Labour, Health and Social Services and Regions. The Agency also coordinates health research programs financed by the Ministry of Labour, Health and Social Services or by the Regions. The National Fund against Accidents created on 1883, took the name of INAIL on 1933. INAIL took up the management of compulsory insurance against occupational diseases in the industrial and agricultural sector, diseases caused by X-rays and radioactive substances; compulsory insurance has also been extended to "housewives". It produces and distributes information on occupational diseases. The INPS, established in 1933, is the large Italian public body that pays out old-age pensions to workers, after receiving contributions from them throughout their working lives, and manages the types of assistance provided for by the "social state", sickness, maternity and unemployment benefits, invalidity payments and social payments for citizens who are in need. INPS is one of the biggest public body in Europe, produces and distributes information that describes National Health Service.

In view of the geography of the Italian territory and the distribution of the population we analyzed the data considering three macro-areas which include different regions, i.e. the regions of Northern Italy: Piedmont, Emilia Romagna, Liguria, Friuli Venetia Giulia, Veneto, Trenton Alto-Adige, Lombardy and Valle d'Aosta; the regions of Central Italy: Tuscany, Umbria, Latium, Marche, Abruzzi, Molise and Sardinia; the regions of Southern Italy: Campania, Puglia, Basilicata, Calabria and Sicily.

For each Region we considered the following indicators in order to assess a possible plan of screening campaign of colorectal cancers: global population, mean age and population older than 65 years; relationship between Gross Domestic Product (GDP) and per capita income; incidence of colorectal cancer and possible screening campaign on the territory; index of patients' emigration and reimbursement through Diagnostic Related Group (DRG) of the pathology as a ratio versus the unit value represented by Italy as a system.

The second part of the paper is the object of the article: the implement of particular methodologies in order to determine which COL is cost-effective in the mass CCS programme. In this chapter a method for efficiency measurement in CCS programme has been described.

First an overview of efficiency measurements applicable is given. Calculation methods is described and examples of inputs and outputs are provided.

A method to measure efficiency is proposed. This method proves to be particularly successful in cost-efficiency analysis, when the performance indicators are numerous and hard to aggregate. The results show that there are two cost-effective strategies after a positive FOBT: COL.

We performed an explorative study to efficiency measurement in CCS. To construct an efficiency measure or measures for the CCS programme, literature has been searched for different types of efficiency measures used in healthcare. Hence a selection of criteria and methods is made which tend to be suitable to evaluate which COL is cost-effective in the mass CCS programme.

Besides Italian CCS programme were carried out to gain understanding of the care process for CRC patients. The proper knowledge of the process it is useful to choose suitable performance indicators.

3. Results

Out of a population of 60.387.000 inhabitants (data updated at 2010), the incidence of colorectal cancers was almost of 49.000 cases, with a prevalence of over 310.000 cases and mortality higher than 18.000 cases (data updated at 2006). The analysis of the abovementioned three macro-areas is characterized by strong differences both in general and in particular terms.

There are considerable imbalances between the Northern, Central and Southern areas considering their input, output and outcome.

http://dx.doi.org/10.5772/52310

Data in terms of distribution of population, mean age and population older than 65 years are distributed in the different macro-areas according to the distribution recorded by the Italian Institute of Statistics which depicts particular realities partially due to the industrial development and the local health level. We can differentiate in detail the following data for each Region (see Tables 1-3).

	Population (pop)	Mean age	% pop ≥ 65 years	GDP/ capita index	Incidence colorectal cancer	Screening plans	Migration Index	DRG Index
Piedmont	4.432.571	44,9	22,6	1,09	90,79 64,11	4 plans sigmoidoscopy	8,43	1,01
Emilia Romagna	4.337.979	45,0	22,8	1,21	139,58 82,86	11 plans (100% territory)	6,31	1,06
Liguria	1.615.064	47,3	26,7	1,03	104,16 82,5	1 plan	11,19	1
Friuli-Venetia Giulia	1.230.936	45,4	22,7	1,11	140,17 95,52	Global regional plan	6,4	1,22
Veneto	4.885.548	42,9	19,3	1,15	124,02 83,94	17 plans	5,31	1,17
Trenton Alto-Adige	1.018.657	41,3	17,8	1,25	113,60 76,14	Global regional plan TRENTO	10,56	1
Lombardy	9.742.676	43,0	19,6	1,30	107,93 74,5	15 plans (100% territory)	3,9	0,81
Valle d'Aosta	127.065	43,6	20,3	1,32	82,83 60,04	Global regional plan	22,17	1
ITALY	60.387.000	42,8	19,9	1	107,8 69,64	L.D. 138 2004 art. 2 bis Sof > 50 years	--	1

Table 1. Macro-area: Northern Italy

Piedmont is a Region with a large-size population with mean age and rate of elderly population higher than the Italian average. It has at its disposal a bit more resources than the Italian average and its screening campaign covers only some provinces; the incidence of the disease is lower than the Italian average; the emigration index is low and the refund of the health expenditure is a little bit higher than the national average. Emilia Romagna is a large-size population with mean age and rate of elderly persons higher than the Italian average. It has at its disposal more resources than the national average and its screening campaign covers all the provinces, the incidence of the disease is higher than the Italian average; the emigration index is low and the refund of the health expenditure is a little bit higher than the national average. Liguria has a middle-size population with mean age and rate of elderly definitely higher than the Italian average. It has at its disposal a little bit more resources than the Italian average and its screening campaign covers only one province; the incidence of the disease is lower than the National average; its emigration index is high and the refund of the health expenditure is on the average. Friuli Venetia Giulia Region has a middle-size population with mean age and rate of elderly persons higher than the Italian average. It has at its disposal more resources than the Italian average and its screening campaign covers all the provinces with a regional plan; the incidence of the disease is higher than the national average; its emigration index is low and the refund of the health expenditure is higher than the national average.

Veneto Region has a large-size population with mean age and rate of elderly in line with the Italian average. It has at its disposal more resources than the Italian average and its screening campaign covers all the provinces; the incidence of the disease is higher than the national average, its emigration index is low and the refund of the health expenditure is higher than the national average. Trenton Alto Adige Region has a middle-size population with mean age and rate of elderly persons lower than the Italian average. It has at its disposal more resources than the national average and its screening campaign covers the whole region, the incidence of the disease is higher than the Italian average; its emigration index is high and the refund of the health expenditure is in line with the national average. Lombardy has a large-size population with mean age higher than the average and a rate of elderly slightly lower than the Italian average. It has at its disposal more resources than the national average and its screening campaign covers all its provinces, the incidence of the disease is slightly higher than the Italian average, it has a low emigration index and the refund of health expenditure is lower than the national average. Valle d'Aosta Region has a small-size population with mean age and rate of elderly persons higher than the national average. It has at its disposal more resources than the national average, its screening campaign covers the whole Region, the incidence of the disease is lower than the national average; it has a high emigration index and the refund of health expenditure is in line with the national average.

Tuscany Region has a large-size population with mean age and rate of elderly persons higher than the Italian average. It has at its disposal more resources than the Italian average and its screening campaign covers the whole territory; the incidence of the disease is lower than the national average; its emigration index is mean and the refund of health expenditure is lower than the national average. Umbria Region has a small-size population with mean age and a rate of elderly persons higher than the Italian average. It has at its disposal fewer resources than the Italian average and its screening campaign covers the whole Region; the incidence of the disease is higher than the national average; the emigration index is high and the refund of health expenditure is higher than the national average.

Lazio Region has a large-size population with mean age and a rate of elderly persons lower than the Italian average. It has at its disposal more resources than the Italian average and its screening campaign covers only some provinces; the incidence of the disease is lower than the national average; its emigration index is intermediate and the refund of health expenditure is lower than the national average.

	Population (pop)	Mean age	% pop ≥ 65 years	GDP/ capita index	Incidence colorectal cancer	Screening plans	Migration Index	DRG Index
Tuscany	3.707.818	4,3	23,3	1,09	106,5 61,01	12 plans (100% territory)	5,92	0,79
Umbria	894.222	44,9	23,3	0,95	123,73 78,80	4 plans (100% territory)	11,28	1,72
Lazio	5.626.710	42,6	19,2	1,22	89,06 52,57	4 plans	6,64	0,89
Marche	1.569.578	44,3	22,6	1,00	109,89 67,70	2007 pilot project	10,75	1
Abruzzi	1.334.675	43,4	21,3	0,81	113,25 42,75	6 plans	10,2	1
Molise	320.795	43,6	22,0	0,72	113,29 43,16	Global Regional plan	20,62	1
Sardinia	1.671.001	42,2	17,8	0,80	101,42 54,12	1 plan	4,24	1
ITALY	60.387.000	42,8	19,9	1	107,8 69,64	L.D. 138 2004 art. 2 bis Sof > 50 years	- -	1

Table 2. Macro-area: Central Italy

Marche Region has a middle-size population with mean age and rate of elderly persons higher than the Italian average. It has at its disposal resources in line with the national average and implements no screening campaign; the incidence of the disease is higher than the national average; its emigration index is high and the refund of health expenditure is in line with the national average.

Abruzzi has a middle-size population with mean age and rate of elderly persons higher than the Italian average. It has at its disposal fewer resources than the national average and its screening campaign covers only some provinces; the incidence of the disease is higher than the national average; its emigration index is high and the refund of health expenditure is in line with the national average.

Molise Region has a small-size population with mean age and rate of elderly higher than the Italian average. It has at its disposal fewer resources than the national average and its screening campaign covers the whole Region; its emigration index is high and the refund of health expenditure is in line with the national average.

Sardinia Region has a middle-size population with mean age and rate of elderly lower than the Italian average. It has at its disposal resources in line with the national average and its screening campaign covers only one province; the incidence of the disease is lower than the national average, its emigration index is low and the refund of health expenditure is in line with the national average.

	Population (pop)	Mean age	% pop ≥ 65 years	GDP/ capita index	Incidence colorectal cancer	Screening plans	Migration Index	DRG Index
Campania	5.812.962	39,0	15,4	0,64	60,09 41,07	4 plans	7,55	0,89
Puglia	4.079.702	40,7	17,4	0,66	68,89 35,98	- -	7,64	1
Basilicata	590.601	42,1	20,0	0,70	104,31 35,98	Global regional plan STOP 2007	24,01	1
Calabria	2.008.709	41,1	18,4	0,65	83,08 35,93	4 plans	14,82	1
Sicily	5.037,799	40,7	18,0	0,66	71,15 45,33	- -	6,09	1
ITALY	60.387.000	42,8	19,9	1	107,8 69,64	L.D. 138 2004 art. 2 bis Sof > 50 years	- -	1

Table 3. Macro-area: Southern Italy

Campania Region has a large-size population with mean age and rate of elderly lower than the Italian average. It has at its disposal fewer resources than the national average and its screening campaign covers only some provinces; the incidence of the disease is lower than the national average; its emigration index is intermediate and the refund of health expenditure is slightly lower than the national average.

Puglia Region has a large population with mean age and rate of elderly lower than the Italian average. It has at is disposal fewer resources than the national average and it has no screening campaign; the incidence of the disease is lower than the national average and its emigration index is intermediate. The refund of health expenditure is in line with the national average.

Basilicata has a small-sized population with mean age and rate of elderly higher than the Italian average. It has at its disposal fewer resources than the national average and the screening campaign was discontinued in 2007, the incidence of the disease is lower than the national average, its emigration index is high and the refund of health expenditure is in line with the national average.

Calabria has a middle-sized population with mean age and rate of elderly lower than the Italian average. It has at its disposal fewer resources than the national average and its screening campaign covers only some provinces; the incidence of the disease in lower than the national average; its emigration index is high and the refund of health expenditure is in line with the national average.

Sicily has a large population with mean age and rate of elderly lower than the Italian average. It has at its disposal fewer resources than the national average and has no screening campaign; the incidence of the disease is lower than the national average, its emigration index is intermediate and the refund of health expenditure is in line with the national average.

4. Discussion

The average cost of colo-rectal cancer treatments in Italy has been estimated to be approximately € 9.149,00 per patient per year including chemotherapy [27]. Some authors estimate that for the city of Ferrara the overall cost related to the introduction of a CCS programme was approximately € 1.400.000,00 (from October 2005 until March 2007 with more than 99.000 individuals invited) with a large proportion of these costs related to the implementation and management of the programme [28]. FOBT plus COL, increase cost relative to cheapest strategy. As a consequence of screening, some individuals with low risk receive a recommendation for a follow-up COL. However follow-up colonoscopies will increase the cost consequences of introducing screening, but not the expected colorectal cancer treatment costs. The Italian Observatory on screening Practices has been collecting data on CCS since 2004 [29]. In 2007 there were 71 CRC screening programmes in Italy, covering 46,6% of the total eligible population, with a higher coverage in the North (71,6%), and in the Centre (52,1%) than in the South (7%). The majority of programmes (65) used the guaiac FOBT (gFOBT) as first-line test. Only seven programmes used the flexible sigmoidoscopy (FS), of which three used a combination of FS and gFOBT. The quality and efficacy of the screening programmes are evaluated using ad hoc indicators developed by the Italian Group for Colorectal Screening (GISCoR) [28]. In 2007, on average 79,1% of the eligible population was invited for FOBT screening, with only Lombardy, Umbria, and most of the programmes in Emilia Romagna reaching the 90% target. Among the invited individuals, 46,3% underwent FOBT with significant variations across (from 26,5% in Lazio to 65% in Veneto) and within regions (from 11 to 80%). Among the people invited for the first time, the average percentage of individuals with a positive test was 5,6%, while among people who were recalled it was 4%. The probability of having a positive result was higher for men than for women and increased with age. Among people with a positive test, only 78,7% underwent a COL [2]. The South and Centre had a lower rate of COL attendance than the North. Men were slightly more likely to undertake a COL after a positive FOBT than women, mainly because of the uncomfortable feeling and concern of women having a male physician performing the tests. The risk of bowel perforation and bleeding during COL was negligible. For FS, on average 66,5% of the eligible population was invited with large variations across programmes. Only 27,7% of those invited underwent FS with a slightly higher proportion among men than women. The response rate was higher whenever FS was combined with FOBT [30]. The percentage of FS successfully completed was 88%, with again a higher level among men than women; 14,3% of men and 7,6% of women were sent for a COL for further analysis and 90% of these attended the test. In 2007 overall FOBT and FS detected 20.796 adenoma of which, 2.449 were carcinomas. An additional 295 carcinomas were diagnosed in individuals who underwent further follow-up tests. Most of the adenomas identified were in Stage I, (54.5%), followed by increased widely Stages III and IV (24,9%), and then in Stage II (20,7%). The critical points are: complications of COL (40 programs) with average perforation rate of 0,08% (2,5% operative COL) and average bleeding rate of 0,55%; low coverage and delay in Southern Italy; low compliance; overload on endoscopy facilities.

The role of screening is an extremely topical question even though in the past it was already subject of discussion and until few years ago it was considered to fall within the competence of the central government [31]. Only in the last years we have observed a different interest especially in Italy due to the changed political conditions. Does a convergence really exist between federalism, screening and standard cost? The process which links the federal structure of the nation with the screening is a thin red line which began with the promulgation of the Constitution and over the years it has been fully implemented with Act No. 42 of year 2009 with enforcement of Article 119 of the Constitution which guarantees autonomy of revenues and expenditure of municipalities, provinces, towns and regions and assure principles of support and social cohesion [32]. In particular, it assures the funding of the essential levels of health care (which includes the practice of screening) referring to a benchmark of cost and requirements [32]. In year 2001 an agreement was made between Government and Regions for the guidelines about prevention, diagnosis and assistance in oncology, including indications for the screenings, and the promulgation of Decree of the President of the Council of Ministry No. 26 of November 29th 2001, which defines the Essential Levels of Care (LEA) including the plans of screening for the early diagnosis of colorectal, breast, cervix cancers [33]. Within the 2001 financial budget (law N. 388, 2000) it was decided that target population screening was free of charge [34]. In 2004 the Health Minister redistributed overall € 7.000.000, a minimum of € 50.000 per region, for reducing the gaps in cancer screenings and activating the CCS programme (€ 1.750.000 specifically for CCS). This agreement made these plans to be a right for women and men. The debate about the allocation of resources in regimen of federalism is very lively, in particular regarding the costs of Health Care System. We remind that the allocation of the funds to the Health Care System for the prevention of diseases remained constant at 5% for some years [35]. The criterion of the historical expenditure will be replaced by the standard cost. The standard cost is the tool to assure the LEA funding and consists of the expenditure for the following items: staff, equipment, consumables and general costs of the health performances of the production unit [36]. Moreover, a "direct" cost of production is predicted, i.e. a percentage to cover the general functioning costs of the equipment of the production unit [37]. The characteristics of the colorectal cancers show a strong geographical variability: chronic trend, increase in the incidence and a still too high mortality rate. The increase in the prevalence should be allotted partially to the ageing of the population, but mostly to the diffusion and implementation of screening plans. The cost of the screening campaign is defined by the following factors: first costs of tests, staff, confirmation procedure (selection of population at risk to reduce costs); second assessment of efficacy: sensitivity, specificity, productive value; third non-invasive method: it is addressed to probably healthy subjects; latter possibility of intervention: the disease or condition to be diagnosed should be susceptible of therapy.

In the first years 2000 the Italian Government, in view of the severe unbalanced offer of screening plans, established to allocate further financial resources (52 million euro between 2004 and 2006) for interventions promoting the re-balancing of the offer and the quality of the screening plan of cervix and breast cancers and the diffusion of the screening of colorectal cancer [33]. Even though in year 2008 in oncology the plans of screening of colorectal cancers had a significant increase exceeding the threshold of 50%, unfortunately they are not always able to achieve acceptable levels of efficacy. According to "The screening plans in Italy 2009", the screening campaigns for colorectal cancers carried out in the last years, showed some critical aspects: we observed a progressive increase in the compliance of the first years versus a progressive stabilization or decrease in the compliance afterwards [20]. There are extremely strong differences between Northern, Central and Southern Italy. However, the rate of detection of cancers by using faecal occult blood and endoscopy has always been lower than the acceptable minimum.

In fact, many differences are reported in relation with the ratio between regional and per capita income resulting into a three-speed Italy. This is mirrored also by the incidence of colorectal cancer, which exhibits a different distribution where the highest rate is in the Northern Italy and the minimum rate in the Southern Italy. According to the data of the National Screening Observatory, they are spread not uniformly throughout the territory. According to "The screening plans in Italy 2009", the real extension of colorectal screening plans (faecal occult blood plus endoscopy) for the macro-areas evidenced some critical aspects [20]. We passed from 5% in 2004 to 12% in 2005, then to 30% in 2006, which stabilized at 37% in 2007/2008 as global Italian data. Even though there were significant differences with a positive presence in the Northern Italy versus a delay in the Central Italy and an insufficient presence in the Southern Italy, these data showed a similar annual tendency for each macro-area. However, the rate of identification of cancers by using faecal occult blood and endoscopy has always been lower than the acceptable minimum. After an initial enthusiasm, we observed a progressive decrease in the percentage of compliance with the plan in both macro-areas. Regarding the emigration index, there are notable differences within the three macro-areas, which influence the general index. The value shows that the regions of Northern Italy have more attraction power versus the regions of Southern Italy, whereas the regions of Central Italy have not particularly high emigration indices.

This latter parameter: the DRG index shows clear imbalances within all regions and therefore it is not a useful element to discriminate the different macro-areas.

The lack of homogeneity on the territory, moreover, is still marked with evident consequences on mortality and morbidity [38]. The implementation of federalism poses a question: if these large differences already exist, will the situation be improved or will the disparity become even stronger? On April 29, 2010, the agreement between Government, Regions and Autonomous Provinces of Trento and Bolzano was undersigned. According to this agreement the regions are committed to implement by September 2010, the Regional Plan of Prevention to carry out the interventions established by the National Plan of Prevention: among the macro-areas of interventions there are oncologic screening programs [39]. The critical points are: complications of COL (40 programmes) with average perforation rate of 0.08% (2,5% operative COL) and average bleeding rate of 0,55%; low coverage and delay in Southern Italy; low compliance; overload on endoscopy facilities.

The critical limit to implement the screening campaigns of colorectal cancers is the allocation of own resources to Regions and local bodies and the overcoming of the dichotomy between legislative and administrative (on the territory) competences and derived finance (transfer from Government to territory) [40]. Up to now the Government has been engaged in funding screening campaigns, from now on the Regions will be in charge of it [41]. Unfortunately since there is not yet an assessment of the costs of this procedure, the "promotion campaign", so far implemented, is risking to be reduced [42].

The concept of standard cost versus the historical cost is playing a crucial role in the fiscal federalism. The standard cost will contribute, in fact, to establish the "official" needs of each local body and therefore the contingent equalizing transfer to which it will have the right to in case of insufficient fiscal capacity [43].

Which approach should be used to calculate the standard costs of the federal finance?

There are two models among those currently used: micro-analytical (standard cost of each supplied performance) and macro-analytical (standard cost of easily measurable variables: demographic structure, epidemiological and social characteristics). The first approach is not very consistent with the purposes of the federalist reform (valid only as control mean) while the second model establishes a budget of expenditure resulting from merely political choices and not from the real needs of the population. What is the solution? To calculate the necessary resources the fundamental element to refer to is the efficiency [44-46]. The efficiency measures the economical employment of resources in the productive process. It is defined as the ratio between performances (screening) and resources (budget) according to the formula: efficiency= output/input [47,48].

A better approach, but for some aspects much more complex, could be the one of DEA [49]. Farrell (1957) in his preliminary work "The measurement of productive efficiency" introduced not only the well-known allocation between technique and price or allocative efficiency, but he also proposed a key to measure the comparative efficiency of the productive units which use various inputs to produce different outputs [50]. The efficiency of each unit would be equal to the ratio between real and potential output [51]. More than two decades after Charnes, Cooper and Rhodes (CCR), the idea of Farrell was developed and it was demonstrated that a linear mathematical program could be used to choose the most effective productive unit. The method, known as Data Envelopment Analysis, has been extensively used to measure the efficiency in many economical areas [52].

The analyses are non-parametric and its characteristic is that it can evaluate the relative efficiency of decisional units, and the like, through linear programming techniques without specifying whether the relative importance of the different factors of production or that of the prices [53]. In this sense the results of non-parametric methods are objective, because they do not require prior specifications. On the other hand, however, their disadvantage is that they do not admit errors being deterministic methods; the results could be therefore influenced. The relative efficiency of the responsibility centres is determined according to the following formula:

$$\max_{u,v} h_0(u, v)=\sum_r u_r y_{r0} \, / \sum v_i x_{i0}$$

Now the system of weights adopted strongly influences the efficiency, therefore through an algorithm of Charnes, Cooper and Rhodes (CCR), we try to find the optimal system of weights (among the proposed ones) in order to maximize the efficiency of the responsibility centre and the comparable ideal responsibility centre [54]. This suggests that the standard cost can be calculated in two ways: maximizing the numerator and fixing the denominator (output-oriented method – screening) or, vice versa, keeping the numerator and minimizing the denominator (input-oriented method – prevention budget) [55]. The difference is important since it determines the form of efficiency that we are assessing. Output-effective means there is no other unit that develops a larger screening with the same budget for the prevention [56].

A productive unit is called input-effective if there is no other unit able to obtain the same screening using a lower budget (DMUs).

This methodology assesses the efficiency as the ratio between quality of the screening and available budget. Some weights are obviously introduced to include demographic and health characteristics of the Region. Now for each unit we can obtain the optimal budget to be allocated to the Region for the screening campaign. In this way by adding the sum of every single regional budget, the necessary budget of national expenditure can be obtained to carry out an effective and really sustainable screening campaign.

In view of the above mentioned results, we can assume an equivalent model (Table 4).

The following example of three Regions (large, middle, and small) illustrate how DEA works.

Each Region has exactly 10 COL (the only input), and we are be able to measure a Region CCR programme based on two outputs: number of patients subject to screening, and number of found cancers. The data for these Regions is as follows:

Region "large": 100 COL, 1000 number of recruited patients, 20 number of found cancers;

Region "medium": 100 COL, 400 number of recruited patients, 50 number of found cancers;

Region "small": 100 COL, 200 number of recruited patients, 150 number of found cancers.

Now, the key to DEA is to determine whether we can create a virtual Region that is better than one or more of the real Regions. Any such dominated Region will be an inefficient Region. Consider trying to create a virtual Region that is better than Region "large". Such a Region would use no more inputs than a Region "large", and produce at least as much output. Clearly, no combination of Regions "medium" and "small" can possibly do that. Region "large" is therefore deemed to be efficient. Region "small" is in the same situation. However, consider Region "medium". If we take half of Region "large" and combine it with half of Region "small", then we create a Region that processes different outputs (600 number of recruited patients, 85 number of found cancers) with just input (100 COL). This dominates "medium" (we would much rather have the virtual Region we created than Region "medium"). Region "medium" is therefore inefficient. Another way to see this is that we can scale down the inputs to "medium" (number of COL) and still have at least as much output. If we assume (and we do), that inputs are linearly scalable, then we estimate that we can get by with 63 COL. We do that by taking 0.34 times Region "small" plus 0.29 times Region "medium". The result uses 63 COL and produces at least as much as Region "medium" does. We say that Region "medium"'s efficiency rating is 0.63. Regions "small" and "large" have an efficiency rating of 1.

	Region		
	Large	**Middle**	**Small**
Population size			
Average			
Range			
Input			
Equivalent number of hours of physicians of general medicine			
Equivalent number of hours of endoscopists			
Equivalent number of hours of anaesthetists			
Equivalent number of hours of nurses			
Equivalent number of hours of executives			
Equivalent number of hours of lab physician			
Number of evaluations			
Number of endoscopies			
Number of histological exams			
Equivalent number of hours of pathologists			
Equivalent number of hours of technicians of pathologic anatomy			
Number of histological analyses			
Output			
Number of recruited patients			
Number of patients subject to screening			
Number of found cancers			

Table 4. Example of sustainable screening campaign.

After the definition of the population size and the observed input and output to assess the screening unit (DMUs), it is possible to calculate the index of efficiency by using the above-mentioned formula. This index can be referred to the single Regions or to the system Italy as a whole.

In many states, a larger question may be whether the overwhelming use of COL as the screening method is the appropriate choice.

Determination of the appropriateness of an indication for COL has been advanced as a means to help rationalize the use of endoscopic resources. Current guidelines regarding the appropriateness of COL are relatively inefficient in excluding a clinically meaningful CRC risk for patients, in whom COL is generally not indicated, raising serious concerns about their applicability to clinical practice.

A tailored navigation approach, which determines the particular concerns and barriers of an eligible individual and matches them with the strengths and weaknesses of each strategy to find the one most suitable, may be the optimal way to maximize the number of people who can benefit from COL.

In the end, a test can only provide benefit if it is actually done [57].

5. Conclusions

Nowadays the Italian National Health Service is distributed on extremely diversified regional realities. Needs and inefficiencies of production are inseparably correlated in the health expenditure of the Regions. In the future the issues that are now more critical will have to be adjusted: to implement screening plans, supply the Regions with the objectives related to common LEAs in view of the regional differences. According to the "National Centre for the Prevention and Control of the Diseases" (institution of coordination between Ministry of Health and Regions for the activities of surveillance, prevention and prompt response to the emergencies), it is necessary to "design the interventions of secondary prevention not as performances but rather as "paths" (profiles of care) offered to the citizen within various organizing activities on the territory aiming at the efficiency in the practice". Only in this way the efficiencies can be optimized and the necessary budget minimized for each Region for the screening campaigns. In order to avoid the funding of squandering, a formula of analytical calculation of the needs will be necessary [58]. A further problem in the future will be to make homogeneous the different kinds of screening currently in use on the territory to assure a higher allocative efficiency and COL will clearly has a future, which will expand even if the technology stands still. For a screening programme to be successful, multiple events have to occur, beginning with awareness and recommendation from the primary-care physician, patient acceptance, financial coverage, risk stratification, screening test, timely diagnosis, timely treatment, and appropriate follow-up. If any one of these steps is faulty or is not of high quality, the screening will fail. In this scenario we had to consider the COL as a means than an aim. In this regard DEA, which is an innovative methodology easy to be applied especially in the health care with diversified systems as ours, can be a useful tool to calculate the regional needs in order to carry out screening campaigns.

Author details

Alberto Vannelli[1*], Michel Zanardo[1], Valerio Basilico[1], Baldovino Griffa[2], Fabrizio Rossi[2], Massimo Buongiorno[3], Luigi Battaglia[4], Vincenzo Pruiti[5], Sara De Dosso[6] and Giulio Capriata[1]

*Address all correspondence to: info@albertovannelli.it

1 Division of Oncologic & Gastrointestinal Surgery Valduce Hospital, Como, Italy

2 Division of General Surgery Valduce Hospital, Como, Italy

3 Finance Ca Foscari University, Venice, Italy

4 Division of General Surgery B Foundation Irccs "National Institute of Tumour", Milan, Italy

5 Azienda Ospedaliera Universitaria Policlinico "G. Martino", Messina, Italy

6 Oncology Institute of Southern Switzerland, Bellinzona, Switzerland

References

[1] Descartes, R. Discourse on the Method for Reasoning Well and for Seeking Truth in the Sciences. Translated by Ian Johnston. Vancouver Island University Nanaimo, BC Canada [Revised May (2010). http://records.viu.ca/~johnstoi/descartes/descartes1.htmaccessed 12 July 2012).

[2] Baxter, N. N, Goldwasser, M. A, Paszat, L. F, Saskin, R, Urbach, D. R, & Rabeneck, L. Association of colonoscopy and death from colorectal cancer. Ann Inter Med (2009). , 150(1), 1-8.

[3] The National Advisory Committee on Health and Disability (National Health Committee)Population screening for colorectal cancer Working Party on Screening for Colorectal Cancer http://www.nhc.health.govt.nz/sites/www.nhc.health.govt.nz/files/documents/publications/colorectalcancer.pdfaccessed 12 July (2012).

[4] Lin, G. A, Trujillo, L, & Frosch, D. L. Consequences of not respecting patient preferences for cancer screening: opportunity lost. Arch Intern Med. (2012). , 172(5), 393-4.

[5] Goodwin, J. S, Singh, A, Reddy, N, Riall, T. S, & Kuo, Y. F. Overuse of screening colonoscopy in the Medicare population. Arch Intern Med. (2011). , 171(15), 1335-43.

[6] Sandler, R. S. Colonoscopy and colorectal cancer mortality: strong beliefs or strong facts? Am J Gastroenterol. (2010). , 105(7), 1633-5.

[7] Mcalearney, A. S, Reeves, K. W, Dickinson, S. L, Kelly, K. M, Tatum, C, Katz, M. L, & Paskett, E. D. Racial differences in colorectal cancer screening practices and knowledge within a low-income population.Cancer. (2008). , 112(2), 391-8.

[8] De Jesus, M, Puleo, E, Shelton, R. C, Mcneill, L. H, & Emmons, K. M. Factors associated with colorectal cancer screening among a low-income, multiethnic, highly insured population: does provider's understanding of the patient's social context matter? J Urban Health. (2010). , 87(2), 236-43.

[9] AIRTUM Working GroupItalian cancer figures, report (2010). Cancer prevalence in Italy. Patients living with cancer, long-term survivors and cured patients. Epidemiol Prev. 2010;34(5-6 Suppl 2) 1-188

[10] Von Karsa, L, Anttila, A, Ronco, G, Ponti, A, Malila, N, Arbyn, M, Segnan, N, Castillo-beltran, M, Boniol, M, Ferlay, J, Hery, C, Sauvaget, C, Voti, L, & Autier, P. European Commission Cancer screening in the European Union. Report on the implementation of the Council Recommendation on cancer screening. Luxembourg: European Communities; (2008). http://ec.europa.eu/health/archive/ph_determinants/genetics/documents/cancer_screening.pdfaccessed 12 July 2012).

[11] Zappa, M, Federici, A, & Salmaso, S. Cancer screening programmes in Italy: unification element or factor for further division?. Epidemiol Prev. (2011). Suppl 2) 100-2.

[12] Cislaghi, C, & Arena, V. Performance. Regional differences in the National Health Service. Epidemiol Prev. (2011). Suppl 2) 126-7.

[13] Ned, R. M, Melillo, S, & Marrone, M. Fecal DNA testing for Colorectal Cancer Screening: the ColoSure™ test. PLoS Curr. (2011). RRN1220.

[14] Guzzinati, S, Spitale, A, Miccinesi, G, Zambon, P, & Rosso, S. The database of the Italian cancer registries: estimates of the observed populations. Epidemiol Prev. (2004).

[15] Crocetti, E, Capocaccia, R, Casella, C, Guzzinati, S, Ferretti, S, Rosso, S, Sacchettini, C, Spitale, A, & Stracci, F. Tumino R; Network of the Italian Cancer Registries (AIRT). Population-based incidence and mortality cancer trends (1986-1997) from the network of Italian cancer registries. Eur J Cancer Prev. (2004). , 13(4), 287-95.

[16] Stracci, F, & Sacchettini, C. Italian Network of Cancer Registries. Methods. Epidemiol Prev. (2004). Suppl) , 12-6.

[17] Guzzinati, S, & Spitale, A. The Italian Network of Cancer Registries (AIRT). Epidemiol Prev. (2004). Suppl) , 7-11.

[18] Paci, E, Quaglia, A, Pannelli, F, & Budroni, M. The impact of screening and early diagnosis on survival--results from the Italian cancer registries. Epidemiol Prev. (2001). Suppl) , 9-14.

[19] Mariotto, A, Dally, L. G, Micheli, A, Canario, F, & Verdecchia, A. Cancer prevalence in Italian regions with local cancer registries. Tumori. (1999). , 85(5), 400-7.

[20] Governo italianoPresidenza del consiglio. Conferenze Stato Regioni ed Unificata http://www.statoregioni.it/dettaglioDoc.asp?idprov=8114&iddoc=26500&tipodoc=18&CONF=CSRaccessed 12 July (2012).

[21] Associazione italiana dei registri tumorihttp://www.registri-tumori.it/cms/accessed 12 July (2012).

[22] Centro nazionale per la prevenzione e il controllo delle malattiehttp://www.ccm-network.it/accessed 12 July (2012).

[23] Gazzetta Ufficiale Law 138 of May 26th (2004). http://www.ccm-network.it/documenti_Ccm/normativa/L_pdfaccessed 12 July 2012).

[24] Gazzetta Ufficiale Health Ministry Decree of July 1st (2004). http://www.ccm-network.it/documenti_Ccm/normativa/DM_1-7-2004.pdf)accessed 12 July 2012).

[25] Gazzetta Ufficiale The labourhealth and social policy Ministry Decree of September 18th (2008). http://www.ccm-network.it/documenti_Ccm/normativa/DM_18settembre_2008.pdf)accessed 12 July 2012).

[26] Charnes, A, Cooper, W. W, & Rhodes, E. Measuring the efficiency of decision making units, European Journal of Operational Research. (1978). , 2-429.

[27] Matarese, V. G, Feo, C. V, Lanza, G, Fusetti, N, Carpanelli, M. C, Cataldo, S, Cifalà, V, Ferretti, S, Gafà, R, Marzola, M, Montanari, E, Palmonari, C, Simone, L, Trevisani, L, Stockbrugger, R, & Gullini, S. The first 2 years of colorectal cancer screening in Ferrara, Italy. Eur J Cancer Prev. (2011). , 20(3), 166-8.

[28] Zorzi, M, Bianchi, P. S, & Grazzini, G. Senore C; Gruppo di lavoro sugli indicatori del GISCoR. Quality indicators for the evaluation of colorectal cancer screening programmes. Epidemiol Prev. (2007). Suppl 1) 6-56.

[29] Segnan, N, Armaroli, P, Bonelli, L, Risio, M, Sciallero, S, Zappa, M, Andreoni, B, Arrigoni, A, Bisanti, L, Casella, C, Crosta, C, Falcini, F, Ferrero, F, Giacomin, A, Giuliani, O, Santarelli, A, Visioli, C. B, Zanetti, R, Atkin, W. S, & Senore, C. and the SCORE Working Group. Once-Only Sigmoidoscopy in Colorectal Cancer Screening: Follow-up Findings of the Italian Randomized Controlled Trial--SCORE. J Natl Cancer Inst. (2011). , 103(17), 1310-22.

[30] Lisi, D, & Hassan, C. Crespi M; AMOD Study Group. Participation in colorectal cancer screening with FOBT and colonoscopy: an Italian, multicentre, randomized population study. Dig Liver Dis. (2010). , 42(5), 371-6.

[31] Alberto VannelliLuigi Battaglia, Elia Poiasina e Ermanno Leo. Lo screening dei tumori del colon retto: tra federalismo e costi standard. Convegno AIES Torino (2010). http://www.coripe.unito.it/files/vannellibattagliapoiasinaleo.pdfaccessed 12 July 2012).

[32] Gazzetta Ufficiale Law 42 of May 5th (2009). http://wwwparlamento.it/parlam/leggi/09042l.htm) (accessed 12 July 2012).

[33] Gazzetta Ufficiale Decree of the President of the Council of Ministry Noof November 29th (2001). http://www.fondazionepromozionesociale.it/lex/nazionali/dpcm29novembre2001.pdf)accessed 12 July 2012).

[34] Gazzetta Ufficiale Law 388 of December 23th (2000). http://wwwcamera.it/parlam/leggi/00388l.htm) (accessed 12 July 2012).

[35] Finanziamento del Servizio sanitario nazionale per l'anno (2010). Seduta della Camera 29 luglio 2010 http://www.camera.it/187?slAnnoMese=201007&slGiorno=29&idSeduta=accessed 12 July 2012).

[36] Gazzetta Ufficiale dm of April 15th (1994). artc. 2 http://www.normativasanitaria.it/jsp/dettaglio.jsp?id=10950accessed 12 July 2012).

[37] Gazzetta Ufficiale dm of April 15th (1994). artc. 2 http://www.normativasanitaria.it/jsp/dettaglio.jsp?id=10950accessed 12 July 2012).

[38] Boccia, A, & De Giusti, M. Del Cimmuto A, Tufi D, Villari P. Health care reforms in Italy: towards an health system with national rights and local responsibilities. Ann Ig. (2003)., 15(6), 771-85.

[39] Lega, F, Sargiacomo, M, & Ianni, L. The rise of governmentality in the Italian National Health System: physiology or pathology of a decentralized and (ongoing) federalist system? Health Serv Manage Res. (2010)., 23(4), 172-80.

[40] France, G. The form and context of federalism: meanings for health care financing. J Health Polit Policy Law. (2008)., 33(4), 649-705.

[41] France, G, & Taroni, F. The evolution of health-policy making in Italy. J Health Polit Policy Law. (2005).

[42] Panà, A, & Muzzi, A. Federalism and health care outcomes monitoring]. Ig Sanita Pubbl. (2003).

[43] Dirindin, N. Fiscal federalism and health: how can the health care system be improved?]. Epidemiol Prev. (2001)., 25(2), 55-6.

[44] Magnussen, J, & Nyland, K. Measuring efficiency in clinical departments. Health Policy. (2008)., 87(1), 1-7.

[45] Akazili, J, Adjuik, M, Chatio, S, Kanyomse, E, Hodgson, A, Aikins, M, & Gyapong, J. What are the Technical and Allocative Efficiencies of Public Health Centres in Ghana? Ghana Med J. (2008)., 42(4), 149-55.

[46] Sebastian, M. S, & Lemma, H. Efficiency of the health extension plan in Tigray, Ethiopia: a data envelopment analysis. BMC Int Health Hum Rights. (2010).

[47] Buck, D. The efficiency of the community dental service in England: a data envelopment analysis. Community Dent Oral Epidemiol. (2000). , 28(4), 274-80.

[48] Johnston, K, & Gerard, K. Assessing efficiency in the UK breast screening plan: does size of screening unit make a difference? Health Policy. (2001). , 56(1), 21-32.

[49] Cooper, W. W, Seidorf, L. M, & Tone, K. Data Envelopment Analysis, Boston: Kluwer Academic Publishers; (2000).

[50] Seiford, L. M, & Thrall, R. M. Recent developments in DEA, the mathematical programming approach to frontier analysis. Journal of Econometrics. (1990). , 46-7.

[51] Simar, L, & Wilson, P. W. Statistical Inference in Nonparametric Frontier Models: The State of the Art. Journal of Productivity Analysis. (2000). , 13-49.

[52] Tan JKHBarry Sheps s. Health decision support systems Jones & Bartlett Learning, (1998). , 1998.

[53] Lins, M. E, & Lobo, M. S. da Silva AC, Fiszman R, Ribeiro VJ.The use of Data Envelopment Analysis (DEA) for Brazilian teaching hospitals' evaluation. Cien Saude Colet. (2007). , 12(4), 985-98.

[54] Censis: 45° Rapporto Annuale sulla situazione sociale del Paese (2011). http://wwwistitutoaffarisociali.it/flex/AppData/Redational/Ejournal/Articoli/Files/D. 44e932590fff07417bb3/valutazione_qualita_in_sanita.pdf (accessed 12 July 2012).

[55] Associazione Italiana di Economia Sanitaria (AIES) 15th Convegno Annuale http://wwwaiesweb.it/convegni/co0008/media/pdf/papers/VIa.pdf (accessed 12 July (2012).

[56] Dervaux, B, Eeckhoudt, L, Lebrun, T, & Sailly, J. C. Determination of cost-effective strategies in colorectal cancer screening Rev Epidemiol Sante Publique. (1992). , 40(5), 296-306.

[57] Osservatorio nazionale degli screeningItalian Cancer Trend (1998-2005). http://www.registri-tumori.it/PDF/AIRTUM2009Trend/E&S1_38_colonretto.pdfaccessed 12 July (2012).

[58] Gianino, M. M, Siliquini, R, Russo, R, & Renga, G. Which competences and what managerial training for the health professions. J Prev Med Hyg. (2006). , 47(2), 74-9.

Section 2

Managing Precursor Lesions: Resection Techniques and Beyond

Chapter 4

Evolution and Strategy of Endoscopic Treatment for Colorectal Tumours

Koh Z.L. Sharon, H. Yamamoto and
Tsang B.S. Charles

Additional information is available at the end of the chapter

http://dx.doi.org/10.5772/53342

1. Introduction

1.1. History

Wolff and Shinya published their experience with *therapeutic* colonoscopy in September 1969 in JAMA [2], three months after they had commenced to perform diagnostic fiber colonoscopy. Since then, this has become an increasingly significant arm of minimally invasive colorectal surgery, complementing, even possibly replacing procedures that were once performed using "open" surgical techniques. [1-3]

Following the introduction of the fiber-optic colonoscopy for diagnostic evaluation of the lower gastrointestinal tract, enabling all parts of the colon to the assessed under direct vision and instrumentation as reported by Deyhle and Demling in 1971, and Sakai in 1972, [4-5] mastery of these techniques by Williams and colleagues have enabled therapeutic interventions to be performed endoscopically. [6]

Propelling this "endoscopic therapy" movement is the increasing evidence of the "adenoma-carcinoma" polyp-cancer sequence introduced by Morson and Bussey from 1968 to 1970. [7] This fundamental concept has enabled a form of prevention of colorectal cancer by endoscopic removal of precursor lesions and is the basis of colonoscopic screening for colorectal cancer, resulting in the effective cessation to their progression to cancer.

2. Polypectomy in the colon

Winawer and colleagues in 1993 provided strong evidence that the prevention of colorectal cancer can be achieved by colonoscopic polypectomy. [9] Data and statistics from the National

Polyp Study Workgroup demonstrated that the incidence of colorectal cancer is reduced by colonoscopic polypectomy and provided evidence for the adherence to the principle of searching and subsequent removal of adenomatous polyps in the colon and rectum. They reported on the 6-year follow-up of 1,418 patients after repeated colonoscopy to clear all polyps. While this study did not have a true control arm, the background age and sex specific incidence of colorectal cancer was used as a control group. The removal of all polyps seen during endoscopy prevented the development of 75% of carcinomas. The Veterans Affairs Study conducted by Muller and Sonnenberg published in 1995 found that only 50% of cancers were prevented, but the study was limited, for not all patients had received total colonoscopy in that study. [10] Hurlstone and colleagues postulate that one possible factor responsible for polyp surveillance failing to prevent all colorectal cancers within these studies may be due to the lack of Western experience of flat and depressed lesions within the colon. [11]

The evolution of colonoscopic polypectomies was between the 1950s and 1970s. As neither radiographic imaging via barium studies; nor macroscopic appearance of the polyps gave any definite information about its nature or behavior, histologic assessment was thereby deemed necessary to establish the diagnosis of these polyps and thereafter, their prognosis. Hellwig and Barbosa reported that forceps biopsy gave samples that were inadequate for the exclusion of the presence of malignancy. [12] Also there was no complete removal of the lesion, which is necessary for a full histological study.

In the 1970s, the largest series of colonoscopic polypectomies performed were reported by Wolff and Shinya in 1973. [13] They reported their undertaking of a program to remove colonic polyps endoscopically. Shinya was also responsible for the conception of "snare polypectomy" and with Hiroshi Ichikawa, developed various polypectomy techniques in the 1970s. This was performed after achieving 1600 uncomplicated diagnostic colonoscopies. They removed 303 polyps ranging from 0.5 to 5.0cm in diameter with minimal complication. Major bleeding requiring transfusion was encountered in one patient, and minor bleeding in four others. The other series published were much smaller and were descriptive, mainly by Friend and Ottenjahn in 1972, Dehyle, Demling, Fruhmorgen, Testas and Williams et al in 1973. Morgenthal et al thus concluded in a review published in 2007 that colonoscopic polypectomy may be the most significant of all developments in therapeutic endoscopy. [8]

Already in the early development of colonoscopic polypectomy, several problems were encountered and along with them, limitations with this technique. In 1974, Williams and colleagues reviewed their series of 300 polypectomies in 169 patients. Fundamental principles such as adequate bowel preparation to ensure minimally obstructed view of the polyp to be snared, and to ensure no residual fluid present to dissipate the energy current have been described right from the introduction of colonoscopic polypectomy and are still adhered to today.

2.1. Electrocautery in snare polypectomy and hot biopsy

Williams et al described the use of a diathermy snare loop technique for excision of polyps up to 4.5 cm in diameter. The "hot-biopsy" technique was also introduced and they reported their results in 107 smaller polyps. Their results compared favorably to surgical polypectomies.

They reported a single "closed" perforation that was managed conservatively, and 2 patients who experienced major hemorrhage. [14]

For small sessile polyps, the snare loop was passed over the head of the polyps and tightened at the base. For pedunculated polyps, the snare was closed halfway down the stalk. This was positioned "high" enough to minimize the risk of heat necrosis of the bowel wall, but "low" enough to include areas of mucosal change suspicious of early malignant invasion of the stalk. [14]

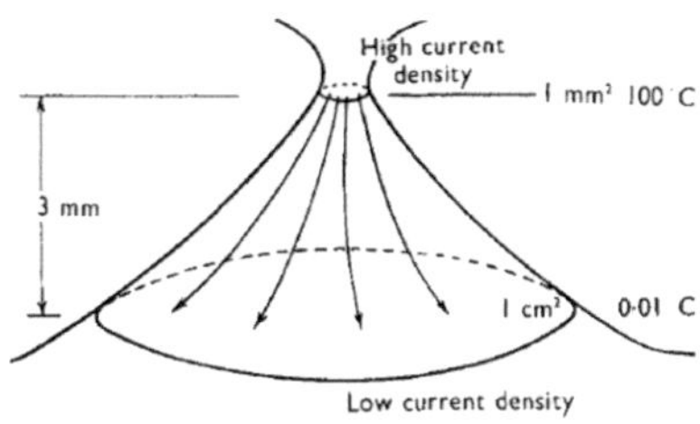

Figure 1. Principle of "current density" in diathermy electrocoagulation – heating effect in the stalk of the polyp (after Curtiss 1973)

The technique of diathermy snare polypectomy was based on the theory of diathermy currents described by Curtiss in 1973. The electrical precautions described then are also still observed today. These are to tighten the snare and elevate the polyp away from the bowel in the direction that the current passes into the smallest possible area of tissue within the stalk, enabling localized heating at the area of highest "current density" (Fig 1). [15] As this is applicable to pedunculated polyps with inherent stalks, Williams and colleagues [14] described the technique of creating a "pseudo-pedicle" in small sessile polyps by lifting the snared polyp forcible. Heat necrosis is avoided by ensuring that the polyp head, upon being lifted up, did not come into contact with the opposite bowel wall during the application of the current. These principles were extended for the same authors described the "hot-biopsy" techniques by which polyps up to 7mm were simultaneously biopsies and also destroyed by the application of a strong coagulating current down the closed jaws of the biopsy forceps. The tissue within the jaws is not heated and therefore preserved, as the current bypasses this area of conductive material.

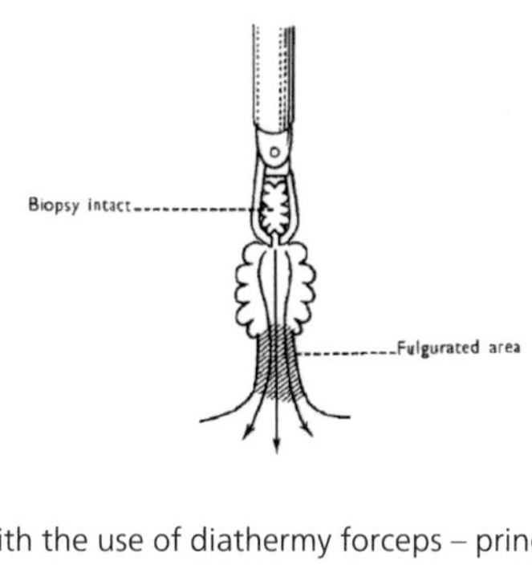

Figure 2. Technique of "hot biopsy" with the use of diathermy forceps – principle of selective coagulation necrosis at the base of the polyp.

Since then, the role of therapeutic colonoscopic polypectomy have grown exponentially as the technical problems of polypectomy and electrosurgery, in comparison to open surgical polypectomy, are more easily mastered and taught. More importantly, these techniques can be learnt not just by the surgeons, but also the gastroenterologists.

2.2. Impact of polypectomy — Review of the technique and histologic outcomes

In the 1980s to 1990s, Williams and Bedenne performed a literature review on what they called "the polyp problem" and carried out a critique of their current practice. They concluded that since the introduction of the adenoma-carcinoma sequence in 1973, there have been no evidence in the literature to disprove this concept that majority of colorectal cancers develop from previous adenomas. Even then, they concluded with the current management of colorectal polyps was "transparently worthwhile" for the ease of the removal of symptomatic or threatening polyps avoids the morbidity of surgery and unnecessary operation. [15]

The concept of the "flat adenoma" was also reviewed, and has been described as precursors of carcinomas especially in inherited colorectal cancers. Jass and colleagues [17] described that this may account for 10% of patients whose carcinoma develop in a "de novo" fashion. These are usually found in the right sided colon and characteristically present as a "firm pale button only 5-15mm in diameter"' that could be missed at endoscopy, especially if bowel preparation of the caecal and right sided colon is inadequate. [18]During this time, colonoscopic techniques were reviewed. [19-20] It was reported that small polyps up to 5-6mm can be conveniently managed with the hot-biopsy technique. Combined with rapid electrocoagulation technique, the histological yield has been reported to be over 95%. There must be some visible eletrocoagulation during this procedure to avoid recurrences of the polyp as simple "cold-biopsy" without electrocoagulation resulted in up to 29% remnant viable tissue. There is however, a significant incidence of complications, namely perforation when coagulation is overdone in the proximal colon. [21-23]

The use of a bipolar electrode, although initially demonstrated promise in localizing heat necrosis to the area within the jaws of the biopsy forceps, was not predictably effective in polyp destruction. This is because the tissue grasped between the jaws were heated and thereby destroyed by the electrical current passing between the jaws, resulting in inability to interpret the histology. [24]For polyps larger than 5-6mm in diameter, Williams et al concluded that it was safer to use conventional snare polypectomy. [16] Retrieval of the specimen was by aspiration into a filtered polyp suction trap commercially available since the late 1980s. [25]

For polyps larger than 1cm (medium to large sized), the principles of sclerotherapy injection with adrenaline in saline for short stalks prior to snaring or after bleeding have been widely practiced. Although some have reported that polyps 3cm or greater in size can be excised by snare polypectomy without employing the injection techniques. [26]

2.3. Advent of endoscopic mucosal resection & submucosa dissection

It is hence, of no surprise when the techniques of submucosal injection with various fluids (ranged from isotonic to hypertonic saline; 50% glucose with epinephrine +/- indigocarmine)

http://dx.doi.org/10.5772/53342

to enable a safer and more reliable removal of relatively large or flat lesions were popularized in the last twenty years as Endoscopic Mucosal Resection (EMR). [28] In general, for lesions larger than 2cm, several endoscopists recognize the challenge in performing an *en bloc* resection, hence piecemeal resection was routinely performed. These had then become accepted as a relatively quick and easy procedure to perform. [29-30] The disadvantages of the lack of a precise histological evaluation and risk of local recurrence were reported and widely accepted. The default staging of the resection automatically becomes Rx as compared to R0 if an adequate en bloc resection had been performed. Hence there was a challenge to perform a single step non piece-meal mucosectomy for large flat lesions.The first such successful procedure in the colorectum for a lesions larger than 2cm was performed by the co-author (H.Y.) and published in 1999. He performed single step resection of a 40mm flat-elevated tumor in the rectum using sodium hyaluronate which enabled a prominent and longer lasting mucosa protrusion. [79-80]

In a recent analysis of 58 lateral spreading tumours (>10 mm in diameter with a low vertical axis extending laterally along the luminal wall) 36 lesions required piecemeal resection due to their maximum diameter exceeding 20 mm, and the majority of recurrences (8/10) detected occurred in this group. These recurrences were successfully managed by further EMR. [11] Re-treatment of recurrent tumors after such piecemeal EMRs were postulated to have added difficulty as the local fibrosis prevented an adequate mucosal lift, hence increasing the risk of perforation and inadequate resection. Hurlstone and colleagues reported their method of addressing these issues. The problem of recurrence that piecemeal or incomplete resection poses may be tackled by utilizing endoscopic submucosal resection (ESD) which has recently been developed by Japanese groups for the endoluminal resection of Paris 0-II lesions of the stomach, gastro-esophageal junction and esophagus using a gastroscope with a distal transparent cap attachment. The technique allows *en bloc* knife dissection after sodium hyaluronic acid or glycerol submucosal infiltration for lesions > 20 mm in diameter. [11]

2.4. Endoscopic microsurgery

In 1987, Buess and colleagues extended the application of endoscopy in the arena of minimally invasive surgery, pushing back their boundaries by introducing the transanal endoscopic microsurgery (TEM) procedure. This enabled two-handed use of surgical instrumentation and suturing techniques via a jumbo proctoscope to enable air insufflation of the rectum and sigmoid colon. He reported the ability to resect large and full thickness lesions up to the distance of 25cm from the anal verge. However, large sessile tumours in the proximal colon will still require surgical management if endoscopic snaring is too risky or if it fails. [31] This eventually resulted in the evolution of the ESD technique, an amulgamation of both endoscopic and surgical principles.

2.5. Strategy of endoscopic treatment for colorectal tumours — Endoscopic submucosal dissection: Technique

ESD is a new endoluminal therapeutic technique involving the use of cutting devices to permit a larger resection of the tissue over the muscularis propria. The major advantages of the technique in comparison with polypectomy and endoscopic mucosal resection are controllable resection size and shape, and en bloc resection of a large lesion or one with ulcerative features. [33-34] Naohisa Yahagi surmised this technique as a "fairly new arrival in the field of endoscopy", but had redefined the whole concept of minimally invasive endoscopic resection for gastrointestinal neoplasms. [35]The technique of endoscopic submucosal dissection (ESD) has extended its applications for en bloc resection of large ulcerative lesions in the stomach for the treatment of early gastric cancer to that of resection of superficial neoplasms of the colon and the rectum for the treatment of early colorectal cancer. [36-39]

ESD has the advantage of permitting en bloc and histologically complete resection. On the other hand, ESD has some disadvantages such as a long operating time, a high frequency of complications, and the need for a high level of technical skill [39-41].

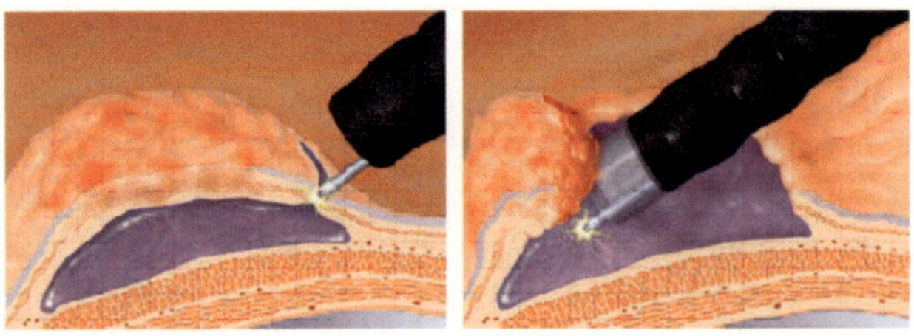

(a) (b)

Figure 3. (a): mucosal incision made 3-5mm outside the tumour edge with Endocut mode. 3(b) Submucosal dissection performed using the ST hood as means of elevation and counter-traction.

The most important aspects of this technique are to incise the mucosa surrounding the lesion (Figure 3a), and to dissect completely the submucosa beneath that lesion (Figure 3b) to achieve reliable en bloc resection regardless of the size or location of the tumor

2.6. Principles of ESD

The technique of endoscopic resection is less invasive than surgical resection [34,39-40]. Its limitation lies in its inability to perform lymph node dissection, hence cure can only be achieved in localized tumors without metastases. [35,39] The risk of lymph node metastases strongly correlates with the depth of invasion of the tumor, the histopathologic type of the lesion and the presence of lymphovascular involvement. [42-46] Hence, the precise staging of the lesion pre-procedure with pit pattern diagnosis using the technique of magnifying endoscopy is strongly recommended for the appropriate selection of tumors for endoscopic resection [47-48].

Detailed pathological examination of the resected specimen is paramount to document the complete resection of the neoplasms, allowing appropriate decisions regarding the need for further surgical intervention. Curative endoscopic resection is defined by confirmation of negative resection margins, differentiated histopathologic type, depth of submucosal invasion to be <1,000 *u*m and no lymphatic or vascular involvement. *En bloc* resection of the entire lesion is necessary to obtain such information.

ESD has demonstrated superiority to EMR for a more reliable en bloc resection of a targeted area of mucosa can be achieved. It has also shown to provide a higher complete resection rate with local recurrence rate as compared to piecemeal EMR. [32,49-51]. It enables the control of the size as well as the shape of the lesion to be resected, those with ulcerative findings can also be resected *en bloc*, leading to a potential cure of the target lesions without resection of that portion of the gastrointestinal tract or organ.

2.7. Indication for colorectal ESD

The characterization and endoscopic staging of each lesion is paramount in determining the suitability and thereby success of this procedure. In general, ESD can be applied to almost all lesions provided that they are within the mucosa and superficial submucosal layer of the colorectal wall. Absolute indications for ESD have been reported to be those that "cannot be resected en bloc by standard available procedures; those that require precise histological evaluation on account of a significant malignant potential. Hurlstone and colleagues describe these to be laterally spreading tumors of the nongranulating types (LST-NG). The use of the snare EMR technique for en bloc resection of larger lesions with features pf LST-NG type, pseudo-depressed type and lesions with type Vi pit pattern with suspicion of carcinoma infiltrating into the submucosal layer (*sm*), or large elevated tumors are deemed difficult.

Other indications described in literature are those with biopsy-induced submucosal fibrotic scars, lesions located at challenging areas: on haustrae and difficult colonic angulations, and large lesions (>20mm), and small rectal carcinoid tumor when *en bloc* resection by conventional methods were deemed impossible. [52-53] Sporadic localized tumors occurring in the background of chronic inflammation such as those seen in inflammatory bowel disease namely ulcerative colitis; and residual early carcinoma post endoscopic resection are also indications for ESD. The success in such cases is dependent on the operability of endoscope, and the skill of the endoscopists - factors that should always be considered in the practice of ESD.

In the past decade, efforts to establish an East-West consensus on the clinicopathological importance of the macroscopic morphology of the colorectal polyp, incorporating the exophytic protruding polyps as well as those that are flat and depressed, have resulted in the introduction of multiple classifications. These are namely, the Paris classification and the modified Kudo criteria. The Cho criterion is used to differentiate tumor stage and nodal disease status by using high-frequency endoscopic ultrasonography. All are used to establish the *exclusion criteria* of ESD, which are: T2/N1 disease, transfixed type IIC component (constant concavity of the lesion regardless of air insufflations or deflation as defined by Kudo). Presence of systemic disease (hepatic metastases) or local nodal metastasis at index computer tomography imaging of abdomen and pelvis excludes ESD as a curative procedure. [58-9]

More recently in Japan, the indications for colorectal ESD have been established by the Colorectal ESD Standardization Implementation Working Group (Table 1). The development of various devices, endoscopes, and accessories for colorectal ESD have increased the safety of colorectal ESD, established its procedures, and simplified its techniques. Consequently, colorectal ESD has been gradually introduced in many institutions, both within Japan and in Asian countries. [59]

Indications for Colorectal ESD - Standardization Implementation Working Group
Lesions larger than 20mm in diameter in which en bloc resection using snare EMR is difficult, although it is indicative for endoscopic treatment
Non granular LST, particularly those of pseudodepressed type
Lesions with V_1 type pit pattern
Carcinoma with submucosal infiltration
Large depressed type lesion
Large lesions with elevated type suspected to be cancer (including granular LST that consisted of large nodules)
Mucosal lesions with fibrosis caused by prolapse due to biopsy of peristalsis of the lesions
Sporadic localized tumors in chronic inflammation such as ulcerative colitis
Local residual early cancer after endoscopic resection

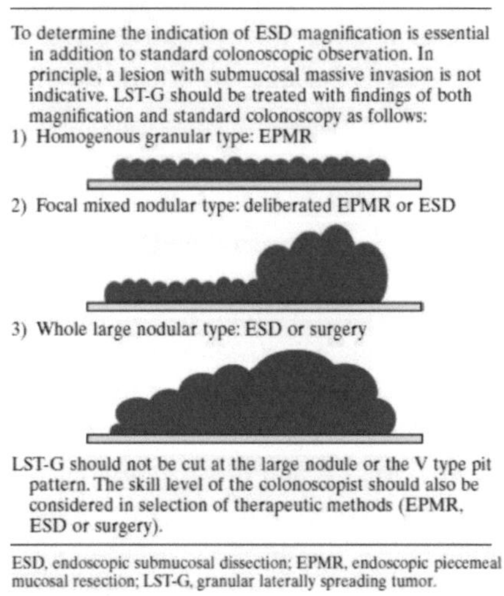

Table 1. Indications of ESD for colorectal neoplasms. The Colorectal ESD Standardization Implementation Working Group, a subordinate organization of the Gastroenterological Endoscopy Promotion Liaison Conference has proposed the Indication Criteria for Colorectal ESD (Tanaka S, Oka S, Chayama K. Colorectal endoscopic submucosal dissection: present status and future perspective, including its differentiation from endoscopic mucosal resection. *J. Gastroenterol.* 2008; 43: 641–51 (Review).

2.8. Assessment of tumour extent

Mucosal neoplasms in the colon and rectum typically have clear margins, which become even more prominent after submucosal injection and/or with the assistance of chromo-endoscopy. Thus in most cases, placing marks around the tumour prior to dissection is not necessary. Chromo-endoscopy with indigo carmine spray with or without the use of crystal violet dye, is useful to enhance the borders of the tumors. Newer imaging techniques, such as narrow band imaging (NBI) and flexible spectral imaging color enhancement (FICE) or Fuji Intelligent Color Enhancement (FICE ®) (Fujifilm Corp., Tokyo, Japan) are also useful to determine the borders of these tumors.

2.9. Preparation and set-up

This aspect of the procedure is important in ensuring optimal conditions during a technically challenging procedure. Optimal vision of the operating field is essential. A well-prepared bowel can also limit the contamination and degree of peritonitis should a perforation occur.

2.9.1. Endoscopes

Thinner endoscopes are preferred for precise control of the tip. Some authors select a single channel upper endoscope for ESD for rectosigmoid and distal left sided lesions. In our case series performed in a local institution, we used a specifically designed colonoscope (EC-450RD5; Fujifilm Corp., Tokyo, Japan; Fig. 4) for ESD in the colon and rectum. It is a single-channel scope with tip size (9.8mm) with a regular shaft size (12.8mm). This enables the usage of the retroflexed approach in any part of the colon and rectum as the tip is thin and short with good angulation ability. A relatively large accessory channel of 3.2 mm and a water jet function with good targeting direction make this scope suitable for ESD. The water jet allows the operator to wash out blood or mucus at the target area from their tips. A mixture of water with simethicon is used as a standard preparation solution for there is marked reduction in adherent residue and enables easier luminal lavage during ESD.

It is paramount to understand that maneuverability of the endoscope is the key factor in successful ESD and this should not be compromised. Hence, some authors report that in the cases of colorectal neoplasms, the application of the upper GI endoscopes is preferable to that of a slim single-channel endoscope. This is especially so when retroflexed manipulation is necessary as an endoscope with a small diameter allows smoother maneuverability in the retroflexed position. Such a position is recommended for large-sized lesions with its oral edge straddling a fold.

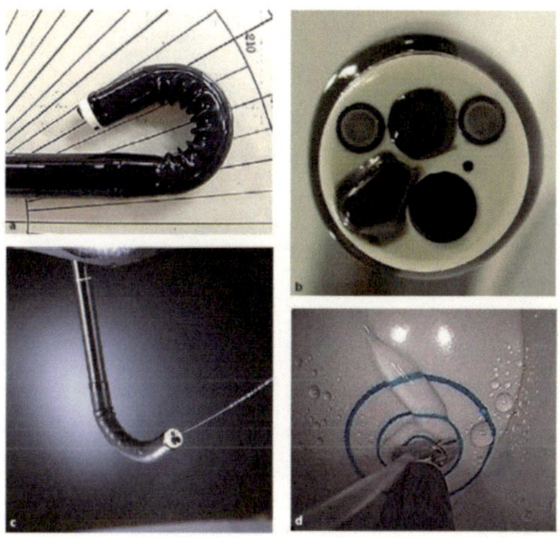

Figure 4. Colonoscope for ESD (EC-450RD5; Fujifilm Corp.). a The bending section of the endoscope tip is thin and short with good angulation capability. b A large accessory channel and a water jet channel are situated close to each other. c Water jet function of the scope. d Good targeting direction of the water jet to the tip of an accessory device.

When a lesion for ESD is located in an unstable part of the colon and paradoxical movements with a standard colonoscope hamper the reliable performance of the ESD procedure, we select a double-balloon colonoscope (EC-450BI5, Fujifilm, Japan; Fig. 5). The double-balloon colonoscope provides precise control of the endoscope tip, even in this situation (Fig. 6). The principle of DBE is well described by the co-author (H.Y.), and this has enabled optimal maneuverability and stability of the endoscope tip especially in the colon with its inherent anatomic variability in comparison to the oesophagus or stomach. Ohya and colleagues [54] highlighted these in their brief article on the use of a balloon over-tube as an endoscopic channel and platform for colorectal ESD in cases whereby access was difficult due to the colon being a longer tubular structure, with folds and formation of loops during intubation resulting in paradoxical movements. These authors report that the use of the balloon over-tube enabled optimal traction on the intestinal wall, and provided a shorter direct access to the lesion.

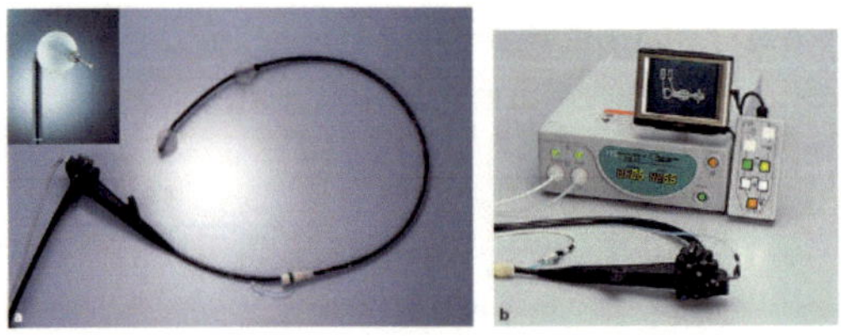

Figure 5. Double-balloon colonoscope (EC-450BI5, Fujifilm Corp.). a Soft balloons are equipped at the tip of the endoscope and the tip of the overtube. b A balloon controller to inflate or deflate the balloons.

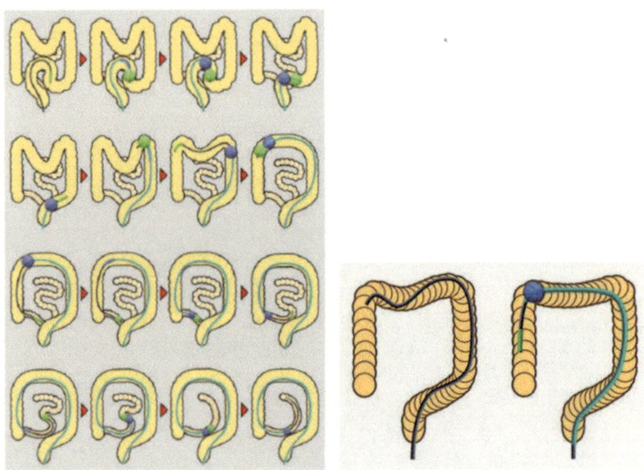

Figure 6. Illustrations demonstrating the sequential maneuvers of the instruments in the double-balloon method: (a) ante grade and (b) retrograde approach. Blue – paradoxical movements with standard colonoscope. Green – Precise control of endoscope tip provided by the double balloon (DB) colonoscope.

2.9.2. Accessories

Several kinds of electrosurgical knives have been developed for ESD. Among the currently available knives, we use a FlushKnife® (1.5mm; DK2618JN15; Fujifilm Corp., Tokyo, Japan) for ESD in the colon for our series. A FlushKnife® is a special needle knife featuring the water jet function through the knife sheath. The water jet function can be used to cleanse the surface of the mucosa and the needle itself. It can also be used for fluid injections directly into the submucosal layer through the FlushKnife® after mucosal incision. This improves is efficacy as it can be used for both injection and dissection. ESD can be performed immediately after the injection without changing the devices. The appropriate length of the needle can be selected from among 1, 1.5, 2, 2.5 and 3 mm sizes, based on the specific situation. (Fig 7)

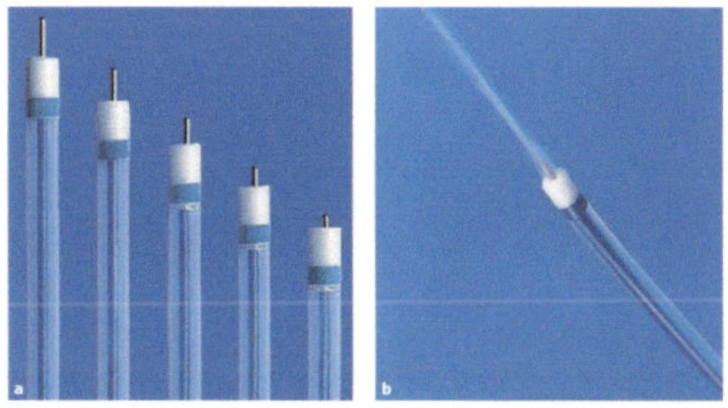

Figure 7. Flush knife (DK2618JN10–30; Fujifilm Corp.). a The appropriate length of the needle can be selected from among 1, 1.5, 2, 2.5 and 3 mm sizes. b Water jet function through the knife sheath.

2.9.3. Hood

A transparent hood attached to the tip of the endoscope is useful to open the incised wound and to maintain a good endoscopic view during the procedure. It also allows precise control of the knife by stabilizing the target with its tip. Use of a hood is substituted for the triangulation used during surgical procedures, which is difficult to apply in endoscopic procedures. We mainly use a transparent hood with a small-caliber tip (ST hood; DH-15GR, DH-16CR; Fujifilm, Japan; Fig 8) for colonic ESD. The ST hood has an aperture small enough to make it easy to widen an incised wound using the edge of the hood, and to allow more accurate adjustment of the depth of incision by the knife point. Using the ST hood, it is easy to create a submucosal tunnel proceeding with submucosal dissection by inserting the tip of the hood into the submucosal layer, which is a useful strategy for effective ESD.

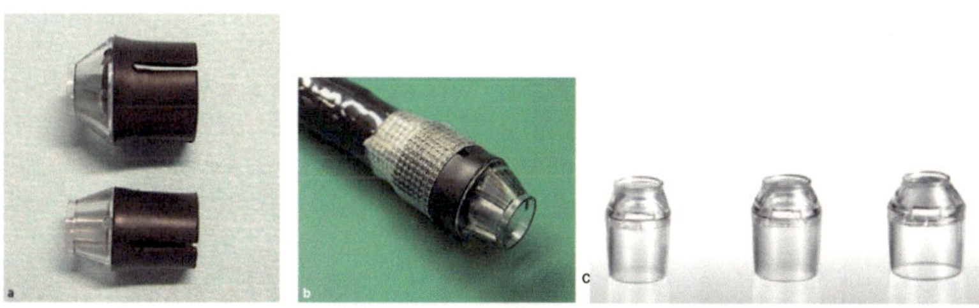

Figure 8. ST hood (DH-15GR, DH-16CR; Fujifilm Corp.). a Two sizes of the hood, DH-15GR for a thin endoscope tip and DH-16CR for a standard colonoscope tip) are available. b ST hood attached to the endoscope. c varying widths and heights for various locations and tissues

2.9.4. Electrosurgical current generator

The current and frequency of the electrosurgical current generator is of great importance to enable a reliable incision with effective control of bleeding and minimum tissue damage. We mainly use the ERBE VIO 300 D (Erbe, Tubingen, Germany). It is set to 'Endo Cut I' mode for mucosal incision, and to 'swift coagulation' or 'dry cut' mode for submucosal dissection. Table 2 is an example of the settings that was used in our case series.

	Device	Cut Mode		Coagulation Mode
Mucosal Incision	Flush knife	Endo Cut I E1/D 4/11	Dry Cut E6 30 W	
Submucosal Dissection	Flush knife	Dry Cut E6 30 W		Swift Coag E4 30 W
Hemostasis	Flush knife Hemostatic Forceps			Spray Coag E2 5 W Soft Coag E6 80 W

Table 2. ERBE VIO 300D settings for ESD procedures (W: watts)

Minor bleeding and small blood vessels can be managed using the knife. However, more reliable hemostasis for a larger vessel can be achieved using hemostatic forceps (HDB2422W; Pentax, Tokyo, Japan). The generator is set to soft coagulation mode for the hemostatic forceps.

Effective control of bleeding during the procedure is a vital factor for successful ESD.

3. ESD technique

ESD for colorectal tumors has been considered more technically demanding as compared to that in the stomach. This can be attributed to these following reasons: (1) thinner and softer colonic wall, (2) endoscopic control is difficult in specific parts of the colon due to paradoxical movement; (3) limitations to the retroflexed approach due to the narrow caliber of the colon; (4) tumours located on or behind a prominent colonic folds, peristalsis, and (5) higher risk of diffuse peritonitis requiring emergency surgical intervention as compared to perforation of the upper gastrointestinal tract. [34]

Several devices have been applied to ESD in the colon and rectum with the principle to use a dissecting technique that allows direct visualization of the submucosal tissue, and to use long-lasting injecting fluid. [79-80]

3.1. Technical method

3.1.1. Approach strategy and technique for mucosal incisions and submucosal dissection

Success of the ESD procedure lies with the maneuverability and stability of the endoscope. Hence, the insertion must be done in a controlled manner to avoid loop formation if possible. Authors have reported that rotation is a key movement. Upon reaching the tumor, the lumen of the intestine is filled with a mixture of water and simethicon to ensure adequate visualization. Chromoendoscopy with indigo carmine is performed to characterize the surface details and extent of the lesion. The borders of the lesion should be clearly visualized. [34]

A good strategy with prior considerations to the angle of approach to the lesion, taking into account the direction of gravity in relation its location is recommended. This can be assessed by observing the direction of the course of the jet stream of water from the water-jet. The position of the patient should be selected to locate the lesion at the top of the colonic lumen with regard to gravity. This enables sufficient opening of the mucosal incision and good visualization of the submucosal tissue during the procedure. Hence, minimal sedation for patient comfort is recommended if possible to allow patients to move positions more readily and report any undue discomfort during the procedure. In cases of unfavorable events such as bleeding and perforation, this positioning is beneficial to avoid or minimize further complications. In this position, bowel contents will not spill or leak into the intraperitoneal cavity and also, in situations of bleeding, blood will flow in the opposite direction (anti-gravity) to that of the lesion and not pool at the area of dissection. For example, if the bleeding point is at the top of the lumen, hemostasis can be performed reliably with accurate identification of the bleeding point because blood flows away from the bleeding point by gravity.

Even in cases of perforation, if the perforation occurs at the top of the lumen with regard to gravity, identification and closing of the perforation is easier, maintaining a good view of the site of perforation. Air, not contaminated intestinal fluid, will flow out from the lumen to the abdominal cavity before closing the perforation, which is important to prevent diffuse peritonitis.

The mucosal incision is made only in the area to be dissected. This is made with a short FlushKnife (1.5 mm; DK2618JN15; Fujifilm Corp., Tokyo, Japan) after sufficient protrusion of the mucosa is obtained with injection of suitable fluid. The Endo Cut mode is used for the mucosal incision. ESD can be performed safely with a FlushKnife as long as adequate thickening of the submucosal layer is present. This maintains a safety margin away from the muscle layer. The dissection should be done parallel to the muscular layer, by sliding the knife from the centre of the tumor toward the mucosal incision on the side, while hooking submucosal fibers with the knife. There are several other types of knives available commercially and several other techniques have been described in literature but these are not described here.

Several newer strategies have been introduced over the last couple of years. As shown in Figure 9(a) [SAFEKnife Horizontal®. DK2518DH1 Fujifilm Corp, Tokyo Japan] newer knives have been designed to enable a different axis of cutting. These are introduced during the submucosal dissection itself during the procedure with the aim to achieve maximal safety and efficacy.

The mucosal incision is made only in the area to be dissected and then dissection of the submucosa from the incised part is promptly started. Circumferential marking around the tumor with the tip of the electrosurgical knife is recommended for lesions in the upper gastrointestinal tract but not for intestinal neoplasms as the colonic wall is thin enough to be perforated in the process.

The development and subsequent maintenance of sufficient mucosal elevation is paramount for safe mucosal incisions and submucosal dissection. For these purposes, 0.4% sodium hyaluronate solution (MucoUp®; Seikagaku Corp, Tokyo, Japan) is the best injection fluid for ESD. [79-80]. The authors have found that the submucosal injection of sodium hyaluronate (0.4%) – commercially known as MucoUp®, (Johnson and Johnson Medical Co., Tokyo, Japan) enables the creation of a long-lasting mucosal protrusion that usually lasts more than 1 hour, providing the longest lasting fluid cushion, [49,79-80] and higher successful en-bloc resection

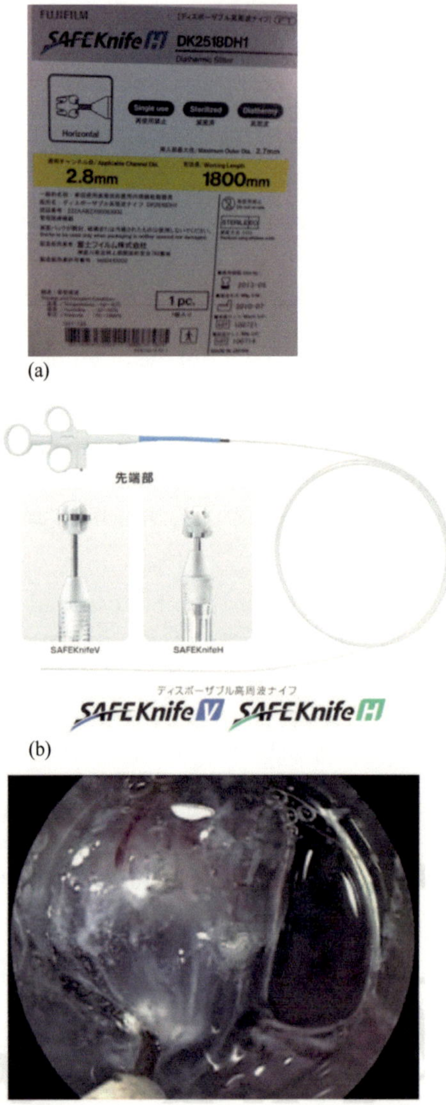

(a)

(b)

(c)

Figure 9. (a): SAFEKnife H ® that cuts in the horizontal plane and (b) SAFEKnife V ® that cuts in the vertical plane – invented by Dr H Yamamoto, manufactured by Fujifilm Corp Japan – 9(c) SAFEKnife V ® has a sandwichlike structure with a central electrode plate placed between 2 insulated plates enablising a safe and effective dieesction of the submucosal layers with a vertical approach

and lower perforation complication rates have been reported using HA, particularly for colorectal ESD [31,44,47,53-54]. However, in view of its high cost and unavailability locally (US $49.50–128.00/mL in the United States), we have created our own solution using (Fig 10a-b) 4 vials of Optovisc Eyedrops® (Ashford, FP Marketing) (Fig 10a) to make up 40mls of solution. 0.4mls of 1:1000 Adrenaline with 4 drops of Indigo carmine solution (Fig 10b).

http://dx.doi.org/10.5772/53342

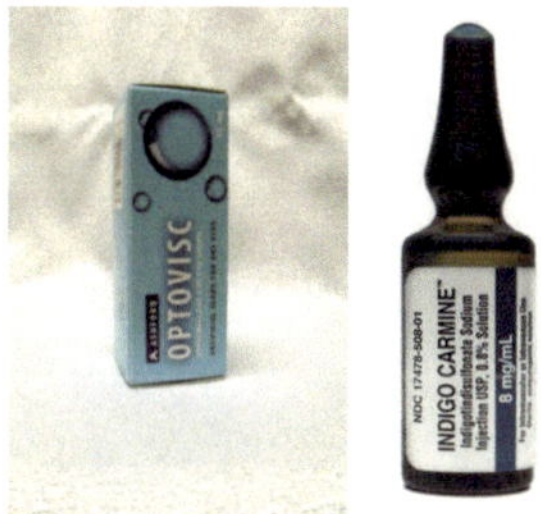

(a) (b)

Figure 10. (a): one vial of Optovisc® (b): Indigo Carmine Solution

This solution is injected into the submucosal layer just outside where the mucosal incision is intended.

3.1.2. Mucosal incision

The mucosal incision is made with a short FlushKnife® (1.5 mm; DK2618JN15; Fujifilm Corp., Tokyo, Japan) after sufficient protrusion of the mucosa is obtained. Only the needle part should be used for the incision, keeping the tip of the sheath touching the surface of the mucosa without pushing the sheath into the submucosal layer. The Endo Cut mode is used for the mucosal incision, at 30 watts. (Table 2)

There is no need for complete marginal cutting of the mucosa before the submucosal dissection. Some authors report that after exposure of the submucosal layer, with the visualization of the blue-stained submucosal connective tissue, further submucosal injection from the exposed submucosal layers may be used to elevate the layer that is to be cut. If the blue submucosal layers is not seen, this may indicate that the muscularis mucosae layers is incompletely cut and the incising line should be traced again until the blue submucosal layer is seen.

3.1.3. Submucosal dissection

ESD can be performed safely with a FlushKnife® as long as adequate thickening of the submucosal layer is present. This maintains a safety margin away from the muscle layer. The dissection should be done parallel to the muscular layer, by sliding the knife from the centre of the tumor toward the mucosal incision on the side, while hooking submucosal fibers with the knife. The submucosal fibres stained blue (indigo-carmine) are very soft and dissected easily with gentle application of the FlushKnife ® using the forced or swift coagulation mode. The knife length may be kept at the same length (<2mm) for both the mucosal incision and submucosal dissection.

A recent "tunneling" method has been introduced to dissect the submucosal layer, starting at the proximal edge of the colorectal tumour, followed by the distal edge.[34] Submucosal dissection is continued to make a tunnel in the submucosal layer by inserting the tip of the endoscope with a transparent hood under the mucosal tumor. This is continued to reach the mucosal incision at the proximal edge. After penetration of the tunnel, which began from both

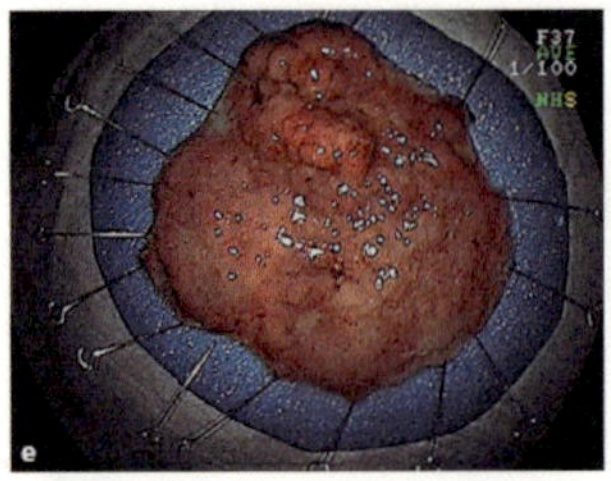

Figure 12. En bloc resection of the entire lesion (68 × 62 mm in diameter). Histopathologic examination confirmed complete curative resection (adenocarcinoma in adenoma, no invasion to submucosa, no lymphatic or vascular involvement); © Photographs courtesy of H Yamamoto 2010

ends, it is widened laterally. The mucosa on both sides of the tumour is then incised laterally and dissected submucosally to complete the dissection. (Fig.11). This tunneling technique enables the endoscope tip to be stabilized, hence a more precise control of the Flushknife® is achieved. This technique also enables a good safety margin for further dissection by stretching the submucosal tissue. Adjusting the approach angle of the knife to be tangential to the wall also is easy with this method because an adjusting force with the endoscope tip can be applied in either direction by pushing the mucosa up or pushing the muscle wall down with the tip of the hood (Fig 11b). This method is particularly useful for large lesions, lesions with fibrosis, and lesions located on a curved wall.

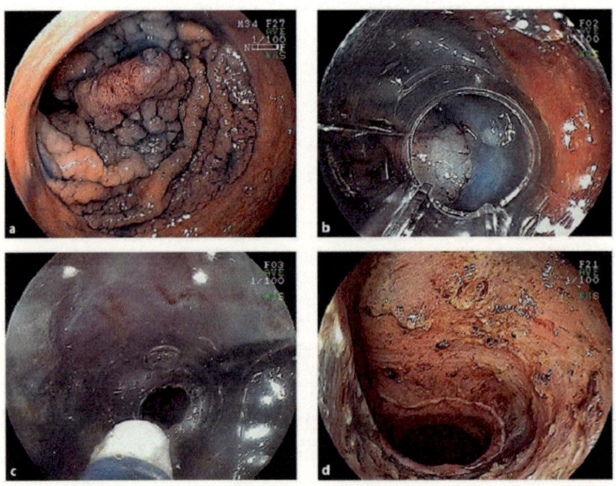

Figure 11. ESD using a tunneling method. a A large granular laterally spreading tumor (LST) in the rectum. b Distal edge of the tumor after submucosal injection of sodium hyaluronate solution. c Penetration of the tunnel in the submucosal layer. d Mucosal defect after the completion of ESD; © Photographs courtesy of H Yamamoto 2010

3.2. Handling of the resected specimen and histopathological assessment

The resected specimen is carefully retrieved per anally without tearing. A small specimen may be retrieved via suction into the soft hood/cap. A Roth net or other retrieval devices may be used for moderate-sized lesions but with larger lesions, an over-tube may be required. The shape and orientation of the specimen is dutifully recorded, and the specimen pinned out on a Styrofoam or corkboard with the oral and anal sides indicated. The preservation of fresh material is ensured by freezing in liquid nitrogen, embedded in OCT prior to freezing, The slice is cut from the middle without warming up to allow a frozen section to be used for further analysis. We recommend the use of formalin soaked needles to fix the specimen, which should be tension-free as there is 20 to 50% shrinkage of the specimen soaked in formalin.

The ESD specimens are regarded as complex specimens and undergo a standardized processing during both macroscopic and microscopic assessment of the specimens. They are photographed with a styrofoam backing board, with the oral side of the specimen "O" at 12 o'clock position, and the anal side "A" at the 6 o'clock position to ensure that the orientation of the specimens are known. (Fig 12)

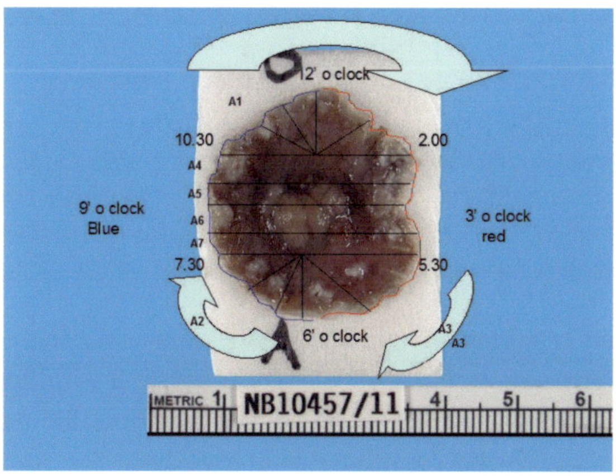

Figure 13. Mounting of a specimen on a Styrofoam board

Since 2009 to 2011, the specimen has been processed as shown below: The principle is to enable a fairly precise assessment of margin involvement. Currently, there are 2 methods of sectioning, each having their advantages and disadvantages. The first is described below whereby each transverse section should be submitted separately. The smaller fragments from the lateral edges should be submitted no more than 2 pieces per block. This has been performed since January 2009. The disadvantage of this method is that rounded irregular edges of such specimen are inadvertently shaved off during each 2mm sectioning and these margins cannot be assessed accurately when the sections happen to be tangential to the edge. The second method of sectioning aims to overcome the above problem. The axis of sectioning is perpendicular to the tangential line drawn at the edge. (Fig 14) This will enable more accurate margin assessment although tissue loss at the apex of each "segment" is inevitable. Inking of the margins is necessary and different colour should be used to represent the respective margins as required.

3.3. Standard operating procedures — Endoscopic Submucosal Dissections (ESD)

Currently all ESD specimens are regarded as complex specimens by the histopathology laboratory. They are photographed with the styrofoam backing board so that the orientation of the specimen is known. The principle of processing the ESD is to be able to tell the clinician fairly precisely where the margin is involved. An example of how the ESD specimen should be grossed and submitted is given below.

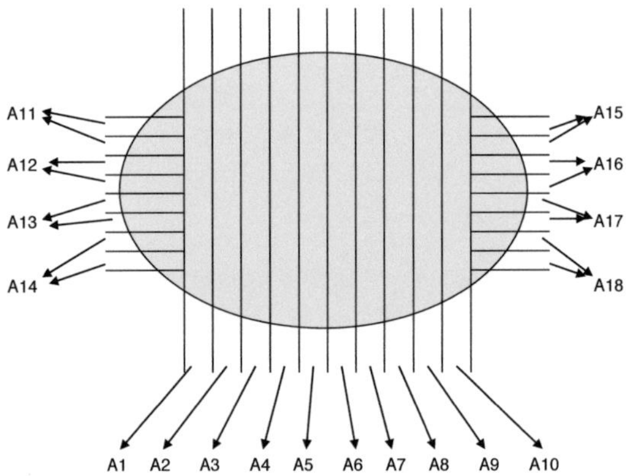

Figure 14. Pictorial diagram of how the specimen is sectioned and labeled

Each transverse section is submitted separately and the smaller fragments from the lateral edges should be submitted no more than 2 pieces per block. It is understood that some ESD specimen may have a rather irregular shape. In this situation, the pathologist or assistant trimmer should discuss with the consultant in charge how the specimen should best be processed so that the margins can be mapped back during microscopy.

An example of how the blocking should be represented in the photograph of the specimen is given below. This will be attached to the back of the report and filed. (Fig 14).

The completeness of the ESD is determined through precise histological evaluation. [56] Any intramucosal carcinoma for which the resection margins are free of tumor is considered radically curative. This is also true for cases where there is submucosal invasion that is limited to 1000 μm or less, or that the invasive front comprises of only highly or well-differentiated tumor. High risk factors for lymph node metastases are generally absent; hence further surgery is deemed unnecessary. [59]

Surgery is recommended for lesions with a high risk of local recurrence or lymph node metastases as seen in these following circumstances: lesions with 1) positive vertical (deep) margin; 2) those with submucosal invasion >1000 μm, 3) presence of vascular infiltration, 4) poorly or undifferentiated cancer front and 5) lesions with budding seen at the deepest part of invasion.

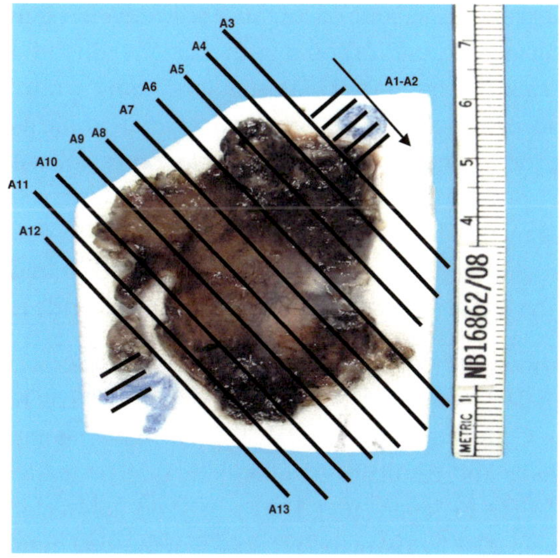

Figure 15. An example of how the trimming should be represented

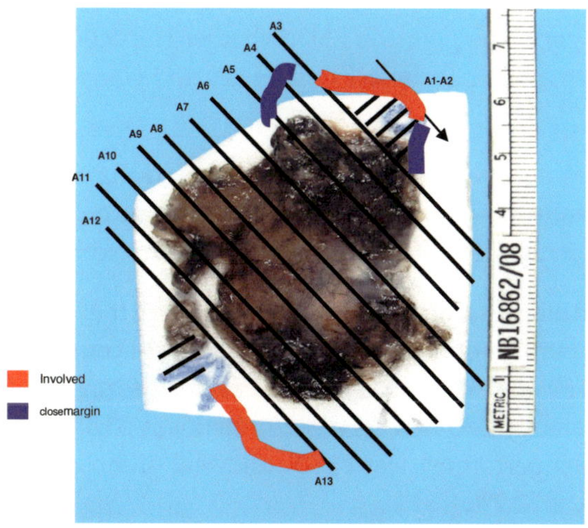

Figure 16. Example of how the margins can be mapped in correlation with microscopy is given below to enable the clinician to be given appropriate information about the margins of concern.

The clinical course after a smooth and uneventful colorectal ESD is usually favorable. Soft food may be started a day after the treatment, presuming no symptoms, and oral intake is then gradually built up. These patients may be discharged from the hospital within 5 days of the treatment, irrespective of resection size. This is to allow identification of delayed complications such as bleeding or perforation. A few days of bowel rest and intravenous administration of antibiotics are recommended for patients who have had a perforation treated with immediate endoscopic closure; for the patient who complains of abdominal discomfort or develops fever.

Immediate surgical intervention is required for those who develop signs of general peritonitis. Patients who have localized peritonitis should be evaluated with radiologic investigation and clinical assessment, as this may be a result of post polypectomy syndrome. Patients who have had esophageal, gastric, or duodenal ESD, a follow-up endoscopic assessment is performed to check the healing process and identify exposed blood vessels with subsequent therapy. However, no such post-procedural examination is necessary after colorectal ESD, as the risk for delayed bleeding is relatively low. In such cases, patients are discharged from the ward within 1 week without checking ulcer healing. They will need to undergo follow-up endoscopies 2 months after the initial ESD to confirm healing and exclude recurrence.

In the recent years, various devices and peripheral equipment, as well as newer techniques, have been described by Japanese endoscopists. Colorectal ESD has henceforth become both safer and simpler. The Colorectal ESD Standardization Implementation Working Group in Japan reported the details and results of a nationwide questionnaire survey on the current situation of colorectal ESD in Japan. [61] They analyzed colorectal ESD performed from January 2000 to September 2008 by 194 of the 391 (28.8% of the total number of those institutions that responded). They reported the prevalence of colorectal ESD in Japan, the total number of colorectal ESD procedures performed during the stipulated period and compared it to the number performed in the last 1 year. They also investigated if those endoscopists that perform colorectal ESDs were performing gastric ESD; whether restrictions were placed upon those operators performing the ESD. Technical differences and equipment preferences were also analyzed.

Outcomes analysis was also performed. It was concluded that there was no observed relationship between the number of cases performed and the time required to complete an en bloc resection. However, operational difficulty was not documented in these comparisons.

The rate of complete en bloc resection of colorectal ESD for all the institutions was 83.8%. When stratified according to number of cases performed, the rate of complete en bloc resection of the institutions where 100 or more colorectal ESD had been performed was 90.2%; that of institutions where 50–99 colorectal ESD had been performed was 83.5%; that of those where 25–49 colorectal ESD had been performed was 85.3%; and that of those where 1–24 colorectal ESD had been performed was 82.2%.

Reported overall incidence of perforation as 4.8% from this survey, a value less than 5.9% reported by Tsuda el al in 2006. Reported rates from other series range from 4 to 10%, higher when compared with EMR (0.3 – 0.5%) [36,61-67]. Small perforations recognized during the procedure can be successfully sealed with endoscopic clips. [56,69,70], larger perforations require urgent salvage surgery to prevent peritonitis and its subsequent complications. [71] It can thus be postulated that the safety of colorectal ESD has increased over the recent years.

The overall incidence of hemorrhage was 1.9%. It is the most common complication of EMR and ESD, with rates reported ranging from 1% to 45%, with an average rate of 10% in larger series. [75-77] Most bleeding episodes are observed during the procedure or within the first 24 hours. [71] Delayed bleeding has been reported in up to 13.9% of patients. [72-73]

http://dx.doi.org/10.5772/53342

Hemostasis may be more difficult to achieve during the procedure as large elevated lesions, lesions that have been resected before and have developed fibrosis, and carcinomatous lesions develop strong neovascularization. Based on their survey, the authors recommended that to acquire a safe colorectal ESD technique, more than a certain number of cases should be performed. However, this "magic number" was not revealed. More importantly, there was no death occurring during this period of assessment in Japan. Table 3 demonstrates the safety and effectiveness of colorectal ESD and in these reports, ESD was performed or colorectal lesions with a median size of 29-37mm with an average procedure time of 90-120min. Niimi et al reports in a study of 310 consecutive patients who underwent ESD for colorectal epithelial neoplasms, overall survival rates were 97.1% at 3 years and 95.3% at 5 years during a median follow up of 38.7 months (range 12.8-104.2 months). Impressively, the disease specific survival rates were 100% at 3 years, leading the co-author (H.Y) to conclude that in expert hands, colorectal ESD is efficacious and safe.

Table 3 | Outcomes of colorectal endoscopic submucosal dissection

Study	Lesions (*n*)	Time (min)	Lesion size (mm)	Specimen size (mm)	*En bloc* resection (%)	Complete *en bloc* (%)	Bleeding (%)	Perforation (%)	Recurrence (%)
Niimi *et al.* (2010)[85]	310	NR	28.9 (6–100)	NR	90.3	74.5	1.6	4.8*	2
Nishiyama *et al.* (2010)[86]	300	NR	26.8	NR	89.2	79.1	0.7	8.1	0.3‡
Saito *et al.* (2010)[28]	145	108±71	37±14	NR	84	NR	1.4	6.2	2
Saito *et al.* (2010)[87]	1,111	116±88	35±18	NR	88	NR	1.5	4.9§	NR
Yoshida *et al.* (2010)[88] Nonelderly	87	92 (20–270)	30.6 (12–80)	NR	93	NR	2.2	9.1	NR
Yoshida *et al.* (2010)[88] Elderly	32	96 (40–290)	32.6 (15–70)	NR	81.2	NR	0	3.1	NR
Yamamoto (unpublished data)	467	60 (5–457)	NR	37 (21–170)	91.3	80.4	1.3	4.3	1.2

*Emergency surgery was required for one case of postoperative perforation. ‡One case of locally recurrent tumour with incomplete resection. §Two immediate perforations with ineffective endoscopic clipping and three delayed perforations required emergency surgery. Abbreviation: NR, not recorded.

Table 3. Summary of outcomes of colorectal ESD

4. Conclusion

ESD has emerged as an important therapeutic modality for superficial colorectal tumors, providing a high en bloc resection rate with lower morbidity as compared to surgical approaches. Both premalignant and early malignant tumors including depressed lesions and those with fibrosis can now be resected with adequate histological assessment. The nature of this procedure for colorectal lesions, with its inherent difficulties, must be recognized and hence a great degree of both skill and patience is required. Colorectal ESD has a higher risk of complication as compared to gastric or esophageal ESD and consequently, requires both a thorough knowledge and specific training to achieve satisfactory performance.

Acknowledgements

Dr Cheng Chee Leong & A/Prof Teh Ming. Department of Pathology, National University Hospital, Singapore

Author details

Koh Z.L. Sharon[1], H. Yamamoto[2] and Tsang B.S. Charles[3]

1 Division of Colorectal Surgery, National University Healthcare System, Singapore

2 Department of Medicine, Head of Division of Gastroenterology & Therapeutic Endoscopy, Jichi Medical University, Togichi, Japan

3 Colorectal Clinic Associates, Mt Elizabeth Novena Specialist Centre Singapore, National University of Singapore Yong Loo Lin School of Medicine, Singapore

References

[1] Wolff, W. I. Colonoscopy: History and development. *Am. J. Gastroenterol.* 84:1017, (1989).

[2] Wolff, W. I, & Shinya, H. Colonofiberscopy. JAMA (1971)., 217, 1509-562.

[3] Shinya, H, & Wolff, W. I. Colonoscopic polypectomy: *Technique and safety. Hosp. Pract.* 24:71, (1975).

[4] Deyhle, P, & Demling, L. Coloscopy: technique, results and indications. *Endoscopy 3,* (1971).

[5] Sakai, Y. The technique of colonofiberoscopy. *Dis Colon Rectum* (1972)., 403-412.

[6] Williams, B, & Teague, R. H. Progress report: colonoscopy. Gut (1973)., 14, 990-1003.

[7] Morson, B. Bussey HJR. Predisposing causes of intestinal cancer *Current Problems in Surgery (February).* (1970). Chicago Year Book Medical Publishers,, 3-50.

[8] Morgenthal, C. B, Richards, W. O, Dunkin, B, et al. The role of the surgeon in the evolution of flexible endoscopy. *Surg Endoc* (2007)., 21, 838-853.

[9] Winawer, S. J, Zauber, A. G, Ho, M. N, et al. Prevention of colorectal cancer by colonoscopic polypectomy. *N Engl J Med* (1993).

[10] Muller, A. D, & Sonnenberg, A. (1995). Prevention of colorectal cancer by flexible endoscopy and polypectomy. A case-control study of 32,702 veterans. *Ann. Intern. Med. 123904910*

[11] Hurlstone, D. P, Sanders, D. S, Cross, S. S, Adam, I, Shorthouse, A. J, Brown, S, Drew, K, & Lobo, A. J. Colonoscopic resection of lateral spreading tumours: a prospective analysis of endoscopic mucosal resection. *Gut 5313341339*(2004c).

[12] Hellwig, A, & Barbosa, E. (1952). How reliable is biopsy of rectal polyps? *Cancer 12,* 620-624.

[13] (1973a) Polypectomy via the fiberoptic colonoscope beyond the reach of the sigmoidoscopy. *New Engl. J. Med. 1973;* 288, 329-332

[14] Christopher, B, Williams, R. H, Hunt, H, Loose, R. H, Riddell, Y, & Sakai, E. T. Swarbrick. Colonoscopy in the management of colon polyps. *Br. J. Surg.*(1974)., 61

[15] Curtiss, L. E. High frequency currents in endoscopy: a review of principles and precautions. Gastrointestinal Endoscopy (1973).

[16] Christopher, B. Williams and Laurent Bedenne. Management of colorectal polyps: Is all the effort worthwhile? *Journal of Gastroenterology and Hepatology Suppl.* 1, 1.(1990)., 14-165.

[17] Jass, J. R. Do all colorectal carcinomas arise in preexisting adenomas? *WorldJ. Surg.* (1989)., 13, 45-51.

[18] Lovli, R. R. Adenomas are precursor lesions for malignant growth in non-polyposis hereditary carcinoma of the colon and rectum. *Surg. Gynae Obst* (1986)., 162, 8-12.

[19] Lee, Y. Early malignant lesions of the colorectum at autopsy. *Dis.* Col. *Rectum* (1988)., 31, 291-7.

[20] Lynch, H. T, & Smyrr, T. Lansiws J Mak. Flat adenomas in a colon cancer-prone kindred. J *Natl Cancer Inst.* (1988). *27882,* 80

[21] Wayi, J. D. Techniques of polypectomy- hot biopsy forceps and snare polypectomy. *Amer. J Gastroenterol.* (1987)., 82, 615-8.

[22] Vanagunas, A, Jacob, P, & Vakil, . . Adequacy of 'hot biopsy' for the treatment of diminutive polyps: a prospective randomised trial. *Amer. J Gastroenterol.* 1989; 84: 383-5.

[23] Church, J. M, Fazio, V, & Jones, W. IT. Small colorectal polyps: are they worth treating? *Dis.* Col. *Rectum* (1988)., 31, 50-3.

[24] Woods, A, Sanowski, R. A, & Wadas, D. Eradication of diminutive polyps: A prospective evaluation of bipolar coagulation versus conventional biopsy removal. *Gastrointest. Endosc.* (1989)., 35, 536-9.

[25] Waye, J. D, Lewis, B, Atchison, M. A, & Talbott, M. The lost polyp: A guide to retrieval during colonoscopy. *Int J Colorect.* Dis. (1988). , 3, 229-31.

[26] Gyorffy, J, & Amontree, S. . Large colorectal polyps: Colonoscopv, pathology and management. *Amer. J. Gustrocrzierol.* 1989; 84: 898-905.

[27] Bertoni, G, & Ricci, E. Conigiiarro. & Bedogni G. Endoscopic removal of large and giant colorectal polyps. *Coloproctology* (1987). , 4, 221-2.

[28] Kudo, S, Tamegai, Y, & Yamano, H. Endoscopic mucosal resection of the colon: the Japanese technique. *Gastrointest Endosc Clin N Am* (2001). , 11, 519-35.

[29] Iishi, H, Tatsuta, M, & Iseki, K. Endoscopic piecemeal resection with submucosal saline injection of large sessile colorectal polyps. *Gastrointest Endosc* (2000). , 51, 697-700.

[30] Tamura, S, Nakajo, K, & Yokoyama, Y. Evaluation of endoscopic mucosal resection for laterally spreading rectal tumors. *Endoscopy* (2004). , 36, 306-12.

[31] Buess, G, Kipfmuller, K, Hack, D, Grussner, R, & Heintz, A. Junginger T: Technique of transanal endoscopic microsurgery. *Surg Endosc* (1988).

[32] Fujishiro, M. Endoscopic submucosal dissection for stomach neoplasms. *World J Gastroenterol* (2006). , 12, 5108-5112.

[33] Kakushima, N, & Fujishiro, M. Endoscopic submucosal dissection for gastrointestinal neoplasms. *World J Gastroenterol* (2008). , 14, 2962-2967.

[34] Yamamoto, H, et al. Endoscopic Submucosal Dissection for Colorectal Tumors. Interventional and Therapeutic Gastrointestinal Endoscopy (2010). , 27

[35] Yahagi, N, Fujishiro, M, Kakushima, N, et al. Endoscopic submucosal dissection for lesions of the esophago-gastric junction and gastric cardia. Gastrointest Endosc. (2004).

[36] Zhou et alEndoscopic Submucosal Dissection for Colorectal Epithelial Neoplasm. Surg Endosc (2009). , 2009, 23-1546.

[37] Kato, M. (2005). Endoscopic submucosal dissection (ESD) is being accepted as a new procedure of endoscopic treatment of early gastric cancer. Intern Med , 44, 85-86.

[38] Ono, H, Kondo, H, Gotoda, T, Shirao, K, Yamaguchi, H, Saito, D, Hosokawa, K, Shimoda, T, & Yoshida, S. (2001). Endoscopic mucosal resection for treatment of early gastric cancer. Gut , 48, 225-229.

[39] Saito, Y, et al. Endoscopic Submucosal Dissection (ESD) for Colorectal Tumors. Digestive Endoscopy ((2009). supp) SS12, 7.

[40] Hurlstone, D. P, et al. Achieving R0 resection in the colorectum using endoscopic submucosal dissection. Br J Surgery (2007). , 94, 1536-1542.

[41] Yoshida, N, et al. Outcomes of endoscopic submucosal dissection for colorectal tumours in elderly people. Int J Colorectal Dis (2009).

[42] Japanese Society for Cancer of the Colon and Rectum ((2005). Colorectal cancer treatment guidelines: the 2005 editionst edt. Kanahara-Shuppan, Tokyo

[43] Tanaka, S, Oka, S, Tamura, T, et al. (2006). Molecular pathologic application as a predictor of lymph node metastasis in submucosal colorectal carcinoma: Implication of immunohistochemical alteration as the deepest invasive margin.

[44] Muto, T, & Mochizuki, H. Masaki T (eds) Tumor budding in colorectal cancer: recent progress in colorectalcancer research. NOVA, Hauppauge, NY, , 171-180.

[45] Tanaka, S, Haruma, K, Oka, S, et al. (2001). Clinicopathologic features and endoscopic treatment of superficially spreading colorectal neoplasms larger than 20 mm. Gastrointest Endosc , 54, 62-66.

[46] Uraoka, T, Saito, Y, Matsuda, T, et al. (2006). Endoscopic indications for endoscopic mucosal resection of laterally spreading tumours in the colorectum. Gut , 55, 1592-1597.

[47] Tanaka, S, et al. Strategy of Endoscopic Treatment for Colorectal Tumor. Recent Progress and Perspective.

[48] Tanaka, S, et al. Colorectal Endoscopic Submucosal Dissection: present status and future perspective, including its differentiation from endoscopic mucosal resection. J Gastroenterol (2008).

[49] Yamamoto, H, Kawata, H, Sunada, K, Sasaki, A, Nakazawa, K, Miyata, T, Sekine, Y, Yano, T, Satoh, K, Ido, K, & Sugano, K. (2003). Successful en bloc resection of large superficial tumors in the stomach and colon using sodium hyaluronate and small-caliber tip transparent hood. Endoscopy , 35, 690-694.

[50] Gotoda, T. (2004). Endoscopic diagnosis and treatment for early gastric cancer. Cancer Rev Asia Pacific , 2, 17-37.

[51] Saito et alClinical outcome of endoscopic submucosal dissection versus endoscopic mucosal resection of large colorectal tumors as determined by curative resection. Surg Endosc (2009).

[52] Hurlstone, D. P, Brown, S, & Cross, S. S. The role of flat and depressed colorectal lesions in colorectal carcinogenesis: new insights from clinicopathological findings in high-magnification chromoscopic colonoscopy. *Histopathology* (2003). , 43, 413-26.

[53] Kudo, S, Shimoda, R, & Kashida, H. Laterally spreading tumor of colon: definition and history (in Japanese with English abstract). *Stomach and Intestine* (2005). , 40, 1721-5.

[54] Tomohiko OhyaKen Ohata, Kazuki Sumiyama, Yousuke Tsuji, Ikuro Koba, Nobuyuki Matsuhashi,Hisao Tajiri. Balloon overtube-guided colorectal endoscopic submucosal dissection. *World J Gastroenterol* (2009). December 28; , 15(48), 6086-6090.

[55] Yamamoto, H, et al. Mucosectomy in the colon with endoscopic submucosal dissection. Endoscopy (2005). , 37, 764-768.

[56] Fujishiro, M, Yahagi, N, Nakamura, M, Kakushima, N, Kodashima, S, Ono, S, et al. Successful outcomes of a novel endoscopic treatment for GI tumors: endoscopic submucosal dissection with a mixture of high-molecular-weight hyaluronic acid, glycerin, and sugar. Gastrointest Endosc (2006). , 63, 243-249.

[57] Tamura, S, Nakajo, K, Yokoyama, Y, et al. Evaluation of endoscopicmucosal resection for laterally spreading rectal tumors. Endoscopy (2004). , 36, 306-12.

[58] Japanese Society for Cancer of the Colon and RectumJapanese Classification of Colorectal Carcinoma. Tokyo: Kanehara, (1997).

[59] Kitajima, K, Fujimori, T, Fujii, S, et al. Correlations between lymph node metastasis and depth of submucosal invasion in submucosal invasive colorectal carcinoma: a Japanese collaborative study. J Gastroenterol (2004). , 39, 534-43.

[60] Shinji TanakaYoshiro Tamegai, Sumio Tsuda, Yutaka Saito, Naohisa Yahagi and-Hiro-o Yamano. Multicenter Questionnaire Survey of Colorectal Endoscopic Submucosal Dissection in Japan. Digestive Endoscopy ((2010). Suppl. 1), SS8, 2.

[61] Tanaka, S, Oka, S, Kaneko, I, et al. Endoscopic submucosal dissection for colorectal neoplasia: possibility of standardization. Gastrointest Endosc (2007). , 66, 100-7.

[62] Oka, S, Tanaka, S, Kaneko, I, et al. Advantage of endoscopic submucosal dissection compared with EMR for early gastric cancer. Gastrointest Endosc (2006). , 64, 877-83.

[63] Fujishiro, M, Yahagi, N, Kakushima, N, et al. Endoscopic submucosal dissection of esophageal squamous cell neoplasms. Clin Gastroenterol Hepatol (2006). , 4, 688-94.

[64] Gotoda, T. A large endoscopic resection by endoscopic submucosal dissection procedure for early gastric cancer. Clin Gastroenterol Hepatol (2005). S, 71-3.

[65] Ono, H. Early gastric cancer: diagnosis, pathology, treatment techniques and treatment outcomes. Eur J Gastroenterol Hepatol (2006). , 18, 863-6.

[66] Fujishiro, M, Yahagi, N, Nakamura, M, et al. Endoscopic submucosal dissection for rectal epithelial neoplasia. Endoscopy (2006). , 38, 493-7.

[67] Inoue, H. Endoscopic mucosal resection for esophageal and gastric mucosal cancers. Can J Gastroenterol (1998). , 12, 355-9.

[68] Yokoi, C, Gotoda, T, Hamanaka, H, & Oda, I. Endoscopic submucosal dissection allows curative resection of locally recurrent early gastric cancer after prior endoscopic mucosal resection. Gastrointest Endosc (2006). , 64, 212-8.

[69] Yoshikane, H, Hidano, H, Sakakibara, A, et al. Endoscopic repair by clipping of iatrogenic colonic perforation. Gastrointest Endosc (1997). , 46, 464-6.

[70] Kim, H. S, Lee, D. K, Jeong, Y. S, et al. Successful endoscopic management of a perforated gastric dysplastic lesion after endoscopic mucosa l resection. Gastrointest Endosc (2000). , 51, 613-5.

[71] Larghi, A, & Waxman, I. State of the art on endoscopic mucosal resection and endoscopic submucosal dissection. Gastrointest Endosc Clin North Am (2007). v., 17, 441-69.

[72] Morales, T. G, Sampliner, R. E, Garewal, H. S, et al. The difference in colon polyp size before and after removal. Gastrointest Endosc (1996). , 43, 25-8.

[73] Lee, S. H, & Park, J. H. Park do H, et al. Clinical efficacy of EMR with submucosal injection of a fibrinogen mixture: a prospective randomized trial. Gastrointest Endosc (2006). , 64, 691-6.

[74] Binmoeller, K. F, Bohnacker, S, Seifert, H, et al. Endoscopic snare excision of "giant" colorectal polyps. Gastrointest Endosc (1996). , 43, 183-8.

[75] Kodama, M, & Kakegawa, T. Treatment of superficial cancer of the esophagus: a summary of responses to a questionnaire on superficial cancer of the esophagus in Japan. Surgery (1998). , 123, 432-9.

[76] Rembacken, B. J, Gotoda, T, Fujii, T, et al. Endoscopic mucosal resection. Endoscopy (2001). , 33, 709-18.

[77] Iishi, H, Tatsuta, M, Iseki, K, et al. Endoscopic piecemeal resection with submucosal saline injection of large sessile colorectal polyps. Gastrointest Endosc (2000). , 51, 697-700.

[78] Stergiou, N, Riphaus, A, Lange, P, et al. Endoscopic snare resection oflarge colonic polyps: how far can we go? Int J Colorectal Dis (2003). , 18, 131-5.

[79] Yamamoto, H, Koiwai, H, et al. A successful single-step endoscopic resection of a 40 millimeter flat-elevated tumor in the rectum: endoscopic mucosal resection using sodium hyaluronate. *Gatrointestinal Endoscopy* 50:5: 701-4. (1999).

[80] Yamamoto, H, Yube, T, Isoda, N, Sato, Y, Sekine, Y, et al. A novel method of endoscopic mucosal resection using sodium hyaluronate. *Gastrointest Endo* (1999). , 50, 251-6.

Chapter 5

Malignant Colorectal Polyps: Diagnosis, Treatment and Prognosis

Luis Bujanda Fernández de Piérola,
Joaquin Cubiella Fernández,
Fernando Múgica Aguinaga,
Lander Hijona Muruamendiaraz and
Carol Julyssa Cobián Malaver

Additional information is available at the end of the chapter

http://dx.doi.org/10.5772/52697

1. Introduction

Adenomatous polyps are non-invasive tumours of epithelial cells arising from the mucosa with the potential to become malignant. The adenoma-carcinoma sequence is well known and it is accepted that more than 95% of colon adenocarcinomas arise from adenoma [1]. The World Health Organisation (WHO) classifies adenomas into tubular (<20% villous architecture), tubulovillous and villous (80% villous architecture), with approximately 87% of adenomas being tubular, 8% tubulovillous and 5% villous [2].

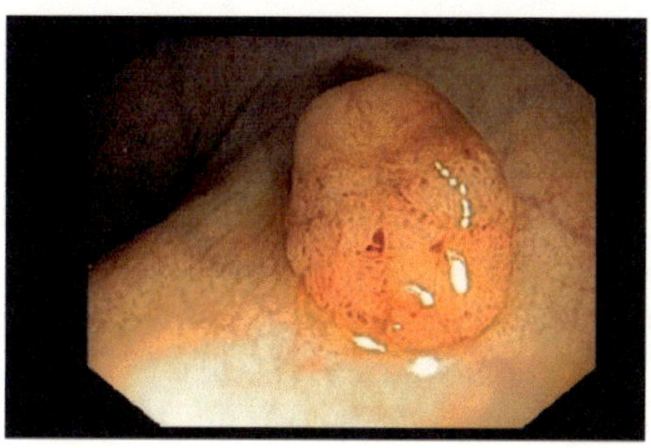

Figure 1. Polyp in colon

Only 5% of adenomas are in danger of becoming malignant. The probability of high grade dysplasia and carcinomatous transformation increases with polyp size, a villous component, when there are many polyps or the age at diagnosis is more than 60 years [2]. The neoplasia is considered to be advanced when polyp size is 1 cm or more, there is a villous component or a high degree of dysplasia. Mixed polyps also have the ability to become malignant, as does hyperplastic polyposis syndrome. More than 25% of advanced polyps are located in the area proximal to the splenic flexure [3].

2. Epidemiology

The prevalence of cancerous polyps in series of endoscopically removed polyps is between 0.2% and 11% [4-6].Currently, screening programs allow the detection and treatment of a great number of adenomas and malignant polyps, and this contributes to a reduction of the mortality by colorectal cancer (CRC) [1,7]. In an asymptomatic population of people over 50 years old who underwent direct colonoscopy, there was a 0.8% prevalence of adenocarcinoma of which 50% were carcinoma “in situ” or in stage I [8,9]. During screening programmes, adenocarcinomas have been detected in between 3% - 4.6% of those who undergo colonoscopy following a positive immunological faecal occult blood test result [10,11].

3. Histology

Carcinoma "in situ", intramucosal carcinoma, high displasia or intraepithelial carcinoma is the stage at which there is no involvement of *the muscularis mucosa.* In general, this tumour stage does not cause metastasis. It is classified as pTis or Stage 0 in the TNM staging system.These terms are defined as non-invasive high grade neoplasia in the Vienna classification [12].Carcinoma in situ or severe displasia or intraepithelial carcinoma corresponds to a carcinoma that is restricted to the epithelial layer without invasion into the lamina propria. Intramucosal carcinoma is a carcinoma characterized by the invasion into the lamina propria.

When the carcinoma spreads to the submucosa, the polyp is considered to have become malignant, being able to spread to lymph nodes or distant sites. The tumours that affect the submucosa are classified as T1 and correspond to Stage I of the TNM staging system. This term is defined as submucosal carcinoma in the classification of Vienna [12].

The term pseudoinvasion refers to the presence of glandular epithelium of the mucosa beneath the muscularis mucosa in colonic polyps. These lesions have no malignant potential and should be management in a similar way to adenomas [13]. However, an inexperienced pathologist can mistake this phenomenon for invasive carcinoma. Pseudoinvasion usually occurs in large polyps (>1 cm), especially those with long stalks, and is most commonly found in polyps of the sigmoid colon. Islands of adenomatous epithelium are displaced through the muscularis mucosa and are found within the submucosa of the stalk. The displaced glandular tissue usually has rounded not infiltrative, contours, carries with it a small amount of lamina propria, and is cytologically identical to the overlying adenomatous component. Hemorrhage and hemosiderin depositions, are commonly seen and are a clue to diagnosis. In addition, inflammation and granulation tissue, can be found.Cystic dilatation of the displaced glands with mucin distention is also not uncommon in pseudoinvasion because mucin produced by the entrapped glands has no means of reaching the lumen. Occasionally, rupture of dilated glands occurs with acellularmucin extravasation and there is a subsequent inflammatory response. Distinction from mucinous (colloid) carcinoma is important and can be difficult. Specifically, in mucinous carcinoma, the mucin pools contain malignant cells, a feature lacking in pseudoinvasion.

For these reasons, it is highly recommended that level sections and second opinions, are obtained in cases of polyps with potential pseudoinvasion [14].

All adenomas have some degree of dysplasia. However, low and high grade dysplasias are artificial subdivisions of a spectrum. There is no definition of "high-grade". Indeed, the WHO book on tumors of the digestive system, does not contain a list of criteria for high-grade dysplasia in adenomas [15,16]. However in general, high-grade dysplasia entails more substantial changes and includes carcinoma "in situ". Among these changes we consider architectural alteration, often resembling the glandular arrangement of adenomas and cytologic abnormalities, principally cellular and nuclear pleomorphism, nuclear hyperchromatism, loss of nuclear polarity, and marked stratification of nuclei. Other authors have considered as features of high grade displasia: loss of normal glandular architecture, hyperchromatic cells with multilayered irregular nuclei and loss of mucin, high nuclear/cytoplasmic ratio, marked nuclear atypia with prominent nuclei and focal cribriform patterns. Not all these features are necessarily present to the same degree in all dysplastic epithelia, while low-grade dysplasia manifests these same changes but to a lesser degree [15,16].

4. Prognostic factors

Many factors have been associated with a higher probability of residual disease or recurrent carcinoma.

4.1. Morphology

Morphology is described as polypoid (pedunculated or sessil) and nonpolypoid (flat or ulcerated) subtypes according to the Paris classification [17]. The type of polyp and its morphology can guide the endoscopist towards its potential malignancy [2,18,19]. These features include the size, the presence of depressed ulceration, irregular contours, deformity, a short and immobile stalk and the inability to elevate a sessile polyp when a submucosal bleb is formed. In such suspicious lesions, as well as in flat or depressed lesions, diagnosis can be carried out using chromoendoscopy and magnification techniques that can highlight abnormalities of glandular cytoarchitecture and reveal information concerning the extent of submucosal invasion [20,21].

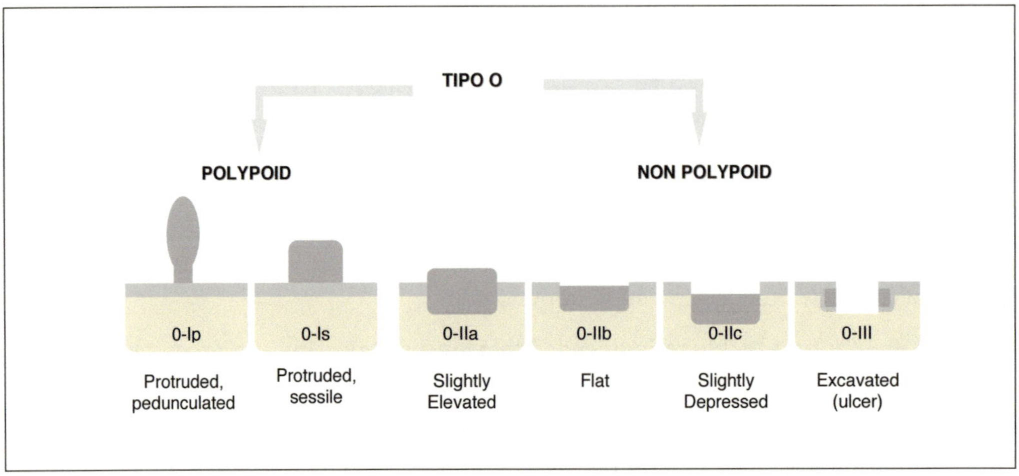

Table 1. The Paris Endoscopy Classification of superficial neoplastic lesions [17]

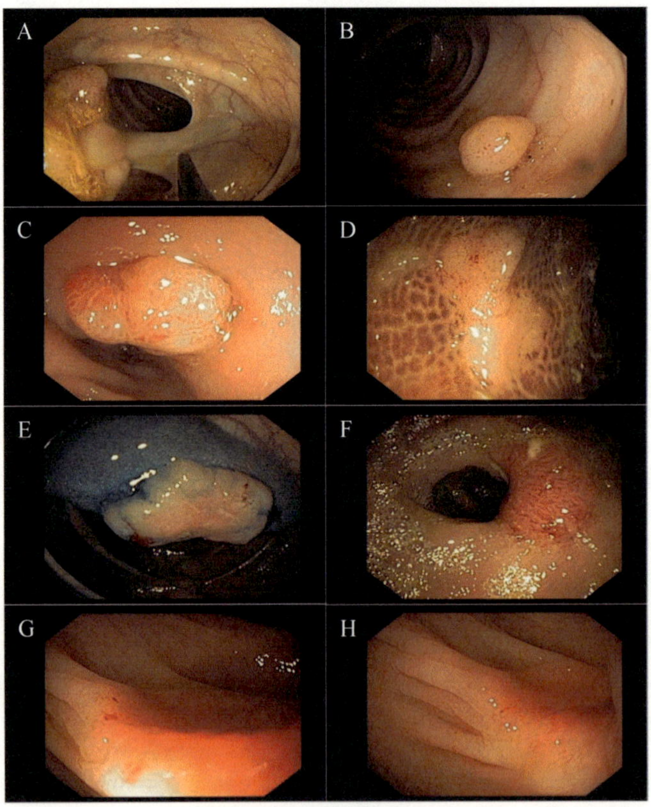

Figure 2. Polyps in colon: Pedunculated polyp 0-Ip (A), sessile polyp 0-Is (B y C), flat polyp 0-IIb (D y F), superficial elevated with central depression 0-IIa + IIc (E) and excavated polyp 0-IIc (G y H).

Kudo et al. [22] developed the pit pattern classification for colon polyps with six classes of surface pattern depicted by magnifying endoscopy after indigo carmine staining. Class 5 of this pit-pattern classification or an unstructured surface has been shown to correlate well with a diagnosis of malignancy, and can provide important additional information prior to endoscopic treatment. However, endoscopic ultrasound using high frequency transendoscopicminiprobes currently appears to be the most accurate method for defining submucosal or further bowel wall invasion, enabling direct referral for surgical intervention in those cases with deeper infiltration who are at the greatest risk of lymphatic spread [23].

4.2. Type of resection

The success of treatment of a malignant polyp depends on the complete resection by polypectomy or surgical intervention. When en-bloc removal of a polyp is performed, it is possible to assess the depth of infiltration of the tumour cells and whether the margin is affected. Pedunculated malignant polyps are easily removed using a loop snare. However, this technique frequently results in piecemeal removal when applied to sessile and flat malignant polyps. Nevertheless, around one-third of malignant polyps are removed in this way [24]. En-bloc removal is advantageous because it allows full histological evaluation of the complete resection and is associated with lower recurrence rates than piecemeal removal [25]. Endoscopic submucosal dissection (ESD) has been found to be particularly useful for the removal of sessile or flat adenomatous lesions. It has an advantage over other endoscopic techniques in that it allows en-bloc removal of large (>2 cm) colonic lesions. In ESD an electrosurgical cutting device is used to carefully dissect the deeper layers of the submucosa to remove neoplastic lesions in the mucosa. In a meta-analysis it was found that ESD en-bloc resection is achieved in 84.9% of lesions, and clear vertical and lateral margins are achieved in 75.3% of cases [26].

4.3. Level of invasion of adenocarcinoma into the polyp and polypectomy resection margin

Haggitt et al. [27] have assigned levels of invasion to each malignant polyp. In this study, level 1 described invasive adenocarcinoma limited to the polyp head, level 2 included involvement of the neck, level 3 corresponded to adenocarcinoma cells in the stalk, and level 4 to invasion, adenocarcinoma cells infiltrating the submucosa at the level of the adjacent bowel wall. In this system, invasive adenocarcinoma in a sessile polyp by definition had level 4 invasion. However, precise histological evaluation of Haggitt's level may be difficult. Properly marked and orientated specimens are essential.

More recently, some authors have proposed an additional histological classification system based on the grade of cell differentiation at the lesion margins and on the size and depth of invasion of the submucosa. Submucosal invasion has been classified into three types based on the depth of invasion. When less than one-third of the submucosa is invaded the stage is sm1, and if more than two-thirds is invaded the stage is sm3, while stage sm2 is intermediate with invasion of cancer into the middle third. It has been shown that penetration of cancerous cells is associated with a risk of lymphatic spread [29-32]. Research based on large patient series has shown a 1-3% risk for lymph node metastases in sm1 cancers, 8% in sm2 cancers and 23% in sm3 cancers [29].

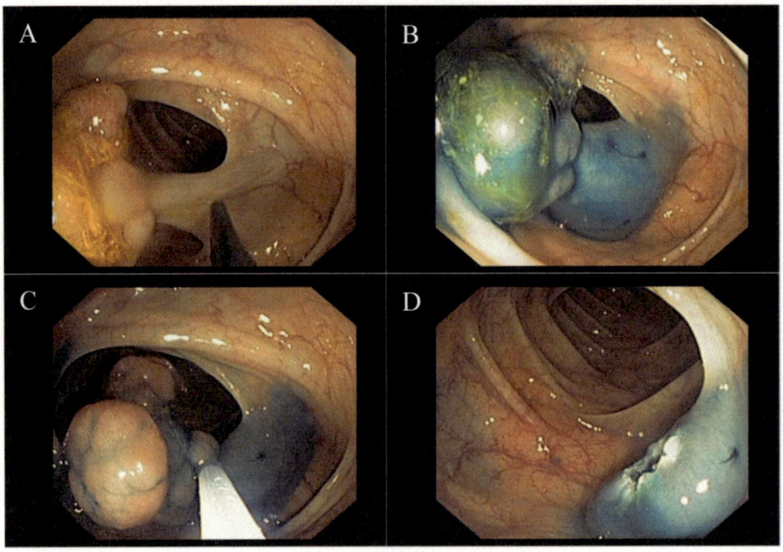

Figure 3. Resection of a pedunculated polyp with an endoscopic snare (A-D).

In sessile polyps, it is essential that the pathologist identifies the stalk or the depth of the diathermy burn. The risk of relapse ranges from 0% to 2% in malignant polyps with a margin of resection greater than 1 mm. If the resection margin is involved, or is less than 1 mm, the percentage of relapse ranges between 21% and 33% [30]. Most authors believe that a resection margin of more than 1 mm is safe and that in such cases the probability of residual disease or recurrent carcinoma is low [4,5,30,31].

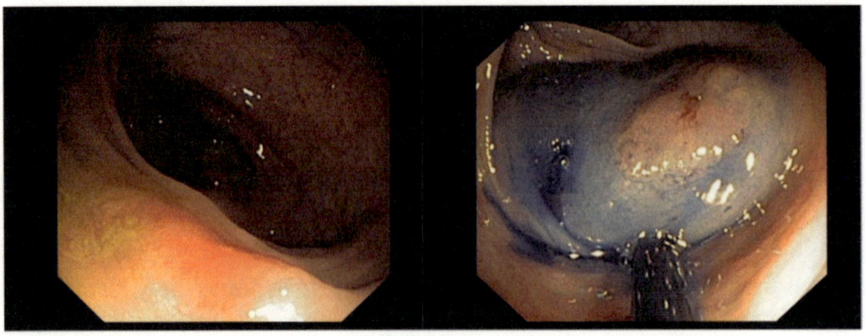

Figure 4. Elevation of a superficial elevated polyp (0-IIb) with Indigo Carmine

4.4. Stage of differentiation

Four grades were considered [32]:

Grade 1: Corresponded to a well-differentiated intestinal-type adenocarcinoma with well-formed glands and open lumina or with more than 95% glandular differentiation.

Grade 2: Moderately differentiated intestinal-type adenocarcinoma containing solid nests showing only focal glands or with 50-95% glandular differentiation.

Grade 3: Carcinoma is poorly differentiated intestinal–type. Signet ring cell or mucinous adenocarcinoma, composed of hyperchromatic cells arranged into solid sheets and forming absorptive glands, with 5% to 50% glandular differentiation.

Grade 4: Undifferentiated tumours which have less than 5% glandular differentiation.

Undifferentiated carcinoma: Medullary carcinomas with high microsatellite instability.

The prognosis correlates with the histological grade [32]. For example, Grade 3 of differentiation is seen in 5.7 to 9.2% of patients and the risk of residual lesions or relapse in these cases is of the order of 36-38% [30].

4.5. Lymphatic invasion

Lymphatic invasion is defined as tumour cells within a true endothelial-lined channel in the absence of red blood cells [33]. The risk of lymphatic spread has been estimated by histological study of resected specimens. Since lymphatics do not penetrate much beyond the muscularis mucosae, focal cancer that has not invaded through this layer appears to present little or no risk of lymph node spread [34]. The near absence of lymphatics within the mucosa has been proposed as the reason for the observed lack of malignant potential (lymph node metastasis) observed in polyps showing only intramucosal carcinoma. However, this theory has been challenged by studies using more sensitive techniques to detect lymphatic vessels. Studies using the relatively new antibody D2-40, which stains lymphatic but not blood vessel endothelium, have shown that lymphatic present in the stalk and mucosa of adenomas and undergo proliferation, are early invasive cancers. Lymphatic channels are often present near nests of infiltrating tumours in malignant polyps [35,36].

Detecting lymphatic invasion by expert pathologists using light microscopy is difficult. There are no recognized guidelines for establishing the presence of lymphatic invasion (for example, the number of sections or immunostains needed to identify lymphatic vessels). For example, in a study in which five pathologists assessed the lymphatic invasion of 140 malignant polyps, they agreed (4 out of 5 observers) on only 17 cases [37].The intra and inter-observer variability in the interpretation of samples received among even the most expert histopathologists can be high and often leads to diagnostic uncertainties [37]. The use of immunohistochemistry for D2-40 may help identify lymphatic channels. However, its use is not yet routine, and technical issues such as loss of a suspicious focus in level sections limits the usefulness of special stains in this setting. The presence of lymphatic invasion has been proposed by some researchers as an indication for colectomy. However, few malignant polyps with lymphatic invasion have been reported, and most of them have had positive margins, grade 3 invasive adenocarcinoma (as defined above), or both [5].

4.6. Vascular invasion

The presence of vascular invasion is defined as cancer in an endothelial-lined channel surrounded by a smooth muscle wall [35]. However, it is difficult to recognise it. Vascular markers (CD31, CD34 and factor VIII) may help. These markers strongly stain blood vessel endothelium, and to a lesser extent lymphatic endothelium [14].The prevalence of venous invasion in malignant polyps varies greatly, ranging from 3.5% to 39% [37].Often venous invasion is associated with lymphatic invasion and/or tumours which have a resection margin of less than 2 mm and/or are poorly differentiated. In contrast, Talbot et al. [38] observed that venous invasion was not associated with poorer prognosis.

4.7. Risk of residual disease or recurrent carcinoma in favourable and unfavourable histology

Favourable histology is defined as grade 1 or 2 differentiated adenocarcinoma in which carcinoma cells are at least 1 mm from a clearly visualized margin, resection is carried out en bloc and there is an absence of vascular or lymphatic invasion.

Unfavourable histology is defined as polyps with biopsy margin ≤1 mm, tumour within the cauterized region constitutes a positive margin, piecemeal removal, poorly differentiated tumour (grade 3) or lymphatic or vascular invasion.In these cases, surgical resection is indicated because of the increased risk of lymph node metastasis or residual disease [14]. On the other hand, in the absence of unfavourable features, polypectomy is considered curative. Sometimes, specimens do not lend themselves to proper analysis for any reason (piecemeal removal or poor orientation) result in a default decision to resect.

In 1995, Volk et al [5] reviewed 20 studies in which 858 malignant polyps were analysed. They observed residual disease or recurrent carcinoma in 89 patients (10%). However, there were relapses or tumours in the area of the resection in only 8 (1%) patients with favourable histological criteria. Subsequent studies have also reported an incidence of less than 1% [37,39]. Only one study described incidence higher than 5% in malignant polyps with favourable histology [40] and the study itself has been widely criticized from subsequent reviews [5]. By contrast, in malignant polyps with unfavourable histology, the risk of relapse or residual lesions ranges between 10% and 39% [5,14,29,39].

4.8. Marking with India Ink

In 1975, Ponsky and King [41] published the first case in which marking with India ink was used with the purpose of locating the polyp during the surgical procedure. Sometimes to locate the base of the polyp after polypectomy or during surgery is extremely difficult.

All the endoscopicallyunresectable polyps in patients in whom surgery would be considered, should be tattooed. Endoscopicallyresectable polyps that could have become malignant should also be tattooed. Among the criteria that should hint the endoscopist about the presence of malignancy in the polyps is size, an irregular surface or a flat or excavated morphology [2,18,42,43].

The size of the polyp is an important factor that indicates malignancy [42,44-46]. The probability of dysplasia could be up to 38,5% in those larger than 1 cm [47].The flat or ulcerated lesions have a higher risk of high-grade dysplasia or carcinoma [22,48-50]. The probability of cancer or severe dysplasia increases from 4% in small flat lesions, up to 6% in small polyps, 16% in large polyps and 29% in long, flat lesions, and up to 75% in depressed lesions [51].

However, tattooing in suspicious polyps at first colonoscopy, in our experience is still low, 17.6%. We study a retrospective series that include 74 patients. Our endoscopists usually marked large polyps, polyps resected in a fragmented manner and polyps with proximal location. However, in a multivariate analysis only proximal location was significant associated with marking. It is known that flat polyps, with a greater potential for malignancy, are most frequently located in the right colon [37,39]. In our series, 16.2% of the polyps were proximal; of these, 58.3% were marked; on the other hand, only 9.7% of the distal polyps were marked. The factors that could have a greater influence when it comes to marking proximal polyps more frequently was their potential to become malignant in this location and the difficulty of finding the polypectomy scar in subsequent controls or in surgery.

We agree with other authors [52-57] that tattooing is one of the best methods for tumor location, either if the patient is following-up by colonoscopy or is undergoing for surgical resection [42,58].

5. Treatment

Prior to removal of the polyp, it is difficult to know whether the polyp is malignant or not. Some features, as we have mentioned earlier, can give some indication of the degree of malignancy. Regardless of the morphological characteristics, a polyp is normally removed when detected.

Polypectomy should be performed en bloc, since this is essential to establish and define favourable or unfavourable histological criteria. In just a few cases, only polyp biopsies are performed, such a lack of coagulation data, polyp could be difficult to remove at that point in time, or the patient being on antiplatelet drugs or anticoagulants.

The indication for a malignant polyp with sessile morphology, regardless of favourable histological criteria, is surgery [10], especially in patients younger than 50 years old, who tend to present fewer surgical complications [59]. Surgical treatment is recommended for malignant polyps with pedunculated morphology which have unfavourable histological criteria (partial polyp resection, poorly differentiated carcinoma, vascular or lymphatic invasion, or lesions ≤1 mm from the polypectomy) [10]. On the other hand, for malignant polyps with pedunculated morphology but with favourable histological criteria, polypectomy is considered to be curative (Figure 7). Non-invasive high grade neoplasia regardless of their morphology, are considered to be cured with polypectomy. Indeed, according to some authors, polyps harbouring "in situ" or "intramucosal" cancer should not be regarded or treated as malignant polyps [59].

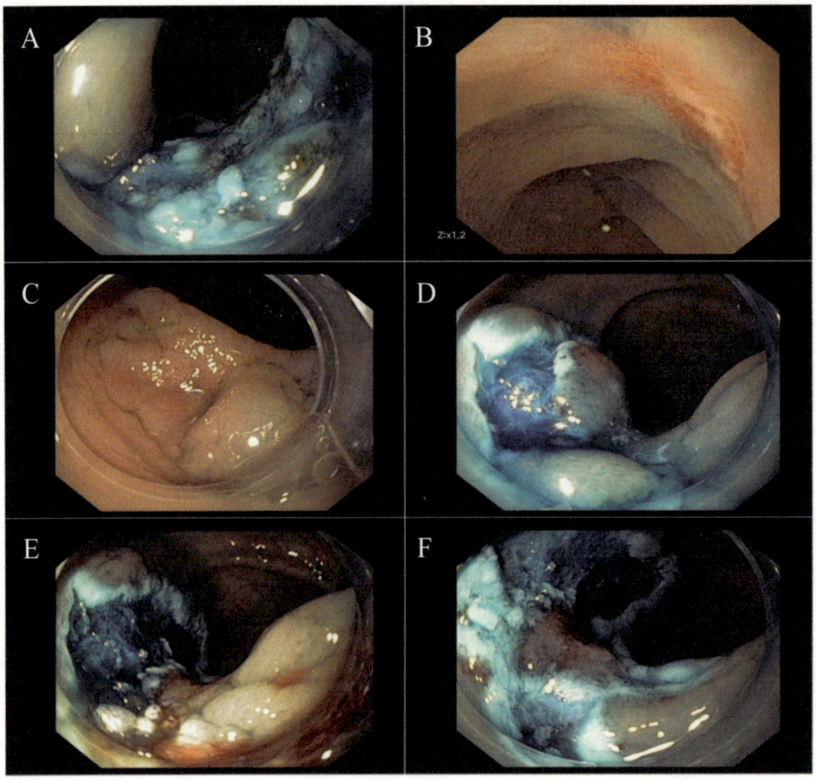

Figure 5. Endoscopic Mucosal Resection in a 0-IIa + Is polyp in colon (A-E), with control of the base after one month (F).

However, until now in many pathology reports were not reported histological criteria. For example at the University of Minnesota between 1987 and 2000, 83% of the reports are not angiolymphatic vessel invasion, 69% not reported the depth of invasion by cancer cells and 22% no stated the degree of tumour differentiation [60]. Beside the agreement among experienced pathologists was poor with respect to histological grade of differentiated carcinoma and angiolymphatic vessel invasion [60].

Endoscopic submucosal dissection (ESD) has emerged as a possible technique to successfully resect malignant colonic polyps en bloc [26,61]. The technique makes it possible to treat and cure large (>2 cm) sessile and flat polyps enabling pathological evaluation in most patients, also can be an alternative to surgery for older patients and for those suffering from associated conditions that contraindicate surgery.

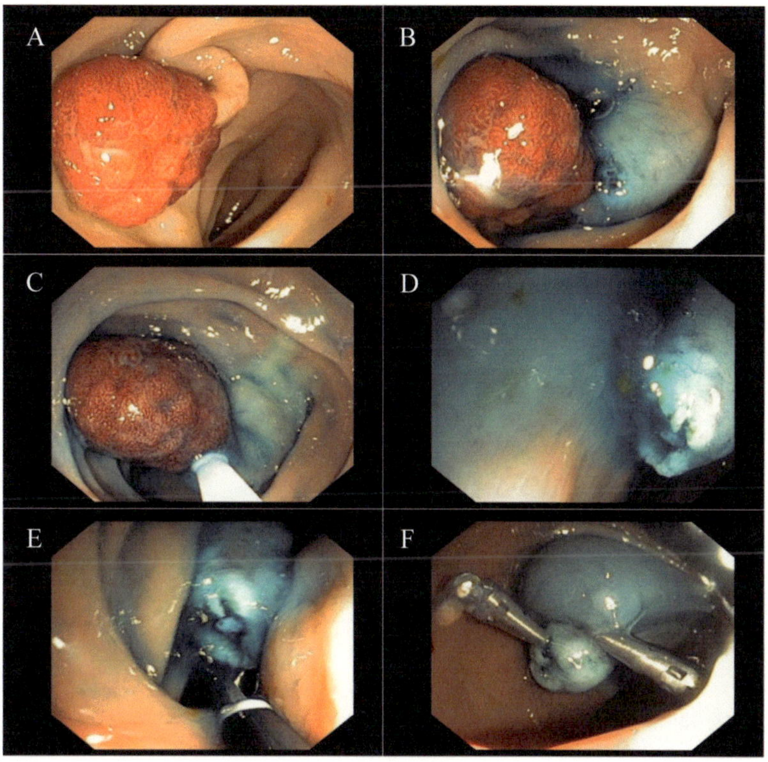

Figure 6. Polypectomy of pediculated polyp 0-Ip. Submucosal injection was performed using indigo carmine (A,B), polypectomy was made with electrosurgical knives (C), After polypectomy, a large non bleeding vessel was visualized (D) and cauterized using coagulation forceps (E) and obliterated with an endoclip (F) to reduce the risk of delayed bleeding

An exception to these guidelines is patients with malignant polyps, with sessile or flat morphology, that are located in the rectum. The occurence of distant metastases is correlated to T-stage and, after radical resection of T1 tumours, the 5-year rate of metastases is about 10% [62], similar to other locations of malignant polyps. About 50% of the local recurrences following local resection are curable if the patients are included in an intensive follow-up programme. Local resection should be offered to patients whenever the individually calculated risk of short-term mortality after major surgery exceeds twice the additional risk of local recurrence added by local procedures. An adequate preoperative evaluation of the patient's general health is essential before deciding the modality of treatment for the individual T1 rectum cancer patient.

In recent years, various serum markers been identified in an effort to establish which patients could benefit from surgical treatment and from a more strict follow up. These markers include metalloproteinase 7, vascular adhesion proteins, vascular endothelial growth factors and cytokeratins [63-66]. The majority of markers have been studied in patients operated on for colon cancer with infiltration of the lamina propria (equivalent to or higher than T2), so these results cannot readily be extrapolated to malignant colorectal polyps.

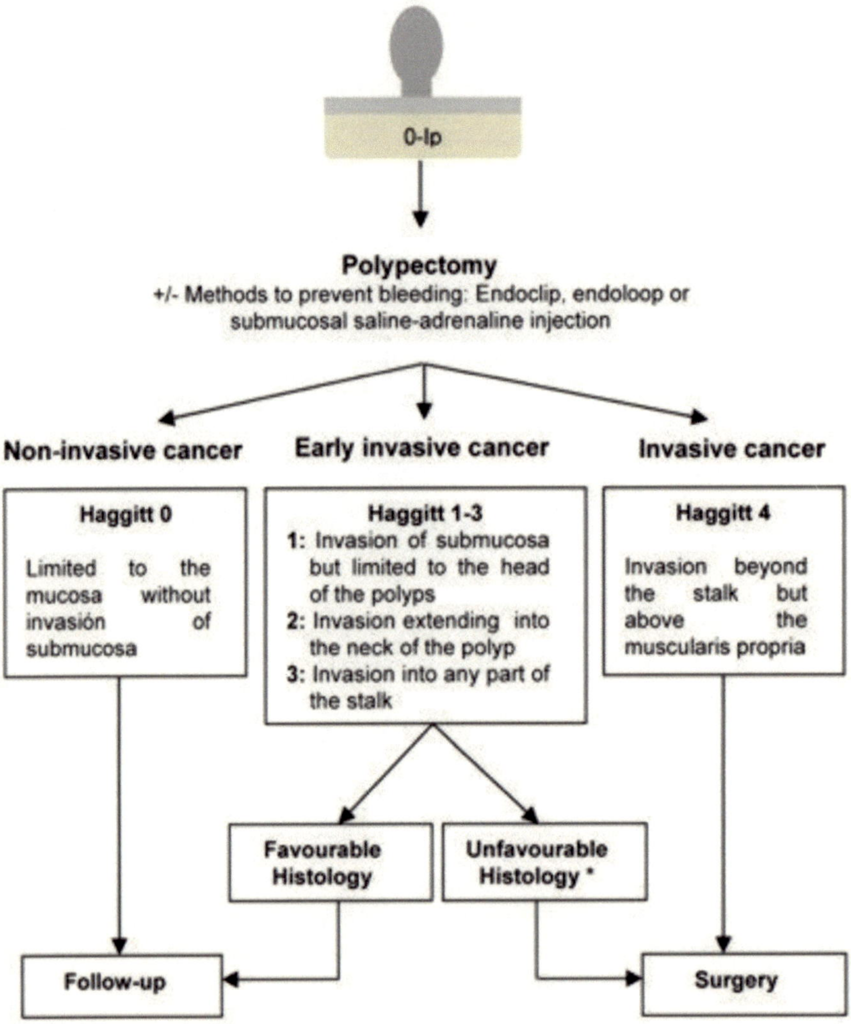

* Biopsy margin ≤ 1 mm, piecemeal removal, poorly differentiated tumour, lymphatic or vascular invasion

Figure 7. Therapeutic algorithm of pedunculated (0-Ip) polyps.

http://dx.doi.org/10.5772/52697

6. Follow-up

In cases of non-invasive high grade neoplasia and malignant polyps with pedunculated morphology and favourable histological criteria, it is recommended that a colonoscopy be carried out three months after taking the biopsy [1,43].If this is normal, a further check-up is advised after one year, three years and five year [43]. Some authors suggest that if the results within three months are negative, subsequent monitoring should be the same as that offered to patients with non-malignant adenomas [35,44]. However, recent studies estimate that 11.8% of patients who have undergone polypectomy will develop a metachronic advanced adenoma and 0.6% an invasive carcinoma. Associated risk factors include age, number of polyps (5 or more), size (greater than 1 cm), villous architecture, proximal location, and being male. Smoking, body mass index, family history of CRC, and degree of dysplasia were not found to be associated with higher risks of advanced adenoma or cancer [45].

There have been reports of cases of malignant pedunculated polyps with unfavourable histological criteria which, despite no findings of residual carcinoma in the intestine wall or lymph node involvement, are found on follow up to have distant metastasis, even five years after surgery [4,5].

7. Conclusion

En brief, the adenoma-carcinoma sequence is well known and polypectomy has proven to reduce the incidence of CRC. However, the success of treatment depends on the complete resection and the future follow up of the base of polypectomy.

Acknowledgments

CIBERehd is funded by the Instituto de Salud Carlos III (Carlos III Health Institute).

Author details

Luis Bujanda Fernández de Piérola[1], Joaquin Cubiella Fernández[2],
Fernando Múgica Aguinaga[1], Lander Hijona Muruamendiaraz[1] and
Carol Julyssa Cobián Malaver[1]

1 Department of Gastroenterology, Donostia Hospital, Centro de Investigación Biomédica en Red en Enfermedades Hepáticas y Digestivas (CIBERehd), University of Basque Country (UPV/EHU), San Sebastian, Gipuzcoa, Spain

2 Department of Gastroenterology, Complexo Hospitalario de Ourense, Ourense, Spain

References

[1] Winawer SJ. Prevention of colorectal cancer by colonoscopic polypectomy. The National Polyp Study Workgroup. N Engl J Med 1993;329: 1977-1981.

[2] O'Brien MJ. National Polyp Study Workgroup. The National Polyp Study. Patient and polyp characteristics associated with high-grade dysplasia in colorectal adenomas. Gastroenterology 1990;98: 371-379.

[3] Liu HH. Prevalence of advanced colonic polyps in asymptomatic Chinese. World J Gastroenterol 2005;11: 4731-4734.

[4] Netzer P. Risk factor assessment of endoscopically removed malignant colorectal polyps. Gut 1998;43: 669-674.

[5] Volk EE. Management and outcome of patients with invasive carcinoma arising in colorectal polyps. Gastroenterology 1995;109: 1801-1807.

[6] Nusko G. Invasive carcinoma in colorectal adenomas: multivariate analysis of patient and adenoma characteristics. Endoscopy 1997;29: 626-631.

[7] Edwards BK. Annual report to the nation on the status of cancer 1975 – 2006, featuring colorectal cancer trends and impact of interventions (risk factors, screening and treatment) to reduce future rates. Cancer 2010;116: 544-573.

[8] Regula J. Colonoscopy in colorectal-cancer screening for detection of advanced neoplasia. N Engl J Med. 2006;355(18): 1863-1872.

[9] Bokemeyer B. Screening colonoscopy for colorectal cancer prevention: results from a German online registry on 269000 cases. Eur J Gastroenterol Hepatol 2009;21:650-655.

[10] Castells A. Prevención del cáncer colorrectal. Actualización 2009. Gastroenterol Hepatol 2009;32: 717.e1-717.e58.

[11] Guittet L. Performance of immunochemical faecal occult blood test in colorectal cancer screening in average-risk population according to possitivity threshold and number of samples. Int J Cancer 2009;125(5): 1127-1133

[12] Schlemper RJ. The Vienna classification of gastrointestinal epithelial neoplasia. Gut 2000;47: 251-255.

[13] Greene FL. Epithelial misplacement in adenomatous polyps of the colon and rectum. Cancer 1974;33: 206-217.

[14] Robert ME. The malignant colon polyp: diagnosis and therapeutic recommendations. Clin Gastroenterol Hepatol 2007;5 :662-667.

[15] Appelman HD. High-grade dysplasia and villous features should not be part of the routine diagnosis of colorectal adenomas. Am J Gastroenterol 2008;103: 1329-1331.

[16] Riddell RH. Epithelial neoplasms of the intestines, atlas of tumor pathology, tumors of the intestines, American Registry of Patholgy, Wahington, DC, 2002: p85-100.

[17] The Paris endoscopic classification of superficial neoplastic lesions: esophagus, stomach, and colon: November 30 to December 1, 2002. Gastrointest Endosc 2003;58(6 Suppl): S3-4

[18] Binmoeller KF. Endoscopic snare excision of "giant" colorectal polyps. Gastrointest Endosc 1996; 43:183-198.

[19] Lieberman D. Polyp size and advanced histology in patient undergoing colonoscopy screening: implication for CT colonography. Gastroenterologyy 2008;135: 1100-1105.

[20] Konishi K. A comparison of magnifying and nonmagnifying colonoscopy for diagnosis of colorectal polyps: a prospective study. Gastrointest Endosc 2003;57 :48-53.

[21] Eisen GM. High-resolution chromoendoscopy for classifying colonic polyps: a multicenter study. Gastrointest Endosc 2002;55: 687-694.

[22] Kudo S. Diagnosis of colorectal tumorous lesions by magnifying endoscopy. Gastrointest Endosc 1996;44: 8-14.

[23] Waxman I. High frequency probe EUS-assisted endoscopic mucosal resection: a therapeutic strategy for submucosal tumors of the GI tract. Gastrointest Endosc 2002;55: 44-49.

[24] Dell'Abate P. Endoscopic treatment of colorectal benign-appearing lesions 3 cm or larger: techniques and outcome. Dis Colon Rectum 2001;44: 112-118.

[25] Church JM. Avoiding surgery in patients with colorectal polyps. Dis Colon Rectum 2003;46: 1513-1516.

[26] Puli SR. Successful complete cure en-bloc resection of large nonpedunculated colonic polyps by endoscopic submucosal dissecion: a meta-analysis and systemic review. Ann Surg Oncol 2009;16: 2147-2151.

[27] Haggitt RC. Prognostic factors in colorectal carcinomas arising in adenomas: implications for lesions removed by endoscopic polypectomy. Gastroenterology 1985;89: 328-336.

[28] Park YJ. Histo-clinical analysis of early colorectal cancer World J Surg 2000;24: 1029-1035.

[29] Tytherleigh MG. Management of early rectal cancer. Br J Surg 2008;95: 409-423.

[30] Cooper HS. Endoscopically removed malignant colorectal polyps: clinico-pathologic correlations. Gastroenterology 1985;108: 1657-1665.

[31] Cunningham KN. Long-term prognosis of well-differentiated adenocarcinoma in endoscopically removed colorectal adenomas. Dig Dis Sci 1994;39: 2034-2037.

[32] Hamilton ST. Carcinoma of colon and rectum. In: hamilton Sr, Aaltonen LA, eds. Pathology & genetics. Tumours of the digestive system, Lyon, France: World Health Organization Classification of Tumours, IARC Press, 2000; p111-112.

[33] Cranley JP. When is endoscopic polypectomy adequate therapy for colonic polyps containing invasive carcinoma? Gastroenterology 1986;91: 419-427.

[34] Fenoglio CM. Distribution of human colonic lymphatics in normal, hyperplastic, and adenomatous tissue. Its relationship to metastasis from small carcinomas in pedunculated adenomas. Gastroenterology. 1973;64: 51-66.

[35] Fogt F. Identification of lymphatic vessels in malignant, adenomatous and normal colonic mucosa using the novel immunostain D2-40. Onco Rep 2004;11: 447-450.

[36] Walgenbach-Bruenagel G. Detection of lymphatic invasion in early stage primary colorectal cancer with the monoclonal antibody D2-40. Eur Surg Res 2006;38: 438-444.

[37] Cooper HS. Endoscopically removed malignant colorectal polyps: clinicopatologic correlations. Gastroenterology 1995;108: 1657-1665.

[38] Talbot IC. The clinical significance of invasion of veins by rectal cancer. Br J Surg 1980;67: 439-442.

[39] Whitlow C. Long-term survival after treatment of malignant colonic polyps. Dis Colon Rectum 1997;40: 929-934.

[40] Colacchio TA. Endoscopic polypectomy: inadequate treatment for invasive colorectal carcinoma. Ann Surg 1981;194: 704-707

[41] Ponsky JK. Endoscopic marking of colonic lesions. Gastrointest Endosc 1975;22: 42-43.

[42] Louis MA. Correlation between preoperative endoscopic and intraoperative findings in localizing colorectal lesions. World J Surg. 2010;34: 1587-1591.

[43] Martínez ME. Adenoma characteristics as risk factors for recurrence of advanced adenomas. Gastroenterology 2001;120: 1077-1083.

[44] Lieberman DA. Five-year colon surveillance after screening colonoscopy. Gastroenterology 2007;133: 1077-1085.

[45] Spencer RJ. Treatment of small colorectal polyps: A population-based study of the risk of subsequent carcinoma. Mayo Clin Proc 1984;59: 305-310.

[46] Butterly LF. Prevalence of clinically important histology in small adenomas. Clin Gastroenterol Hepatol 2006;4: 343-348.

[47] Gschwantler M. High-grade dysplasia and invasive carcinoma in colorectal adenomas: a multivariate analysis of the impact of adenoma and patient characteristics. Eur J Gastroenterol Hepatol 2002;14: 183-188.

[48] Ross AS. Flat and Depressed Neoplasms of the Colon in Western Populations. Am J Gastroenterol 2006;101: 172-180.

[49] Rembacken BJ. Flat and depressed colonic neoplasms: a prospective study of 1000 colonoscopies in the UK. The Lancet 2000;355: 1211-1214.

[50] Soetikno RM. Prevalence of nonpolypoid (flat and depressed) colorectal neoplasms in asymptomatic and symptomatic adults. JAMA 2008;299: 1027-1035.

[51] Walsh RM. Endoscopic resection of large sessile colorectal polyps. Gastrointest Endosc 1992;38: 303-309.

[52] Cho YB. Tumor localization for laparoscopic colorectal surgery. World J Surg 2007;31: 1491-1495.

[53] Nizam R. Colonic tattooing with India ink: benefits, risks, and alternatives. Am J Gastroenterol 1996;91: 1804-1808.

[54] Hilliard G. The elusive colonic malignancy. A need for definitive preoperative localization. Am Surg 1990;56: 742-744.

[55] Hammond DC. Endoscopic tattooing of the colon. An experimental study. Am Surg 1989;55: 457-461.

[56] McArthur CS. Safety of preoperation endoscopic tattoo with india ink for identification of colonic lesions. Surg Endosc 1999;13: 397-400.

[57] Arteaga-González I. The use of preoperative endoscopic tattooing in laparoscopic colorectal cancer surgery for endoscopically advanced tumors: a prospective comparative clinical study. World J Surg 2006;30: 605-611.

[58] Park JW. The usefulness of preoperative colonoscopic tattooing using a saline test injection method with prepackaged sterile India ink for localization in laparoscopic colorectal surgery. Surg Endosc 2008;22: 501-505

[59] Hassan C. The colorectal malignant polyp: Scoping a dilemma. Digest Liver Dis 2007;39: 92-100.

[60] Komuta K. Interobserver variability in the pathological assessment of malignant colorectal polyps. Br J Surg 2009;91: 1479-1484.

[61] Repici A. Endoscopic mucosal resection for early colorectal neoplasia: pathologic basis procedures and outcomes. Dis Colon Rectum 2009;52: 1502-1515.

[62] Endreseth BH. Rectal Cancer Group. Transanal excision versus major surgery for T1 rectal cancer. Dis Colon Rectum 2005;48: 1380-1388.

[63] Martínez-Fernandez A. Serum matrilysin levels predict outcome in curatively resected colorectal cancer patients. Ann Surg Oncol. 2009;16: 1412-1420.

[64] Toiyama Y. Circulating form of human vascular adhesion protein-1 (VAP-1): decreased serum levels in progression of colorectal cancer and predictive marker of lymphatic and hepatic metastasis. J Surg Oncol. 2009;99: 368-372.

[65] Alabi AA. Preoperative serum vascular endothelial growth factor-a is a marker for subsequent recurrence in colorectal cancer patients. Dis Colon Rectum. 2009;52: 993-999.

[66] Wang JY. Multiple molecular markers as predictors of colorectal cancer in patients with normal perioperative serum carcinoembryonic antigen levels. Clin Cancer Res. 2007;13: 2406-2413.

Chapter 6

The Malignant Polyp: Polypectomy or Surgical Resection?

Josef M. Taylor and Kenneth B. Hosie

Additional information is available at the end of the chapter

http://dx.doi.org/10.5772/52865

1. Introduction

Endoscopic resection of colorectal polyps is a well-recognised therapy for the prevention of colorectal carcinoma. Roughly 10% of resected polyps contain foci of carcinoma and are often termed malignant polyps or polyp cancers. Their incidence is increasing in line with the increasing use of colonoscopy.[1] A proportion of these will have progressed to nodal disease before presentation and a further oncological resection should be considered for high risk patients.[2]

The risk of nodal disease at presentation can be stratified by histology but definitive staging information can currently only be obtained by oncological resection, a procedure which can cause significant morbidity and mortality, especially in the elderly. This is of particular relevance as the majority of patients do not have nodal disease, even for the most dangerous categories of polyp.[3] There is a real risk of causing excess morbidity by over treating the majority in order to adequately treat the minority.

2. Malignant polyps

Not all polyps are created equal. The adenoma carcinoma sequence has long been recognised as the natural history of colorectal carcinoma and it is therefore logical that some adenomas will be discovered with foci of malignancy within them.

For those confined to the mucosa, polyps showing foci of potentially malignant cells are often termed *carcinoma in situ*. The lack of lymphatics in the mucosa prevents distant spread and, as these lesions are neither regarded as malignant or treated as malignancies, the term high grade mucosal neoplasm is now preferred. [4]

The definition of colorectal carcinoma is dysplasia crossing the *muscularis mucosa,* so when high grade dysplasia in these polyps crosses this barrier the lesion is termed a malignant polyp. A malignant polyp is essentially a macroscopically benign lesion that contains malignant foci on further examination. When the totality of the polyp is comprised of malignancy the term polypoid carcinoma is often used.

T1 lesions are therapeutically significant as they are the first lesions where nodal and distant metastases must be considered. The management of these polyps is based on the belief that the risk of spread can be stratified according to the histology of the resected polyp.[5] In the past authors used various criteria to define favourable or unfavourable histology and guide management.[1,2,6,7] For a large part, this has involved dividing patients into two groups. A "low risk" group, who are safe without further treatment and a "high risk group", for whom surgery should be considered.[8,9] Unfortunately published studies disagree about the factors that are most significant.[3,10-12]

3. Factors affecting risk of nodal disease

3.1. Morphology

The Paris classification[13] of gastro-intestinal tumours recognises that adenomas may be polypoid or non polypoid. Non polypoid (0-II, 0-III) lesions are not usually removed endoscopically as they are more challenging to remove and are recognised to have high malignant potential.

0-I: Polypoid	0-Ip: Pedunculated
	0-Is: Sessile
0-II : Non-Polypoid, Non Ulcerated	0-IIa: Slightly elevated
	0-IIb: Flat
	0-IIc: Slightly depressed
0-III: Ulcerated	

Table 1. Paris Classification of Superficial Tumours of the Colon and Rectum.[13]

Polypoid lesions can be pedunculated (Type 0-1p) or sessile (Type 0-1s). Due to their shape malignant sessile polyps are harder to remove with clear margins and have more ready access to the deeper portions of the submucosa. They are therefore more likely to be classified as high risk. Seitz et al[9] presented a series of 114 endoscopically removed malignant polyps. Overall 46% of these polyps were sessile, but 65% of "high risk" (ie. requiring surgical removal) polyps were sessile. Conversely only 23% of "low risk" polyps were sessile.

An earlier literature series of 741 malignant polyps reported that 58.3% of sessile polyps had "high risk features" (Grade 3-4, vascular or lymphatic invasion, positive resection margin) whereas only 10% of pedunculated polyps were similarly classified.[11] One meta-analysis reported positive resection margins in 56.8% of sessile lesions verses 18.7% in polypoid lesions (P < 0.0001).

Size and tubular or villous architecture are also well known to affect the malignant potential of polyps. However, in a similar fashion to flat or depressed areas of dysplasia, very large polyps are seldom excised endoscopically and are not relevant to the current topic.

3.2. Grading

Polyps are defined by dysplasia and the varying degree displayed by different polyps is thought to explain a large degree of their different metastatic potential.[14]

Negative for Intraepithelial neoplasia.	
Indefinite for Intraepithelial neoplasia.	
Low-grade Intraepithelial neoplasia.	Adenoma/dysplasia
High-grade neoplasia (intraepithelial or intramucosal)	Adenoma/dysplasia (4-1
	Noninvasive carcinoma (4-2)
	Suspicious for invasive carcinoma (4-3)
	Intramucosal carcinoma (lamina propria invasion) (4-4)
Submucosal carcinoma	

Table 2. Revised Vienna classification of epithelial neoplasla for esophagus, stomach, and colon. [13]

The revised Vienna classification is widely used to define the degree of dysplasia colorectal polyp. By definition malignant polyps are 4-4. For colorectal carcinomas the WHO classification recognises 4 grades of differentiation, with G1 representing well differentiated, through moderate (G2) and poorly differentiated (G3) to undifferentiated (G4). G1-2 are conventionally regarded as low grade and G3-4 as high grade.

In a meta-analysis of published series, Hassan *et al.*[1] reported a 3.9 (1.9-8.4) odds ratio for nodal metastasis with regard to high vs low grade malignant polyps. The odds ratio for mortality was reported as 9.2 (4.7-18.2). Determining the exact risk from high grade dysplasia is complicated by their relative rarity. One study of 80 malignant polyps found only 2 poorly differentiated polyps.[12] In a meta-analysis 7.2% of 1612 malignant polys were high grade.[1]

It is interesting to note that despite poor differentiation being recognised as an important determinant of nodal disease, no universally accepted definition exists. Indeed in studies where the prevalence of highly dysplastic lesions was lower, the risk of nodal disease in these polyps was increased. (See Table 3). This suggests that poor differentiation, when a rigorous definition is used is an extremely important predictor of nodal disease. Those studies that did not find the degree of dysplasia to be significant are hampered by the very small number of highly dysplastic lesions in their sample.

Study	Number Of T1 Tumours	Incidence of G3 Poorly Differentiated/% (No. of Cases)	Incidence of Nodal Involvement / % (No. of Cases)
Yamamoto et al 2004	301	0.1 (4)	-
Tominaga et al 2005	155	1.3 (2)	50.0 (1)
Kurokawa et al 2005	180	1.1 (2)	50.0 (1)
Whitlow et al 1997	59	1.7 (1)	0 (0)
Haggitt et al 1985	64	3.1 (2)	0 (0)
Geraghty et al 1991	81	2.5 (2)	-
Suzuki et al 2003	65	3.1 (2)	100 (2)
Sakuragi et al 2003	278	2.5 (7)	57.1 (4)
Seitz et al 2004	116	3.4 (4)	-
Wang et al 2005	159	4.4 (7)	85.7 (6)
Morson et al 1984	61	5 (3)	-
Cooper et al 1995	140	5.7 (8)	-
Netzer et al 1998	62	8.1 (5)	40.0 (2)
Hackelsberger et al 1995	87	11.5 (10)	-
Hassan et al 2005	380	14.7 (56)	23.2 (13)
Nascimbeni et al 2002	344	34.0 (117)	-
Nascimbeni et al 2004	144	39.6 (57)	-

Table 3. Incidence of G3 Poorly Differentiated T1 Colorectal Carcinoma and Incidence of Nodal Involvement. In those studied with a higher incidence of G3 carcinoma, incidence of nodal disease in those carcinomas falls. From[3]

3.3. Depth of invasion

Haggitt's classification is based on the greatest anatomical depth of invasion in pedunculated polyps.[5] Haggitt 0 lesions are confined to the mucosa. Haggitt grades 1-3 breach the submucosa within the polyp, and they are confined to the head, neck and stalk of the polyp respectively. Only Haggitt 4 lesions invade past the stalk into the submucosa of the wall. Most authors would agree that only Haggit 4 lesions require further treatment. If adequately excised, Haggitt 0-3 lesions have a risk of recurrence (<1%) which is lower than the predicted mortality of an oncological resection.[15,16] Conversely, for level 4 lessions, Haggitt reported nodal disease rates of almost 13%.

All sessile lesions are Haggitt 4 by definition, but other authors have treated selected sessile lesions with polypectomy alone to good effect. Kudo produced a refinement for sessile polyps by dividing the submucosa into thirds.[13] This has become known as the Kikuchi classification. [2] Lesions confined to the superficial third of the submucosa (called Sm1) demonstrated very low rates of nodal disease and many authors recommend no further treatment after polypectomy for Sm1. In the absence of other risk factors most would agree for Sm2 lesions as well.[7]

The Kikuchi classification has been widely accepted for the assessment of T1 colorectal tumours but can be difficult to perform on endoscopy specimens as the *muscularis propria* is not usually included in the specimen.[2]

Difficulty is also encountered when the *muscularis muscosa* cannot be identified. A large collaborative Japanese study used Haggit level 2 (i.e. the border between the head and neck of the polyp) as a baseline for pedunculated polyps. Provided that there was no lymphatic invasion, they found no nodal disease if the depth of invasion from here was <3mm. For sessile polyps the superficial aspect of the lesion was used and again no nodal disease discovered if the invasion was <1mm, regardless of other lymphatic invasion. [17] Other Japanese studies have also found good correlation between quantitative measures of submucosal invasion and risk of lymph node metastasis.[18,19]

Although the study included operative specimens as well as endocsopically removed malignant polyps, Ueno[14] showed that the width of tumour invasion is also an important factor.

3.4. Incomplete or piecemeal resection

Involved resection margins have been shown to be strongly associated with poor outcomes. These patients have higher mortality, local recurrence and rates of residual disease. In one, all be it small, study 75% of incompletely resected polyps were associated with an adverse outcome.[20] It should be noted that even when incomplete resection is reported, absence of residual disease in the surgical specimen is the rule (94% in one study) rather than the exception[21]. This is likely due to diathermy electrofulguration of the remnant.

The European recommendations state that tumour cells within 1mm of the margin represents a positive margin[22], with some authors arguing then >2mm represents the true safe margin[21].

Incomplete removal is failure of primary therapy and requires further resection. Piecemeal removal of the polyp prevents proper histological assessment and surgery is mandated in all cases. For this reason endoscopic mucosal resection by the strip biopsy method is discouraged for the removal of potentially malignant lesions.

3.5. Lymphatic and vascular invasion

Lymphatic invasion has been sighted by some authors as an important predictor of nodal disease. Controversy exists however as reported cases are rare and usually associated with poorly differentiated tumours or incomplete resection. Inter-observer variability and the ease of mistaking retraction artefact for lymphatic invasion also make interpretation difficult.[6,12]

Lymphatic invasion is usually associated with other high risk factors and in those cases with adverse outcomes, almost invariably so. Many authors would regard its status as an independent risk factor is unclear.[20] However a large multi-centre retrospective study from Japan found lymphatic involvement to be highly significant for nodal metastases (odds ratio 4.69 P<0.0001) in a multivariate analysis of risk factors.[17] They also found that in a small number of cases adverse outcomes were seen from cases of lymphatic invasion, despite invasion being confined to the head of the polyp (Haggit 1).

Vascular invasion is also considered difficult to identify, but where present, it is strongly associated with nodal disease. Yasuda[18] studied T1 rectal tumours, including specimens from primary resections and resections after polypectomy. The odds ratio for the nodal metastasis with reference to the presence or absence of vascular invasion was 12.023 (3.751–116.751 p=0.001). Another study of sessile T1 colorectal carcinomas found that vascular invasion was a significant factor in both univariate and multivariate analysis. However they admit that the small number of cases of vascular invasion were found in lesions with deeper Sm3 invasion.[23]

An odds ratio of 7 (2.6–19.2) for lymph node metastasis was reported in the only meta-analysis looking specifically at malignant polyps and the presence of vascular invasion.[1] However, the same analysis demonstrated no such increased risk in polyps that would otherwise be considered low risk. It may well be that vascular invasion carries no special significance in itself and should not be emphasised in decision making.

3.6. Tumour budding

Tumour budding is the presence of microscopic islands of tumour cells out ahead of the main front of tumour invasion. At present there is no defined agree standard to reporting the phenomenon but several authors have found it to be highly significant. Yasuda reported an odds ratio of 11.11 (3.64–146.03)[18] for predicting nodal disease but until further study occurs it is difficult to make firm recommendations.

3.7. Location

T1 rectal tumours seem to be particularly likely to cause nodal disease, especially when located in the lower third.[15,23] However at this stage there have been no studies looking at this relationship specifically in malignant polyps.

4. "The low risk polyp"

Several authors, starting with Morson in 1984[24], have developed the concept of the low risk polyp. That is, a polyp which can be safely treated with polypectomy alone, as there is minimal risk of nodal disease. The concept has been incorporated into the American College of Gastroenterology guide lines[25]. They recommend no further treatment if:

The polyp is considered to be completely excised by the endoscopist and is submitted *in toto* for pathological examination.

In the pathology laboratory, the polyp is fixed and sectioned so that it is possible to accurately determine the depth of invasion, grade of differentiation, and completeness of excision of the carcinoma.

The cancer is not poorly differentiated.

There is no vascular or lymphatic involvement.

The margin of excision is not involved. Invasion of the stalk of a pedunculated polyp, by itself, is not an unfavourable prognostic finding, as long as the cancer does not extend to the margin of stalk resection.

The European recommendations, while noting the potential of tumour budding and lymphatic and vascular invasion as prognostic factors, decline to provide a guideline as they have not been statistically significant in all cases.[22]

Another perspective is given by Nicholls,[7] who instead offered an algorithmic approach. He differentiates between colonic and rectal polyps. For rectal lesions judged to be adenoma prior to resection he recommends that all poorly differentiated lesions be removed. For colonic polyps he suggested further resection solely for Haggit 4 polyps (including by definition all sessile polyps) with a depth of invasion >1000 μm.

Systematic review of studies which selected low risk polyps using methodology broadly similar to the American criteria has demonstrated very low rates of nodal recurrence. (See Table 4). Mortality from oncological resection varies greatly by age and co-morbidity but is usually quoted around 3-5%.[26-28] Therefore, for these lesions, the safest course of action is surveillance rather than further resection.[8,29]

It should be noted that these criteria take no account of the depth of invasion and that these guidelines would encourage the removal of some lesions that have been safely treated by endoscopy. It may be that they are documenting many of the same characteristics but in a different way. It is not hard to imagine that Sm3 lesions are less likely to be excised with clear margins and are more likely to show poor differentiation. Indeed a large study of surgically resected sessile T1 colorectal tumours found Sm3 invasion in 68% of G3+4 tumours and on 33% in G1+2 (P=0.001). This study also found tumour grade not to be significant on multivariate analysis.[23]

Given Japanese experience it maybe be better to refine the criteria for a low risk polyp as any polyp lacking all of these features:

High grade (G3-4) lesions.

Incomplete resection or other factors preventing adequate histological assessment of the lesion.

Piecemeal resection

Depth of invasion greater than 2mm from *muscularis mucosa*

Width of invasion greater than 4mm.

The utility of including lymphatic invasion, vascular invasion or tumour budding is unclear at this time. Further work should be done to examine the risk from polyps of the lower third of the rectum, especially as these can often require a permanent stoma if oncological resection is performed.

Study	No. Of Polyps	Unfavourable Outcome	Unfavourable outcome in low risk group
Bernard et al. 1988	19	3	0
Christie 1988	88	6	0
Conte et al. 1987	30	4	0
Cooper et al. 1995	140	16	0
Cranley et al. 1986	39	10	0
Cunningham et al. 1994	36	2	0
Eckardt et al. 1988	61	11	0
Fried et al. 1984	22	0	0
Geraghty et al. 1991	80	5	0
Hackelsberger et al. 1995	86	8	0
Kikuchi et al. 1995	78	9	0
Kyzer et al. 1992	42	1	0
Morson et al. 1984	60	2	0
Netzer et al. 1998	70	16	0
Rossini et al. 1988	66	4	0
Shatney et al. 1975	28	1	0
Speroni et al. 1988	30	2	0
Sugihara et al. 1989	25	3	0
Volk et al. 1995	47	10	0
Whitlow et al. 1997	59	4	0
Seitz et al. 2004	114	16	0
Total	1,227	135	0

Table 4. Incidence of Adverse Outcome in Low Risk Polyps. Low risk = Low risk = excision complete with resection margins of at least 2 mm, no Grade 3 carcinoma, and no vascular invasion. (From Sitz et al. 2004)

http://dx.doi.org/10.5772/52865

5. "The high risk polyp"

Polyps that do not meet the low risk criteria should be considered for surgical removal even if there has been total excision of the primary lesion. Indeed, it is unusual to find residual tumour in the surgical specimen, especially if the lesion had clear histological margins.[6] The justification for surgery is the desire for regional control as the risk of nodal disease is much higher in these patients and oncological resection is required to obtain regional control in a similar manner to other colorectal malignancies. The dilemma is that only a minority of these patients have nodal disease requiring control and these patients are only reliably identified after resection. Especially in elderly, the decision to resect has the possibility to cause considerable harm without producing a benefit to the patient.

5.1. "First do no harm..."

It is an old surgical adage that surgery is only indicated if the natural history of the cure is better than the natural history of the disease. In situations of uncertainly like this it is useful to examine the possible outcomes of proposed courses of action in order to see were the survival advantage lies.

The outcomes of the decision to operate will be a function of the risk of nodal disease and the risk of operative mortality and morbidity. We feel it is useful to consider these decisions with reference to a 2x2 table of results

		Nodal disease	
		Yes	*No*
Further Resection	*Yes*	Survival similar to resested Stage IIIa disease (roughly 75%)	Operative mortality (Variable)
	No	Survival as for stage IV disease (Roughly 5%)	Curative procedure, without operative mortality (Roughly 100%)

Table 5. 2x2 Table of outcomes from the decision regarding further resection of high risk malignant polyps.

5.2. Nodal disease and oncological resection

We see no reason to regard these patients as any different from patients who had proceded straight to oncological resection and post operatively were staged either IIIa to IIIc (TNM v5). In the SEER data from 1998 to 2000 there is a huge difference between those with regard to five year survival (73% vs. 28% respectively). Clearly this stage differentiation has huge implications for the advisability of surgery. It has been suggested that T1-2N2 tumours have a better survival that T3-4N2 tumours and the TNMv6 classification has been changed to reflect this. Newer SEER data shows five year survival of 87.7% for T1-2N1 disease and 75% for T1-2N2 disease. [30]

To our knowledge there is no current method of estimating the extent of nodal disease from polypectomy histology.

5.3. Nodal disease and no further resection

For those patients with nodal disease who do not have it resected the prognosis is likely to be compromised. Intensive surveillance is likely to detect continued disease progression.

The role of chemotherapy and or radiotherapy has not been clearly defined in this group but is likely to be palliative in nature.

5.4. Absence of Nodal disease

The survival of patients after endoscopic removal of T1 lesions and no nodal disease is excellent. The mortality in these groups will be limited to the operative mortality from further resection.

5.5. Risk of Nodal disease

Various figures have been quoted in the text for the risk of nodal disease in high risk patients. This can partly be explained by the differing criteria used to define risk by various authors. Further stratification within the "high risk group" may become apparent with further study.

The St Mark's Lymph Node Positivity Model[31] can be used to predict the individual risk of nodal metastasis after local resection of rectal tumours. However it makes no distinction within T1 tumours. Such assessment of individual risk factors to produce a personalised risk is not possible based on the current evidence. Further studies using multivariate analysis will be required to tease out the importance of individual risk factors.

For our analysis we have chosen to present data based on Sm depth as this has shown to be a reproducible predictor of nodal disease. Both Kikuchi and Nascimbeni reported rates of roughly 5, 10 and 25% for Sm 1, 2 and 3 respectively.[23,32]

Risk Factor	**Incidence of nodal disease**
Depth of invasion	Haggit 1.2.3 = <1%[9] Kikuchi SM1 = 5% Kikuchi Sm2 = 10% Kicuchi Sm3 = 25%[23, 32]
Poorly differentiated	25-100%. *Not found to be important in multivariate analysis.*[14, 17]
Lympho-vascular Invasion	41% *Poor reproducibility.*[18]
Incomplete resection	75%[20]

Table 6. Incidence of nodal disease by risk factor

http://dx.doi.org/10.5772/52865

5.6. The risk of further resection

Oncological resection of colorectal lesions is performed via segmental resection of the affected potion of the bowel and its draining lymph node basin. Harvesting these nodes gains local control and definatively stages the disease. It is a major undertaking with considerable risks. In the case of very low rectal tumours an abdomino-perinal excision of rectum (APER) results in permanent stoma formation.

In the UK at least, operative mortality has fallen in recent years. 30 day mortality was 6.8% in 1999, falling to 3.7% in 2009/10.[33,34] Rates from Scandinavia (4.8%)[26] and the US (3.1%)[27] are broadly similar. This remains considerably higher than the rate of nodal disease in the low risk malignant polyps. The 90 day mortality rate, considered by some authors to be a more accurate measure of operative mortality is higher still, is 5.6% in the UK.[34]

This baseline rate is affected by both tumour and patient factors. Patients over the age of 80 are over ten times more likely to die than those under 50 (15% vs 1.2% 30 day mortality).[28,33] Comparing ASA1 and ASA4 patients, the odds ratio for death at 30 days is 14.06. Patients with rectal tumours do better than those with colonic tumours, though this seems to be due to high mortality for patients undergoing subtotal or total colectomy. Female sex, affluence, high volume surgical centres and elective rather than emergency surgery all also have a beneficial effect.[33]

On top of mortality, anastomotic leaks, wound complications, cardiovascular complications, defecatory disorders and the psychological impact of stoma formation must also be considered when deciding whether or not to resect. Morbidity rates of up to 35% have been reported in the past.[15] These seem to affect laparoscopic surgery as much as open resections, but hospital discharge and return to work occurs sooner following laparoscopic procedures. [35,36]

A more accurate individualised operative risk can be estimated from risk scoring systems. CR-POSSUM uses patient and operative parameters to estimate operative risk on an individual basis and has been well validated.[37,38] Cardiopulmonary exercise testing is also useful in predicting complications and the length of hospital stay. Both these tools can be of great use to the surgeon and patient when used thoughtfully during surgical planning. [39]

5.7. The special case of rectal tumours

There has been considerable interest in recent years in local resection of early rectal tumours to avoid stoma formation. This is relevant as malignant polyps in the rectum are a variety of early rectal tumour. Transanal Endoscopic Microsurgery (TEMS) allows full thickness excision of rectal lesions below the peritoneal fold, with excellent rates of local recurrence.[15] Its ability to harvest local lymph nodes is limited, and as such it is not generally a suitable second procedure for high risk lesions. It may have a role as secondary procedure for incompletely removed polyps which otherwise show favourable features. In its guidance the ACPGBI recommended full classical resection of rectal tumours that show the high risk features described earlier.[40]

The anatomical location of the draining nodes in rectal lesions has also encouraged more extensive use of imaging to predict local nodal metastases. Endoanal Ultrasound and MRI both have the ability to detect enlarged local nodes; however distinguishing between the commonly found reactive nodes and metastases can be difficult. Micrometastases have also been detected in radiologically normal nodes. The use of new contrast agents may improve accuracy but currently histological examination remains the gold standard for detecting nodal disease. [15]

For locally excised T1 and T2 tumours adjuvant chemoradiotherapy has been used with success to prevent local recurrence if further surgery is not deemed appropriate. The role of adjuvant therapy in malignant polyps is unexplored at this time.

5.8. Calculating the survival advantage

As the nodal status of these patients is unknown prior to surgery, mortality is a composite of the mortality of those with and without nodal disease. The contribution from each group will be in proportion to the risk of nodal disease.

cM = R.NM + (1-R).nM

Where cM= Composite mortality

R =Risk of nodal disease

NM =Mortality of those with nodal disease

nM =Mortality of those without nodal disease

The best course of action can be discerned by calculating the difference between cM with and without surgery. Tables 7-9 contain sample composite survival figures and number needed to treat at five years for various stages of malignant polyp.

Using this method we can see that for a patient with a Sm3 lesion (25% of nodal disease) and a predicted operative mortality of 2% there will be an absolute risk reduction of mortality at 5 years of 16% (NNT 6.25) if 5 year survival of node positive patients is 75% and a 4.5% reduction (NNT 21.05) if 5 year survival of node positive patients is 27%. In stage IIIa (75% five year survival) disease the absolute risk is reduced by 10% (NNT 1), but this disappears for stage IIIc. There has been considerable debate regarding the need to resect Sm2 lesions. In this model the benefit from resection disappears once operative mortality reaches 5% for IIIa lesions and 10% for IIIc lesions. Clearly careful though needs to be given to risk when choosing to operate on these patients.

Obviously this model makes no account of operative morbidity. For patients with IIIc disease and Sm3 lesions there is a survival advantage to operating; however the decision to subject 40 patients to major surgery to save 1 life at five years needs careful consideration.

http://dx.doi.org/10.5772/52865

	Patient A	Patient B	Patient C	Patient D
Age	55	55	80	60
Lesion	Kikuchi Sm3	Haggit level 1	Kikuchi Sm2	Kikuchi Sm1
Risk of nodal disease	25%	<1%	10%	5%
Operative Mortality	1%	1%	10%	5%
Compsite Survival without further resection	81.00	"/>99%	90.50	95.25
Compsite survival with resection	94.20	99%	88.50	94.00
Survival advantage	13.20	-	-	-

Table 7. Examples of using composite survival to inform decision making in patients with malignant polyps

6. Conclusion

This problem has been known and debated for over 30 years.[41] As the role of endoscopy has grown and developed, guidelines have been formulated to help clinicians make beneficial choices. Unfortunately the small scale and heterogeneity for published work had prevented any guidelines from gaining universal acceptance. The focus on tumour grade in the American guidance has been challenged by work from Japan that emphasises the importance of quantitative measures of the depth of invasion. Japanese work has also shown lymphatic invasion, vascular invasion and tumour budding to be of high prognostic significance, but concerns about reproducibility have prevented their universal adoption. It is also unclear which observed prognostic factors are truly significant and which are cofounding. None of the prognostic factors identified are highly specific and clinicians must still make difficult decisions based on the balance of risk.

The solution to this problem will surely come from improved pre-operative staging. Endo-anal ultra sound and targeted contrast MRI have both shown promise for rectal tumours. Sentinel node mapping in the colon has also been investigated but remains experimental. [42]

Until highly accurate pre-operative staging of nodal disease is possible effort must be made to refine the classification of malignant polyps to identify the truly significant prognostic factors. It is the opinion of the authors that an individualised prediction model comparing operative surgical risk and risk of progressive disease should be used to counsel patients regarding future strategies. Creation of a national or international database would facil;itate better predictive models.

Risk Of Nodal Disease/%		Operative Survival/ %				
		99	98	95	90	85
5	No Resectio /%	95.25	95.25	95.25	95.25	95.25
	Resection/%	98.45	97.50	94.65	89.90	85.15
	Survival Advantage/%	3.20	2.25	-	-	-
	NNT	**31.25**	**44.44**	-	-	-
10	No Resection/%	90.50	90.50	90.50	90.50	90.50
	Resection/%	97.90	97.00	94.30	89.80	85.30
	Survival Advantage/%	7.40	6.50	3.80	-	-
	NNT	**13.51**	**15.38**	**26.32**	-	-
15	No Resection/%	85.75	85.75	85.75	85.75	85.75
	Resection/%	97.35	96.50	93.95	89.70	85.45
	Survival Advantage/%	11.60	10.75	8.20	3.95	-
	NNT	**8.62**	**9.30**	**12.20**	**25.32**	-
20	No Resection/%	81.00	81.00	81.00	81.00	81.00
	Resection/%	96.80	96.00	93.60	89.60	84.00
	Survival Advantage/%	15.80	15.00	12.60	8.60	3.00
	NNT	**6.33**	**6.67**	**7.94**	**11.63**	**33.33**
25	No Resection/%	76.25	76.25	76.25	76.25	76.25
	Resection/%	96.25	95.50	93.25	89.50	85.75
	Survival Advantage/%	20.00	19.25	17.00	13.25	9.50
	NNT	**5.00**	**5.19**	**5.88**	**7.55**	**10.53**
30	No Resection/%	71.50	71.50	71.50	71.50	71.50
	Resection/%	95.70	95.00	92.90	89.40	85.90
	Survival Advantage/%	24.20	23.50	21.40	17.90	14.40
	NNT	**0.04**	**0.04**	**0.05**	**0.06**	**0.07**

Table 8. 5 year survival, survival advantage with further resection and number needed to treat if 5 year survival for node positive patients is 88% after resection.

http://dx.doi.org/10.5772/52865

Risk Of Nodal Disease/%		**Operative Survival/ %**				
		99	98	95	90	85
5	No Resection/%	95.25	95.25	95.25	95.25	95.25
	Resection/%	97.80	96.85	94.00	89.25	84.50
	Survival Advantage/%	2.55	1.60	-	-	-
	NNT	**39.22**	**62.50**	-	-	-
10	No Resection/%	90.50	90.50	90.50	90.50	90.50
	Resection/%	96.60	95.70	93.00	88.50	84.00
	Survival Advantage/%	6.10	5.20	2.50	-	-
	NNT	**16.39**	**19.23**	**40.00**	-	-
15	No Resection/%	85.75	85.75	85.75	85.75	85.75
	Resection/%	95.40	94.55	92.00	87.75	83.50
	Survival Advantage/%	9.65	8.80	6.25	2.00	-
	NNT	**10.36**	**11.36**	**16.00**	**50.00**	-
20	No Resection/%	81.00	81.00	81.00	81.00	81.00
	Resection/%	94.20	93.40	91.00	87.00	83.00
	Survival Advantage/%	13.20	12.40	10.00	6.00	2.00
	NNT	**7.58**	**8.06**	**10.00**	**16.67**	**50.00**
25	No Resection/%	76.25	76.25	76.25	76.25	76.25
	Resection/%	93.00	92.25	90.00	86.25	82.50
	Survival Advantage/%	16.75	16.00	13.75	10.00	6.25
	NNT	**5.97**	**6.25**	**7.27**	**10.00**	**16.00**
30	No Resection/%	71.50	71.50	71.50	71.50	71.50
	Resection/%	91.80	91.10	89.00	85.50	82.00
	Survival Advantage/%	20.30	19.60	17.50	14.00	10.50
	NNT	**4.93**	**5.10**	**5.71**	**7.14**	**9.52**

Table 9. 5 year survival, survival advantage with further resection and number needed to treat if 5 year survival is 75% after resection.

Risk Of Nodal Disease/%		Operative Survival/ %				
		99	98	95	90	85
5	No Resection/%	95.25	95.25	95.25	95.25	95.25
	Resection/%	95.30	94.35	91.50	86.75	82.00
	Survival Advantage/%	0.05	-	-	-	-
	NNT	**2000.00**	-	-	-	-
10	No Resection/%	90.50	90.50	90.50	90.50	90.50
	Resection/%	91.60	90.70	88.00	83.50	79.00
	Survival Advantage/%	1.10	0.20	-	-	-
	NNT	**90.91**	**500.00**	-	-	-
15	No Resection/%	85.75	85.75	85.75	85.75	85.75
	Resection/%	87.90	87.05	84.50	80.25	76.00
	Survival Advantage/%	2.15	1.30	-	-	-
	NNT	**46.51**	**76.92**	-	-	-
20	No Resection/%	81.00	81.00	81.00	81.00	81.00
	Resection/%	84.20	83.40	81.00	77.00	73.00
	Survival Advantage/%	3.20	2.40	0.00	-	-
	NNT	**31.25**	**41.67**	-	-	-
25	No Resection/%	76.25	76.25	76.25	76.25	76.25
	Resection/%	80.50	79.75	77.50	73.75	70.00
	Survival Advantage/%	4.25	3.50	1.25	-	-
	NNT	**23.53**	**28.57**	**80.00**	-	-
30	No Resection/%	71.50	71.50	71.50	71.50	71.50
	Resection/%	76.80	76.10	74.00	70.50	67.00
	Survival Advantage/%	5.30	4.60	2.50	-	-
	NNT	**18.87**	**21.74**	**40.00**	-	-

Table 10. 5 year survival, survival advantage with further resection and number needed to treat if 5 year survival in node positive patients is 27% after resection.

Author details

Josef M. Taylor and Kenneth B. Hosie*

*Address all correspondence to: kenneth.hosie@nhs.net

Department of Surgery, Derriford Hospital, Plymouth, United Kingdom

References

[1] Hassan C, Zullo A, Risio M, Rossini FP, Morini S. Histologic risk factors and clinical outcome in colorectal malignant polyp: a pooled-data analysis. Dis Colon Rectum 2005;48 1588-1596.

[2] Bujanda L, Cosme A, Gil I, Arenas-Mirave JI. Malignant colorectal polyps. World J Gastroenterol 2010;16 3103-3111.

[3] Ueno H, Hashiguchi Y, Kajiwara Y, Shinto E, Shimazaki H, et al. Proposed objective criteria for "grade 3" in early invasive colorectal cancer. Am J Clin Pathol 2010;134 312-322.

[4] Risio M. The Natural History of pT1 Colorectal Cancer. Front Oncol 2012;2 22.

[5] Haggitt RC, Glotzbach RE, Soffer EE, Wruble LD. Prognostic factors in colorectal carcinomas arising in adenomas: implications for lesions removed by endoscopic polypectomy. Gastroenterology 1985;89 328-336.

[6] Mitchell PJ, Haboubi NY. The malignant adenoma: when to operate and when to watch. Surg Endosc 2008;22 1563-1569.

[7] Nicholls RJ, Zinicola R, Binda GA. Indications for colorectal resection for adenoma before and after polypectomy. Tech Coloproctol 2004;8 Suppl 2 s291-294.

[8] Volk EE, Goldblum JR, Petras RE, Carey WD, Fazio VW. Management and outcome of patients with invasive carcinoma arising in colorectal polyps. Gastroenterology 1995;109 1801-1807.

[9] Seitz U, Bohnacker S, Seewald S, Thonke F, Brand B, et al. Is endoscopic polypectomy an adequate therapy for malignant colorectal adenomas? Presentation of 114 patients and review of the literature. Dis Colon Rectum 2004;47 1789-1796; discussion 1796-1787.

[10] Cooper HS, Deppisch LM, Gourley WK, Kahn EI, Lev R, et al. Endoscopically removed malignant colorectal polyps: clinicopathologic correlations. Gastroenterology 1995;108 1657-1665.

[11] Coverlizza S, Risio M, Ferrari A, Fenoglio-Preiser CM, Rossini FP. Colorectal adenomas containing invasive carcinoma. Pathologic assessment of lymph node metastatic potential. Cancer 1989;64 1937-1947.

[12] Geraghty JM, Williams CB, Talbot IC. Malignant colorectal polyps: venous invasion and successful treatment by endoscopic polypectomy. Gut 1991;32 774-778.

[13] The Paris endoscopic classification of superficial neoplastic lesions: esophagus, stomach, and colon: November 30 to December 1, 2002. Gastrointest Endosc 2003;58 S3-43.

[14] Ueno H, Mochizuki H, Hashiguchi Y, Shimazaki H, Aida S, et al. Risk factors for an adverse outcome in early invasive colorectal carcinoma. Gastroenterology 2004;127 385-394.

[15] Tytherleigh MG, Warren BF, Mortensen NJ. Management of early rectal cancer. Br J Surg 2008;95 409-423.

[16] Kyzer S, Begin LR, Gordon PH, Mitmaker B. The care of patients with colorectal polyps that contain invasive adenocarcinoma. Endoscopic polypectomy or colectomy? Cancer 1992;70 2044-2050.

[17] Kitajima K, Fujimori T, Fujii S, Takeda J, Ohkura Y, et al. Correlations between lymph node metastasis and depth of submucosal invasion in submucosal invasive colorectal carcinoma: a Japanese collaborative study. J Gastroenterol 2004;39 534-543.

[18] Yasuda K, Inomata M, Shiromizu A, Shiraishi N, Higashi H, et al. Risk factors for occult lymph node metastasis of colorectal cancer invading the submucosa and indications for endoscopic mucosal resection. Dis Colon Rectum 2007;50 1370-1376.

[19] Sakuragi M, Togashi K, Konishi F, Koinuma K, Kawamura Y, et al. Predictive factors for lymph node metastasis in T1 stage colorectal carcinomas. Dis Colon Rectum 2003;46 1626-1632.

[20] Netzer P, Forster C, Biral R, Ruchti C, Neuweiler J, et al. Risk factor assessment of endoscopically removed malignant colorectal polyps. Gut 1998;43 669-674.

[21] Jang EJ, Kim DD, Cho CH. Value and interpretation of resection margin after a colonoscopic polypectomy for malignant polyps. J Korean Soc Coloproctol 2011;27 194-201.

[22] Quirke P, Risio M, Lambert R, von Karsa L, Vieth M. Quality assurance in pathology in colorectal cancer screening and diagnosis-European recommendations. Virchows Arch 2011;458 1-19.

[23] Nascimbeni R, Burgart LJ, Nivatvongs S, Larson DR. Risk of lymph node metastasis in T1 carcinoma of the colon and rectum. Dis Colon Rectum 2002;45 200-206.

[24] Morson BC, Whiteway JE, Jones EA, Macrae FA, Williams CB. Histopathology and prognosis of malignant colorectal polyps treated by endoscopic polypectomy. Gut 1984;25 437-444.

[25] Bond JH. Polyp guideline: diagnosis, treatment, and surveillance for patients with colorectal polyps. Practice Parameters Committee of the American College of Gastroenterology. Am J Gastroenterol 2000;95 3053-3063.

[26] Frederiksen BL, Osler M, Harling H, Ladelund S, Jorgensen T. The impact of socioeconomic factors on 30-day mortality following elective colorectal cancer surgery: a nationwide study. Eur J Cancer 2009;45 1248-1256.

[27] Dimick JB, Cowan JA, Upchurch GR, Colletti LM. Hospital volume and surgical outcomes for elderly patients with colorectal cancer in the United States1 1 Presented at

the Annual Meeting of the Association for Academic Surgery, Boston, MA, November 7th–9th, 2002. The Journal of surgical research 2003;114 50-56.

[28] Latkauskas T, Rudinskaite G, Kurtinaitis J, Janciauskiene R, Tamelis A, et al. The impact of age on post-operative outcomes of colorectal cancer patients undergoing surgical treatment. BMC Cancer 2005;5 153.

[29] Ruiz-Tovar J, Jimenez-Miramon J, Valle A, Limones M. Endoscopic resection as unique treatment for early colorectal cancer. Rev Esp Enferm Dig 2010;102 435-441.

[30] Gunderson LL, Jessup JM, Sargent DJ, Greene FL, Stewart AK. Revised TN categorization for colon cancer based on national survival outcomes data. J Clin Oncol 2010;28 264-271.

[31] Risk Prediction in Surgery. http://www.riskprediction.org.uk/ (Accessed 1st August 2012)

[32] Kikuchi R, Takano M, Takagi K, Fujimoto N, Nozaki R, et al. Management of early invasive colorectal cancer. Risk of recurrence and clinical guidelines. Dis Colon Rectum 1995;38 1286-1295.

[33] Morris EJ, Taylor EF, Thomas JD, Quirke P, Finan PJ, et al. Thirty-day postoperative mortality after colorectal cancer surgery in England. Gut 2011;60 806-813.

[34] National Bowel Cancer Audit Report 2011. http://www.ic.nhs.uk/webfiles/Services/NCASP/audits%20and%20reports/Bowel_Cancer_Audit_Report_2011_interactive.pdf (Accessed 1st August 2012)

[35] Leung KL, Kwok SP, Lam SC, Lee JF, Yiu RY, et al. Laparoscopic resection of rectosigmoid carcinoma: prospective randomised trial. Lancet 2004;363 1187-1192.

[36] Lourenco T, Murray A, Grant A, McKinley A, Krukowski Z, et al. Laparoscopic surgery for colorectal cancer: safe and effective? - A systematic review. Surg Endosc 2008;22 1146-1160.

[37] Al-Homoud S, Purkayastha S, Aziz O, Smith JJ, Thompson MD, et al. Evaluating operative risk in colorectal cancer surgery: ASA and POSSUM-based predictive models. Surg Oncol 2004;13 83-92.

[38] Bromage SJ, Cunliffe WJ. Validation of the CR-POSSUM risk-adjusted scoring system for major colorectal cancer surgery in a single center. Dis Colon Rectum 2007;50 192-196.

[39] Struthers R, Erasmus P, Holmes K, Warman P, Collingwood A, et al. Assessing fitness for surgery: a comparison of questionnaire, incremental shuttle walk, and cardiopulmonary exercise testing in general surgical patients. Br J Anaesth 2008;101 774-780.

[40] ASGBI Guidelines for the Management of Colorectal Cancer 3rd Edition. www.acpgbi.org.uk/assets/documents/COLO_guides.pdf (Accessed 1st August 2012)

[41] Morson BC, Bussey HJ, Samoorian S. Policy of local excision for early cancer of the colorectum. Gut 1977;18 1045-1050.

[42] Cahill RA, Leroy J, Marescaux J. Could lymphatic mapping and sentinel node biopsy provide oncological providence for local resectional techniques for colon cancer? A review of the literature. BMC Surg 2008;8 17.

Chapter 7

Desmoplastic Reaction in Biopsy Specimens of T1 Stage Colorectal Cancer Plays a Critical Role in Defining the Level of Sub-Mucosal Invasion

Shigeki Tomita, Kazuhito Ichikawa and Takahiro Fujimori

Additional information is available at the end of the chapter

http://dx.doi.org/10.5772/51900

1. Introduction

Observation of the mucosal crypt patterns using chromoendoscopy with magnification has been reported to be the most reliable method for determining whether a colorectal cancer (CRC) is early or advanced tumour. Moreover, brand-new endoscopic system have the capability to enhance visibility by the capillary pattern, which may prove to be reliable for detection of deep submucosal invasive CRC.

Early CRC is defined as a tumour whose invasion is limited to the mucosa or submucosa. The endoscopic mucosal resection and endoscopic mucosal dissection (EMR/ESD) have become useful for early CRC. However, EMR/ESD is applicable only to intramucosal carcinoma, and additional surgery is required if the resected lesion reveals submucosal invasion by pathological diagnosis. Therefore, endoscopist and surgical pathologist considered that it would be very useful to predict the depth of invasion of submucosal invasive CRC before EMR/ESD. On the other hand, desmoplastic reaction (DR) which is characterized by the infiltration of eosinophilic myofibroblasts in the stroma of invasive carcinoma is suggested to be a prognostic marker in CRC patients.

Here we describe that detection of DR in pre-treatment biopsy specimens is useful for predicting the depth of submucosal invasion and evaluation of submucosal depth with head invasion or stalk invasion in post EMR/ESD specimen is useful for predicting the lymph node metastasis and discuss relevant issues in arriving at the correct differential diagnosis based on histological findings for gastrointestinal endoscopist and surgical pathologist.

2. Correlations between lymph node metastasis and early colorectal carcinoma

The endoscopic mucosal resection and endoscopic submucosal dissection (EMR/ESD) have become useful for early CRC which is defined as a T1 stage tumour whose invasion is limited to the mucosa or submucosa according to the T categories for colorectal cancer of the American Joint Committee on Cancer (AJCC) staging system (Table 1).

Tx: No description of the tumor's extent is possible because of incomplete information.
Tis: The cancer is in the earliest stage (in situ). It involves only the mucosa. It has not grown beyond the muscularis mucosa (inner muscle layer).
T1: The cancer has grown through the muscularis mucosa and extends into the submucosa.
T2: The cancer has grown through the submucosa and extends into the muscularis propria (thick outer muscle layer).
T3: The cancer has grown through the muscularis propria and into the outermost layers of the colon or rectum but not through them. It has not reached any nearby organs or tissues.
T4a: The cancer has grown through the serosa (also known as the visceral peritoneum), the outermost lining of the intestines.
T4b:The cancer has grown through the wall of the colon or rectum and is attached to or invades into nearby tissues or organs.

Table 1. T categories for colorectal cancer of the AJCC staging system.

The endoscopic mucosal dissection (EMR: endoscopic mucosal resection and ESD: endoscopic submucosal dissection) of intramucosal carcinoma is accepted as curative, as there is almost negative of lymph node metastasis. [1-4]. However, the reported prevalence rates of lymph node metastasis range from 6 to 12% of all patients with submucosal invasive colorectal carcinoma (SICC) [3-6]. Therefore, the endoscopic mucosal dissected cases of SICC with lymph node metastasis, and after EMR/ESD, surgical resection accompanied with lymph node dissection is necessary.

It has been known that we should be considered be additional resection is required due to the risk of lymph node metastasis following findings (1) massive submucosal invasion: (2) lymphatic/vessel invasion; or (3) poorly differentiated component in resected EMR/ESD specimens [7, 8]. There has been no standard method of measurement of submucosal invasion depth. Therefore, Japanese Society for Cancer of the Colon and Rectum has recently demonstrated definite for method of measurement of submucosal invasion depth.

3. Ip type (pedunculated lesion) and non-Ip type (nonpedunculated lesion) of early colorectal carcinoma

Macroscopic type (endoscopic finding) was assessed according to the macroscopic classification of early stomach carcinoma, with minor modifications. In shortly, SICCs were divided into two lesions: pedunculated (Ip type) (Figure. 1, Figure. 2(a)) and nonpedunculated (Non-Ip type) (Figure. 1b, Figure. 2(b)). Nonpedunculated lesion were subclassified as semipedunculated lesion (Isp type) and sessile lesion (Is type). Respectively. Ip type (pedunculated lesion) has typically head with stalk (Figure. 1, Figure 2).

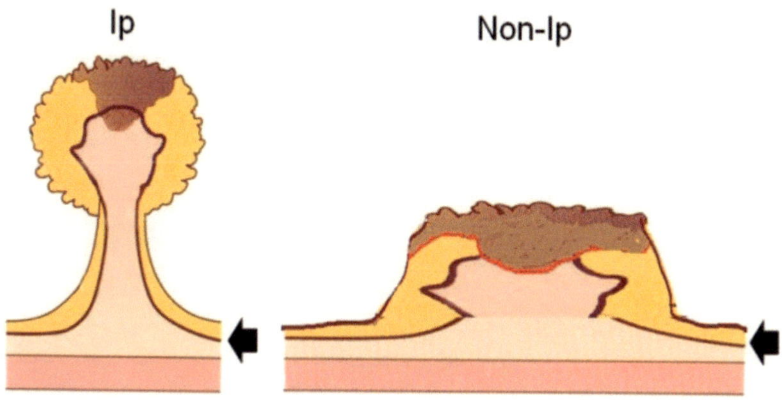

Figure 1. Schema of macroscopic (endoscopic) classification of SICCs: pedunculated(Ip type) and nonpedunculated(Non-Ip type). Arrowhead: muscularis mucosae.: 0 μm

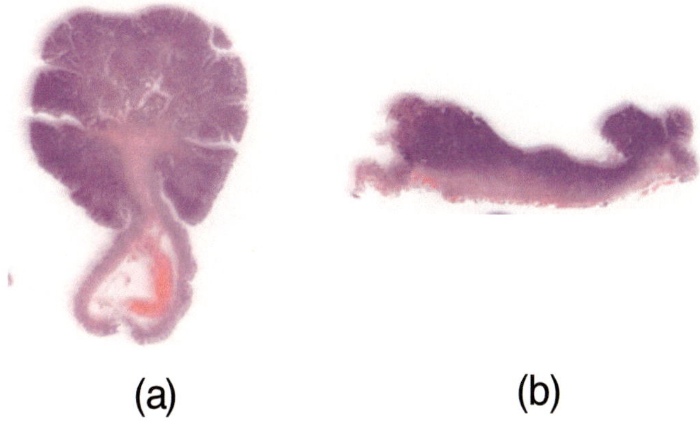

Figure 2. Histological appearance of pedunculated(Ip type) (a) and nonpedunculated(Non-Ip type) (b) on Hematoxylin and Eosin staining section.

The method used for measurement of submucosal invasion depth (Figure. 3)

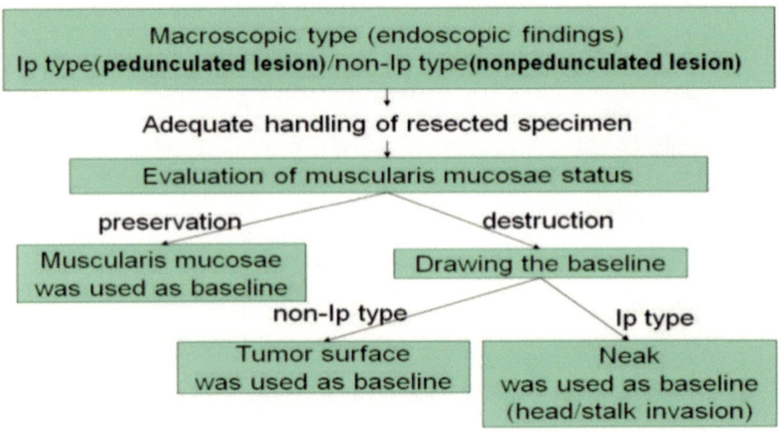

Figure 3. Algorithm of measurement of submucosal invasion depth.

Firstly, EMR/ESD resected specimens are divided into pedunculated(Ip type) and nonpedunculated(Non-Ip type). For pedunculated SICC, level 2 according to Haggitt's classification [9] was used as the baseline (so-called Haggitt's line), and submucosal invasion depth was measured as the vertical distance from this line to the deepest site of invasion. The baseline to distinguish between head invasion, (Figure. 4(a)) and stalk invasion, (Figure. 4(b)). In head invasion, submucosal invasion depth was regarded as 0 μm. When the deepest portion of invasion was located below the baseline, the case was defined as a stalk invasion and the vertical distance from this line to the deepest portion of invasion was utilized as submucosal invasion depth.

http://dx.doi.org/10.5772/51900

On the other hand, nonpedunculated and when the muscularis mucosae could be identified in hematoxylin and eosin stain, the muscularis mucosae was used as baseline and the vertical distance from this line to the deepest site of invasion represented submucosal invasion depth, (Figure. 4(c))., however, when the muscularis mucosae could not be identified, the superficial aspect of the SICC was used as baseline, (Figure. 4(d)).

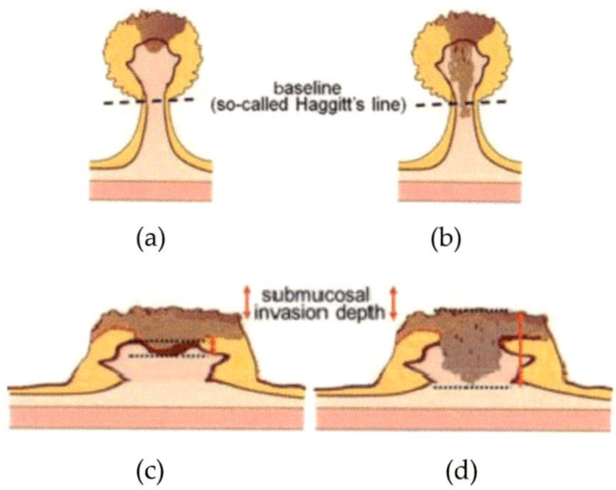

Figure 4. Schema of measurement of submucosal invasion depth. Ip type with head invasion (a) and stalk invasion (b), non-Ip type with musucular mucosae (c) and without musucular mucosae (d).

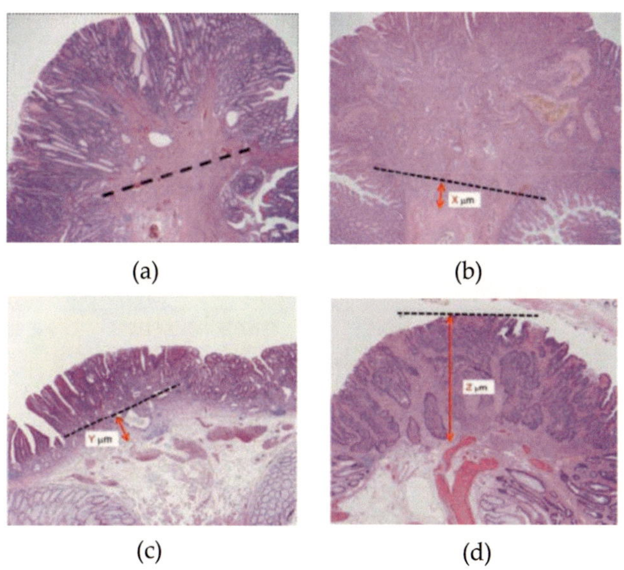

Figure 5. Histological findings with depth of submucosal invasion (μm). Ip type with head invasion: 0 μm (a) and stalk invasion: X μm (b), non-Ip type with musucular mucosae: Y μm (c) and without musucular mucosae: Z μm (d) on Hematoxylin and Eosin staining section

4. Correlations between lymph node metastasis and depth of submucosal invasive colorectal carcinoma

The Japanese collaborative retrospectively study for 865 SICCs. This nationwide survey not only represents a first for Japan, but reviewing the literature using PubMed revealed no similar surveys from anywhere in the world at that time [3] This study reported that pedunculated (Ip type) SICC, rate of lymph node metastasis was never in head invasion cases and stalk invasion cases with submucosal invasion depth < 3000 μm if lymphatic invasion was negative (Table 2).

And, For nonpedunculated (non-Ip type) SICC, rate of lymph node metastasis was also 0% if submucosal invasion depth was <1000 μm (Table 3). In multivariate analysis, SM depth <1000μm (P <0.006), sprouting (P <0.002), and lymphatic invasion (P<0.0001) represented significant risk factors, with odds ratios of 5.404, 2.276, and 4.691, respectively. Several priviously reports suggested that prognosis in patients with early colorectal carcinoma based on Haggitt's classification, finding that level 4 which is carcinoma invading the submucosa of the bowel wall below the stalk of the polyp but above the muscularis propria, represented the most important factor for lymph node metastasis [9, 10]. Therefore, these results revealed that submucosal invasion could be an important of predicting lymph node metastasis potential.

					Histological type at the deepest portion	
	LNM (+)	Ly (+)	V (+)	Sp (+)	wel, mod	por
SM depth (μm)	(%)	(%)	(%)	(%)	(%)	(%)
X=0 (n=53)	3 (5.7)	15 (28.3)	9 (17.0)	15 (28.3)	51 (96.2)	2 (3.8)
0 <X<500 (n=10)	0 (0)	2 (20.0)	0 (0)	3 (33.3)	10 (100)	0 (0)
500≤X<1000 (n=7)	0 (0)	1 (14.3)	0 (0)	2 (28.6)	7 (100)	0 (0)
1000≤X<1500 (n=11)	1 (9.1)	2 (18.2)	3 (27.3)	7 (63.6)	11 (100)	0 (0)
1500≤X<2000 (n = 7)	1 (14.3)	4 (57.1)	0 (0)	5 (71.4)	7 (100)	0 (0)
2000 ≤X<2500 (n= 10)	1 (10.0)	4 (40.0)	3 (30.0)	1 (10.0)	9 (90.0)	1 (10.0)
2500≤X< 3000 (n= 4)	0 (0)	0 (0)	2 (50)	1 (25.0)	4 (100)	0 (0)
3000 ≤X<3500 (n= 9)	2 (22.2)	4 (44.4)	3 (33.3)	5 (55.6)	8 (88.9)	1 (11.1)
3500 ≤X (n= 30)	2 (6.7)	9 (30.0)	10 (33.3)	10 (33.3)	28 (93.3)	2 (6.7)

SICC, submucosal invasive colorectal carcinoma; SM depth, depth of submucosal invasion of SICC; LNM, lymph node metastasis; Ly, lymphatic invasion; V, venous invasion; Sp, sprouting; wel, well-differentiated adenocarcinoma; mod, moderately differentiated adenocarcinoma; por, poorly differentiated adenocarcinoma

Table 2. Relationship between clinicopathological factors and the rate of lymph node metastasis according to SM depth in pedunculated (Ip type) SICC (adapted from [3])

					Histological type at the deepest portion		Status of muscularis mucosae	
	LNM (+)	Ly (+)	V (+)	Sp (+)	wel, mod	por	Identified	Not identified
SM depth (μm)	(%)	(%)	(%)	(%)	(%)	(%)	(%)	(%)
0 <X<500 (n=65)	0 (0)	5 (7.7)	3 (4.6)	9 (13.8)	64 (98.5)	1 (1.5)	64 (98.5)	1 (1.5)
500≤X<1000 (n=58)	0 (0)	12 (20.7)	7 (12.1)	7 (12.1)	58 (100)	0 (0)	51 (87.9)	7 (12.1)
1000≤X<1500 (n=52)	6 (11.5)	16 (30.8)	12 (23.1)	16 (30.8)	51 (98.1)	1 (1.9)	36 (69.2)	16 (30.8)
1500≤X<2000 (n = 82)	10 (12.2)	27 (32.9)	16 (19.5)	37 (45.1)	82 (100)	0 (0)	48 (58.5)	34 (41.5)
2000 ≤X<2500 (n= 84)	13 (15.5)	28 (33.3)	21 (25.0)	42 (50.0)	78 (92.9)	6 (7.1)	31 (36.9)	53 (63.1)
2500≤X< 3000 (n= 71)	8 (11.3)	29 (40.8)	16 (22.5)	38 (53.5)	71 (100)	0 (0)	20 (28.2)	51 (71.8)
3000 ≤X<3500 (n= 72)	5 (6.9)	26 (36.1)	15 (20.8)	35 (48.6)	69 (95.8)	3 (4.2)	16 (22.2)	56 (77.8)
3500 ≤X (n= 240)	35 (14.6)	92 (38.3)	74 (30.8)	133 (55.4)	237 (98.8)	3 (1.2)	48 (20.0)	192 (80.0)

Table 3. Relationship between clinicopathological factors and the rate of lymph node metastasis according to SM depth in nonpedunculated (non-Ip type) SICC (adapted from [3])

Suprisingly, Japanese collaborative retrospectively nationwide survey shows both of Ip type (pedunculated lesion) and non-Ip type (nonpedunculated lesion) of early colorectal carcinoma with rate of lymph node metastasis was also 0% if submucosal invasion depth was <1000 μm (Table 4). It is easy to measure one southern micrometer using by small ruler under microscopy for surgical pathologist. When if submucosal invasion depth was 1000 μm ≤, surgical pathologist should be advice to gastrointestinal endoscopist. And recently Japanese large-scale multicenter retrospectively study for 384 (head invasion: 240, stalk invasion: 144) pedunculated (Ip type) SICCs demonstrated that incidence of lymph node metastasis was 3.5%. the incidence of lymph node metastasis was 0.0% inpatients with head invasion, ascompared with 6.2% in patients with stalk invasion (Tabel 4). Pedunculated type early invasive colorectal cancers pathologically diagnosed as head invasion can be only treated by endoscopic resection.

SM depth X (μm)			Ip type		Non-Ip type	
			n	pN positive (%)	n	pN positive (%)
head invasion (X=0)			53	3(5.7)*		
0	<X<	500	10	0(0)	65	0(0)
500	≤X<	1000	7	0(0)	58	0(0)
1000	≤X<	1500	11	1(9.1)*	52	6(11.5)
1500	≤X<	2000	7	1(14.3)*	82	10(12.2)
2000	≤X<	2500	10	1(10.0)*	84	13(15.3)
2500	≤X<	3000	4	0(0)	71	8(11.3)
3000	≤X<	3500	9	2(22.2)	72	5(6.9)
3500	≤X		30	2(6.7)	240	35(14.6)

Ip type: pedunculated lesion. Non-Ip type: nonpedunculated lesion

*: vessels invasion

Table 4. Relationship between clinicopathological factors and the rate of the lymph node metastasis according to SM depth (summarized of Table 2 and 3, adapted from [11]. English translated version]

	Head invasion	Stalk invasion	Total
Lymph node metastasis n (%)	0/101 (0)	8/129 (6.2)	8/230 (3.5)
95% CI (%)	0.00–3.60P	2.70–11.90	1.50–6.70
		*P = 0.02	
Recurrence n (%)	0/219 (0)	1/121 (0.8)	1/340 (0.3)
95% CI (%)	0.00–1.70	0.02–4.50	0.01–1.60
		**P = 0.72	
Lymphovascular invasion†, n (%)	35/240 (15)	55/144 (38)	90/384 (23)
Lymphatic invasion, n (%)	21 (9)	33 (23)	54 (14)
Venous invasion, n (%)	16 (7)	37 (26)	53 (14)
Poorly differentiated component, n (%)	26/240 (11)	26/144 (18)	52/384 (14)

Lymphatic and/or venous invasion. CI, confidence interval

Table 5. Histopathological characteristics of 384 cases of pedunculated type early invasive colorectal cancer (adapted from [12])

http://dx.doi.org/10.5772/51900

5. The treatment of colorectal carcinoma with submucosal invasion state after endoscopic resection

Many new treatment methods have been developed over the last few decades. The Japanese Society for Cancer of the Colon and Rectum guidelines 2010 for the treatment of colorectal cancer (JSCCR Guidelines 2010 [13]) have been prepared to show standard treatment strategies for submucosal invasive colorectal cancer (Figure. 6).

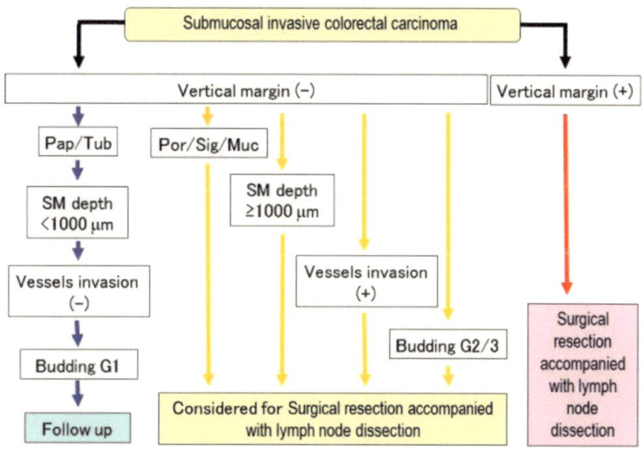

Figure 6. Guide line for the treatment of colorectal carcinoma with submucosal invasion state after endoscopic resection. (adapted from JSCCR Guidelines 2010 [13] with minor modifications);; Pap: papillary adenocarcinoma, Tub: tubular adenocarcinoma, Por: poorly differentiated adenocarcinoma, Sig: signet-ring cell carcinoma, Muc: mucinous adenocarcinoma, SM: submucosal invasion, Budding: tumor budding. The tumor budding denotes that at the invasion front of colorectal adenocarcinomas tumour cells, and the potential of tumour budding as a prognostic factor (G1:Grade 1 to G3: Grade 3) for routine surgical pathology [14,15])

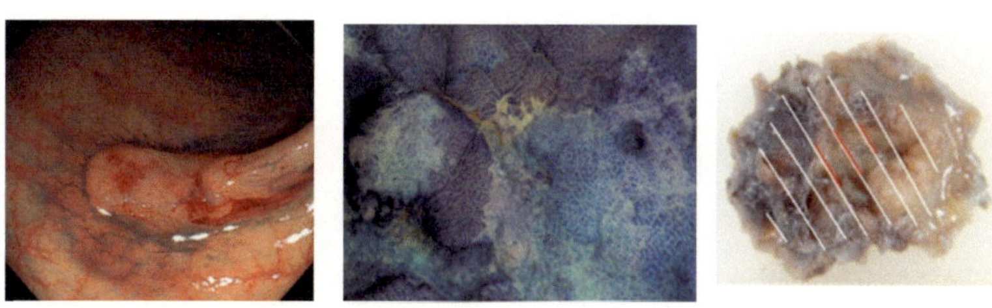

a) Endoscopic finding (b) Stereomicroscopic finding (c) Macroscopic finding

Figure 7. Endoscopic, stereomicroscopic, macroscopic findings of the early colorectal carcinoma. Endoscopic finding of the pedunculated(Non-Ip) type (a), several pits are arranged irregularly in the stereomicroscopic view (b), macroscopic appearance of SICC, post formalin-fixed. Most of the endoscopic detectable lesions were the irregular elevated type macroscopically. (White bar: mucosal invasion, Red bar: submucosal invasion) (c),

6. Detection of desmoplastic reaction in biopsy specimens of colorectal cancer

Early CRC, including submucosal invasive colorectal carcinoma (SICC), is defined as a tumor whose invasion is limited to the mucosa or submucosa. The endoscopic resection (EMR/ESD) have been useful for early CRC. However, endoscopic resection is applicable only to intramucosal carcinoma (Tis stage tumor), and additional surgery is required if the resected specimen reveals submucosal invasion by pathological diagnosis. However, the study of Japanese Society for Cancer of the Colon and Recum have recently demonstrated that the depth of submucosal invasion is closely correlated with the prevalence of lymph node metastasis in patients with SICC (See. Correlations between lymph node metastasis and early colorectal Carcinoma).

Therefore, gastrointestinal endoscopist and surgical pathologist considered that it would be very useful to predict the depth of invasion of SICC before endoscopic resection for case selection. New endoscopic systems are possible to predict submocosal invasion depth without biopsy. However, these developed systems have not been used in everywhere. On the other hand, the stromal change associated with carcinoma invasion has been called desmoplastic reaction (DR), desmoplasia, and cancer-associated fibroblast. Reported incidence of the DR is suggested to be a prognostic marker in CRC patients [16, 17]. Recently, JSCCR studies have been assessed the DR in pretreatment biopsy specimens of SICRC to predict the submucosal depth in retorospective and prospective study.

The DR is characterized by modifications in the composition of stromal cells and extracellular matrix (ECM) components with eosinophilic change [18, 19] (Figure. 8). The main producers of many ECM compounds and represent the major cellular component including DR that often show differentiated phenotype with expression of the smooth muscle actin, platelet derived growth factor receptor- type I collagen [18, 20, 21].

The presence and histological findings of DR in biopsy specimens were evaluated by pathologists at each respective institute and the criteria for assessment of DR established in consensus meeting among JSCCR members including us. (Table 6).

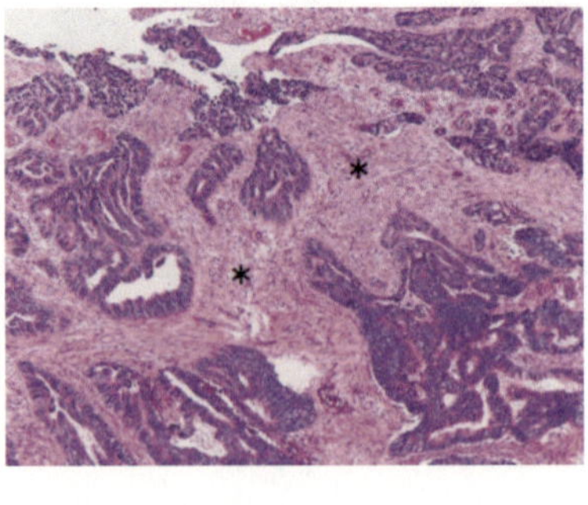

Figure 8. Histological appearance of desmoplastic reaction (DR). Note the growth of eosinophilic spindle cells (myofibroblasts.*) with submucosal invasive carcinoma component on Hematoxylin and Eosin staining section.

http://dx.doi.org/10.5772/51900

1) Existence of carcinoma is required for detection of DR.
2) The histological findings of infiltrating carcinoma do not signify the presence of DR.
3) DR contains areas of collagen fiber accumulation and myofibroblast proliferation, but inflammatory infiltration does not signify the presence of DR.
4) All histological findings were determined by HE stain alone; detection of DR does notrequire the use of any special stains.
DR, desmoplastic reaction.

Table 6. Criteria for detection of desmoplastic reaction (adapted from [22])

A retorospective study for detection of desmoplastic reaction in biopsy specimens of early colorectal cancer reported that 359 patients with SICRCs, who had undergone surgical or endoscopic mucosal resection, were analysed [23]. For pedunculated (Ip type) SICRCs was not significantly related to submucosal depth. However, for nonpedunculated (non-Ip type) the prevalence of DR in pretreatment biopsy specimens was significantly related to submucosal depth. When nonpedunculated(non-Ip type) SICRCs were further divided using a specific cut off value of 1000 μm for submucosal depth, the positivity ratio of DR in pretreatment biopsy specimens was significantly higher in SICRCs with an submucosal depth of 1000 μm than in cases where the submucosal depth was <1000 μm (Table 7). Detection of DR in pretreatment biopsy specimens is useful for the prediction of submucosal depth in nonpedunculated (non-Ip) SICRCs,

Depth of submucosal invasion (μm)	Pedunculated SICRC		Nonpedunculated SICRC	
	DR (-) (%)	DR (+) (%)	DR (-) (%)	DR (+) (%)
X<1000	3 (37.5)	5 (62.5)	30 (65.2)	16 (34.8)
1000 ≤ X < 2000	1 (50.0)	1 (50.0)	25 (56.8)	19 (43.2)
2000 ≤ X < 3000	5 (100)	0 (0.0)	22 (27.5)	58 (72.5)
3000 ≤ X < 4000	3 (33.3)	6 (66.7)	20 (29.9)	47 (70.1)
4000 ≤ X < 5000	0 (0.0)	1 (100)	11 (31.4)	24 (68.6)
5000 ≤ X < 6000	1 (100)	0 (0.0)	10 (43.5)	13 (56.5)
6000 ≤ X < 7000	2 (100)	0 (0.0)	5 (55.6)	4 (44.4)
7000 ≤ X < 8000	0 (0.0)	2 (100)	0 (0.0)	4 (100)
8000 ≤ X < 9000	0 (0.0)	0 (0.0)	4 (44.4)	5 (55.6)
9000 ≤ X < 10000	0 (0.0)	0 (0.0)	0 (0.0)	4 (100)
10000 ≤X	1 (50.0)	1 (50.0)	2 (33.3)	4 (66.7

Table 7. Relationship between depth of submucosal invasion and DR in biopsy specimens of patients with SICRCs - retorospective study - (adapted from [23])

After retorospective study [22], same study group confirmed verification of patients SICRC with 112 nonpedunculated (non-Ip type) cases. Finally, nonpedunculated (non-Ip type) case of the prevalence of DR was significantly correlated with submucosal depth. The sensitivity and specificity of detection of DR for prediction of pSM2 (tumor invasion <1000 μm) in non-pedunculated SICRC were 68.6% and 92.0%, respectively.

Additionally, receiver operating characteristic (ROC), analysis confirmed 950 μm as the best diagnostic cut-off value of submucosal depth for DR detection, and 50 μm, which is the difference between the value of 950 μm as determined by cut off value (COV) and 1000 μm, the defining value of pSM2, is an acceptable measurement error range.

In statistics and diagnostic testing, positive predictive value (PPV) is the proportion of patients with positive test results who are correctly diagnosed, on the other hand, negative predictive value (NPV) is negative test results. Both of PPV and NPV are critical measure of the performance of a diagnostic method. In this studies revealed that PPV:0.93, NPV:0.59 in pedunculated and PPV:0.95, NPV:0.59 in nonpedunculated type. These results provide a basis for assessment of DR as a good indicator of pSM2. (Table 8).

Depth of submucosal invasion	Number of patients	DR–negative	DR–positive
pSM2	54	17	37
pM+ pSM1	27	24	3

pSM2, SM invasion ≧1000 μm; pM + pSM1, SM invasion < 1000 μm.

Sensitivity: (37/37+ 17) x 100 = 68.5%.

Specificity: (24/24+ 3) x 100 = 88.9%.

DR, desmoplastic reaction.

Depth of submucosal invasion	Number of patients	DR–negative	DR–positive
pSM2	51	16	35
pM+ pSM1	25	23	2

pSM2, SM invasion ≧1000 μm; pM + pSM1, SM invasion < 1000 μm.

Sensitivity: (35/35+ 16) x100 = 68.6%.

Specificity: (23/23+ 2) x 100 = 92.0%.

DR, desmoplastic reaction.

Table 8. Relationship between depth of submucosal invasion and DR in biopsy specimens of patients with pedunculated (upper part) and nonpedunculated (lower part) type - prospective study - (adapted from [22])

http://dx.doi.org/10.5772/51900

7. Conclusion

In this issue, we have discussed the a critical role of pathological assessment for T1 stage colorectal cancer, several problems related to the pathological diagnosis of early CRC at increased risk of lymph node metastasis and submucosal invasion. A new endoscopic systems which may prove to be reliable for detection of deep submucosal invasive CRC. Moreover, current endoscopic resection (EMR/ESD) have become useful for early CRC, but, these resection is applicable only to intramucosal carcinoma, and additional surgery is required if the resected lesion reveals submucosal invasion by pathological diagnosis, because prevalence rates of lymph node metastasis about 10% of all patients with submucosal invasive colorectal carcinoma.

We believe that curative endoscopic management for early CRC may be need to accurately pathological diagnosis of submucosal depth. Assessment of DR in pretreatment biopsy specimen nonpedunculated (non-Ip type) and submucosal depth with head invasion or stalk invasion in pedunculated (Ip type) for post endoscopic resection (EMR/ESD) specimen may be useful for the clinicopathological diagnosis of colorectal carcinoma with invasion into the submucosal layer.

Acknowledgment

The authors would like to thank member of Japanese Society for Cancer of the Colon and Recum; Professor Ajioka (Division of Molecular and Functional Pathology, Department of Cellular Function, Graduate School of Medical and Dental Sciences, Niigata University), Dr Ueno (Department of Surgery, National Defense Medical College, Saitama, Professer Ohkura (Department of Pathology, Kyorin University School of Medicine), Professor Kashida (Department of Gastroenterology and Hepatology, Faculty of Medicine, Kinki University), Professor Togashi (Department of Gastroenterology, Fukushima Prefectural Aizu General Hospital), Professor Yao (Department of Human Pathology, Juntendo University School of Medicine) Dr Wada (Department of Pathology, Juntendo Shizuoka Hospital of Juntendo University School of Medicine), Professor Watanabe (Department of Surgical Oncology The University of Tokyo), Dr Ochiai (Pathology Division, Research Center for Innovative Oncology, National Cancer Center Hospital East), Professor Sugai (Diagnostic Pathology, Iwate Medical University, Morioka), Professor Sugihara (Surgical Oncology, Tokyo Medical and Dental University). And we also thank Dr Fujii (Center for Gastrointestinal Endoscopy, Kyoto-Katsura Hospital) for his insightful comments. Moreover, the authors greatly thank Ms C. Sato -Matsuyama, A. Shimizu, M. Katayama, (Department of Surgical and Molecular Pathology, DOKKYO Medical University School of Medicine) for technical assistance and to Ms. S. Kidachi, A. Kikuchi (Department of Surgical and Molecular Pathology, DOKKYO Medical University School of Medicine) for secretarial assistance in preparing the manuscript.

This work was partially supported by the Grant-in-Aid for Scientific Research (C: No 18659101, 23590410) from the Ministry of Education, Culture, Sports, Science and Technology (MEXT) of Japan and DOKKYO Medical University Young Investigator Award (2009, 2011, 2012).

Author details

Shigeki Tomita, Kazuhito Ichikawa and Takahiro Fujimori

*Address all correspondence to: sstomita@dokkyomed.ac.jp

Department of Surgical and Molecular Pathology, DOKKYO Medical University School of Medicine, Tochigi, Japan

References

[1] Morson. BC, Whiteway JE, Jones EA, Macrae FA, Williams CB. Histopathology and prognosis of malignant colorectal polyps treated by endoscopic polypectomy. Gut 1984;25(5): 437-444.

[2] Fujimori T, Kawamata H, Kashida H. Precancerous lesions of the colorectum. Journal of gastroenterology 2001;36(9): 587-594.

[3] Kitajima K, Fujimori T, Fujii S, Takeda J, Ohkura Y, Kawamata H, Kumamoto T, Ishiguro S, Kato Y, Shimoda T, Iwashita A, Ajioka Y, Watanabe H, Watanabe T, Muto T, Nagasako K. Correlations between lymph node metastasis and depth of submucosal invasion in submucosal invasive colorectal carcinoma: a Japanese collaborative study. Journal of gastroenterology 2004;39(6): 534-543..

[4] Al Natour RH, Saund MS, Sanchez VM, Whang EE, Sharma AM, Huang Q, Boosalis VA, Gold JS. Tumor size and depth predict rate of lymph node metastasis in colon carcinoids and can be used to select patients for endoscopic resection. Journal of gastrointestinal surgery 2012;16(3): 595-602.

[5] Cooper HS. Surgical pathology of endoscopically removed malignant polyps of the colon and rectum. The American journal of surgical pathology 1983;7(7): 613-623.

[6] Minamoto T, Mai M, Ogino T, Sawaguchi K, Ohta T, Fujimoto T, Takahashi Y. Early invasive colorectal carcinomas metastatic to the lymph node with attention to their nonpolypoid development. The American journal of gastroenterology 1993;88(7): 1035-1039.

[7] Coverlizza S, Risio M, Ferrari A, Fenoglio-Preiser CM, Rossini FP. Colorectal adenomas containing invasive carcinoma: pathologic assessment of lymph node metastatic potential. Cancer 1989;64(9): 1937-1947.

[8] Netzer P, Forster C, Biral R, Ruchti C, Neuweiler J, Stauffer E, Schönegg R, Maurer C, Hüsler J, Halter F, Schmassmann A. Risk factor assessment of endoscopically removed malignant polyps. Gut 1998;43(5): 669-674.

[9] Haggitt RC, Glotzbach RE, Soffer EE, Wruble LD. Prognostic factors in colorectal carcinomas arising in adenomas: implications for lesions removed by endoscopic polypectomy. Gastroenterology 1985;89(2): 328-36.

[10] Pollard CW, Nivatvongs S, Rojanasakul A, Reiman HM, Dozois RR. The fate of patients following polypectomy alone for polyps containing invasive carcinoma. Diseases of the colon and rectum 1992;35(10): 933-937.

[11] Japanese Society for Cancer of the Colon and Rectum. Japanese Society for Cancer of the Colon and Rectum (JSCCR) guidelines 2005 for the treatment of colorectal cancer. In Japanease, Tokyo, Kanehara: 2005.

[12] Matsuda T, Fukuzawa M, Uraoka T, Nishi M, Yamaguchi Y, Kobayashi N, Ikematsu H, Saito Y, Nakajima T, Fujii T, Murakami Y, Shimoda T, Kushima R, Fujimori T. Risk of lymph node metastasis in patients with pedunculated type early invasive colorectal cancer: a retrospective multicenter study. Cancer science 2011;102(9): 1693-1697

[13] Watanabe T, Itabashi M, Shimada Y, Tanaka S, Ito Y, Ajioka Y, Hamaguchi T, Hyodo I, Igarashi M, Ishida H, Ishiguro M, Kanemitsu Y, Kokudo N, Muro K, Ochiai A, Oguchi M, Ohkura Y, Saito Y, Sakai Y, Ueno H, Yoshino T, Fujimori T, Koinuma N, Morita T, Nishimura G, Sakata Y, Takahashi K, Takiuchi H, Tsuruta O, Yamaguchi T, Yoshida M, Yamaguchi N, Kotake K, Sugihara K; Japanese Society for Cancer of the Colon and Rectum. Japanese Society for Cancer of the Colon and Rectum (JSCCR) guidelines 2010 for the treatment of colorectal cancer. International journal of clinical oncology 2012;17(1): 1-29.

[14] Prall F. Tumour budding in colorectal carcinoma. Histopathology 2007;50(1): 151-162.

[15] Ueno H, Murphy J, Jass JR, Mochizuki H, Talbot IC. Tumour 'budding' as an index to estimate the potential of aggressiveness in rectal cancer. Histopathology 2002;40(2): 127-132.

[16] Nakada I, Tasaki T, Ubukata H, Goto Y, Watanabe Y, Sato S, Tabuchi T, Tsuchiya A, Soma T. Desmoplastic response in biopsy specimens of early colorectal carcinoma is predictive of deep submucosal invasion. Diseases of the colon and rectum 1998;41(7): 896-900.

[17] Tsujino T, Seshimo I, Yamamoto H, Ngan CY, Ezumi K, Takemasa I, Ikeda M, Sekimoto M, Matsuura N, Monden M. Stromal myofibroblasts predict disease recurrence for colorectal cancer. Clinical cancer research 2007;13(7): 2082-2090.

[18] Ban S, Shimizu M. Muscularis mucosae in desmoplastic stroma formation of early invasive rectal adenocarcinoma. World journal of gastroenterology 2009;15(39): 4976-4979.

[19] Karagiannis GS, Petraki C, Prassas I, Saraon P, Musrap N, Dimitromanolakis A, Diamandis EP. Proteomic signatures of the desmoplastic invasion front reveal collagen

type XII as a marker of myofibroblastic differentiation during colorectal cancer metastasis. Oncotarget. 2012;3(3): 267-285.

[20] De Wever O, Demetter P, Mareel M, Bracke M. Stromal myofibroblasts are drivers of invasive cancer growth. International journal of cancer 2008;123(10): 2229-2238.

[21] Kimura R, Fujimori T, Ichikawa K, Ajioka Y, Ueno H, Ohkura Y, Kashida H, Togashi K, Yao T, Wada R, Watanabe T, Ochiai A, Sugai T, Sugihara K, Igarashi Y. Desmoplastic reaction in biopsy specimens of early colorectal cancer: A Japanese prospective multicenter study. Pathology international 2012;62(8): 525-531.

[22] Schmid SA, Dietrich A, Schulte S, Gaumann A, Kunz-Schughart LA. Fibroblastic reaction and vascular maturation in human colon cancers. International journal of radiation biology 2009;85(11): 1013-1025.

[23] Hirose M, Fukui H, Igarashi Y, Fujimori Y, Katake Y, Sekikawa A, Ichikawa K, Tomita S, Imura J, Ajioka Y, Ueno H, Hase K, Ohkura Y, Kashida H, Togashi K, Nishigami T, Matsui T, Yao T, Wada R, Matsuda K, Watanabe T, Ochiai A, Sugai T, Sugihara K, Fujimori T. Detection of desmoplastic reaction in biopsy specimens is useful for predicting the depth of invasion of early colorectal cancer: a Japanese collaborative study. Journal of gastroenterology 2010;45(12): 1212-1218.

Chapter 8

In vivo Optical Diagnosis of Polyp Histology: Can We Omit Pathological Examination of Diminutive Polyps?

Marco Bustamante-Balén

Additional information is available at the end of the chapter

http://dx.doi.org/10.5772/53205

1. Introduction

In the United States colorectal cancer (CRC) is the third more commonly diagnosed cancer in both sexes and it is also the third leading cause of cancer death among men and women [1]. In Europe CRC is the second leading cause of cancer death in both sexes [2]. These figures mean a heavy economic burden for any health system. The national cost of a year of CRC care in the United States has been estimated to be between \$4.5 and \$9.6 billion [3]. In Spain €180.6 million of annual loses in work productivity because of CRC have been reported [4].

Adenomatous polyps are the precursors of CRC in most of the cases. Through a progressive accumulation of mutations and following some of the described carcinogenetic pathways [5], a benign adenomatous polyp develops into an advanced adenoma with high-grade dysplasia (HGD) and then progresses to invasive cancer (Figure 1). Invasive cancers confined to the wall of the colon (TNM stages I and II) are curable by surgery while more advanced cancers are treated by a combination of surgery and chemotherapy.

Detecting cancer at an early stage or, even better, diagnosing and resecting adenomas before a carcinoma has developed improves outcomes. This was first confirmed in the initial report of the National Polyp Study [6] which showed a reduction in the incidence of colorectal cancer of around 76% in patients in which a polypectomy had been performed. Recently, the same group has described in the same cohort of patients a reduction in mortality of 53% in the long term [7]. This is the rationale for population-based screening programs, designed to detect advanced adenomas and CRC at an early and curable stage. For instance, recently the results of a nationwide screening colonoscopy program in Germany have been reported of a nationwide screening colonoscopy program in Germany, showing that 69.6% of diagnosed CRC were stages I and II [8]. Therefore, screening for CRC with removal of adenomas and surveillance colonoscopy of patients who have been treated for adenomas or CCR is recommended by Professional Societies and authorities [9-11]. Surveillance intervals after resection of one or more adenomas are planned based primarily in the number, size and presence of advanced histological features [12]. Polyps larger than 10 mm, with villous component (> 25%) or with high-grade dysplasia are considered advanced adenomas and have a greater tendency to malignancy [13]. Detection and resection of these advanced adenomas is the main objective of the surveillance programs [14,15]. Therefore, submitting all resected polyps to pathologic evaluation is the standard of care.

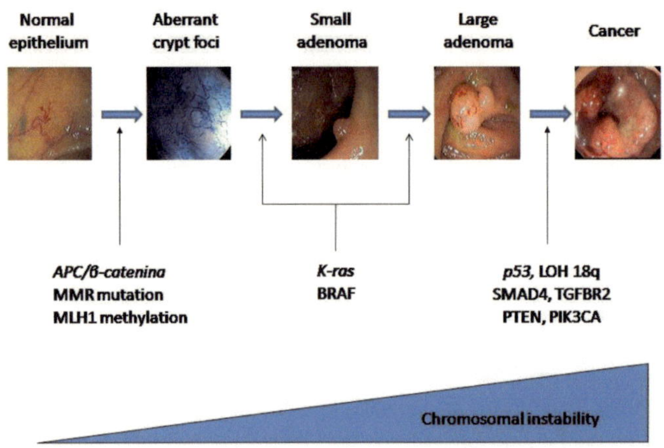

Figure 1. Development of CRC from normal tissue to adenocarcinoma

However, most of the adenomas diagnosed in colonoscopies are 5 mm or less (diminutive polyps). In symptomatic patients the proportion of adenomas larger than 10 mm is between 5 and 15% [16-18]. A report from our group using chromoendoscopy to improve the adenoma detection rate showed that 73% of adenomas were < 5 mm [19]. This is also the situation in screening colonoscopy, with reported proportions of adenomas < 5 mm of around 80% [20]. A significant proportion of diminutive polyps, between 23% and 40%, are not even adenomas [21-24]. Overall, the prevalence of advanced histology in diminutive polyps seems low, although there is some heterogeneity in the literature due to different inclusion criteria (screening versus symptomatic patients; patients only with polyps less than a specific size, etc.), differences in the performed analysis (per-patient, per-polyp) and probably also due to the variability in the pathologic interpretation of dysplasia and proportion of villous component (table 1).

A recent systematic review with stringent inclusion criteria (average-risk asymptomatic population, clear definition of advanced adenoma, definition of the method adopted to assess polyp size, reported prevalence of advanced adenomas according to polyp size, and at least 500 subjects included) showed that the prevalence of advanced lesions among patients whose largest polyp was diminutive (≤ 5 mm), small (6-9 mm) and large (≥ 10 mm) was 0.9%, 4.9% and 73.5% respectively [27]. The most recent study on this topic, a retrospective review of data from three prospective clinical trials has shown that the prevalence of advanced histological features in diminutive polyps is 0.5%.

Study (n patients)	AA ≤ 5 mm	AA 6-9 mm	AA ≥10 mm	HGD ≤ 5 mm	HGD 6-9 mm	HGD ≥10 mm
Unal [22] (n = 5087)	32 (0.6%)	12 (0.2%)	NA	-	-	-
Tsai [21] (n = 5087)	105 (2.1%)	67 (1.3%)	76 (1.5%)	2 (0.04%)	1 (0.02%)	0
Bretagne [25] (n = 2294)	-	-	-	6 (0.26%)	19 (0.82%)	227 (9.9%)
Lieberman [26] (n = 13992)	45 (0.3%)	62 (0.4%)	737 (5.3%)	1 (0.007%)	9 (0.06%)	45 (0.3%)
Gupta [23] (n = 1150)	3 (0.26%)	3 (0.26%)	6 (0.5%)	1 (0.08%)	0	1 (0.08%)

Table 1. Absolute prevalence of advanced adenomas according to the largest polyp size. AA: advanced adenoma; HGD: high-grade dysplasia; NA: non-applicable

Moreover, it remains unclear the practical role of advanced histological features in assessing the individual risk of CRC and in planning the management of patients with colonic polyps. First, there is a substantial interobserver variability in the diagnosis of the villous component and even HGD, with kappa index ranging from 0.35 to 0.48 and 0.38 to 0.69 respectively [28,29]. This problem may be even greater in polyps less than 10 mm [30]. Second, it is not clear that villous component or HGD are independent predictors of the subsequent development of advanced adenomas during follow-up. In the case of villous component the published studies do not separately identify patients whose most advanced polyp is a tubulovillous or villous adenoma < 10 mm in size, therefore the risk of this subgroup of polyps cannot be accurately assessed [31]. High grade dysplasia has not been shown to be an independent risk factor for metachronous advanced neoplasm in the NCI Pooling Project after adjustments for size and histology [32].

Taking all these data as a whole it appears clear that the standard practice of submitting all diminutive polyps found in colonoscopy to pathological assessment may have little clinical impact on the management of patients, and may result in substantial costs. Waiting for the pathological report may induce a delay in informing the patient and in recommending the next colonoscopy surveillance interval. In this context, some authors are recommending a "resect and discard" strategy to be applied to diminutive polyps found anywhere in the colorectum. Following this strategy the histology of a diminutive polyp would be assessed by an appropriate endoscopic method, the assessment would be recorded by means of a high-resolution photograph and the polyp then would be resected and discarded. The endoscopic assessment of histology would be used to make an immediate recommendation regarding the next colonoscopy surveillance interval. Finally, when multiple diminutive rectosigmoid hyperplastic polyps are suspected endoscopically, histology can be established by real-time endoscopic assessment and documented by photography without the need of resection and pathological evaluation [33].

2. Endoscopic assessment of polyp histology

The key factor in adopting the "resect and discard" strategy is the endoscopic evaluation of polyp histology, since this information is necessary to plan the next surveillance interval. Moreover, the presence of suspicious endoscopic features may prompt a polyp to be submitted to pathologic assessment. Therefore, a reliable endoscopic method of evaluating histology is needed.

In recent years several imaging-enhancing technologies have emerged as an adjuvant for diagnosing and evaluating colorectal lesions [34]. High-resolution and magnification endoscopes allow enlarging the image and discriminating details. These endoscopes are often used in combination with chromoendoscopy, which involves the topical application of dyes at the time of endoscopy to enhance tissue characterization. Narrow-band imaging (NBI) is a technology that applies narrow-bandwidth filters to white light endoscopy allowing discrimination of mucosal vascular net. Fuji Intelligent Color Enhancement (FICE) and i-Scan are based on the same physical principles as NBI but are not depending on optical filters but on a postprocessing image system. All these technologies have been evaluated in the prediction of histology of colon polyps.

2.1. High-resolution/magnification endoscopy and chromoendoscopy

The usefulness of this technology in assessing histology is based on the pit-pattern classification proposed by Kudo which is intended to differentiate between non-neoplastic, neoplastic and malignant polyps. Following this classification patterns I and II correspond to non-neoplastic lesions and patterns III to V to neoplastic ones. Type V suggests malignant transformation [35].

Several large case series evaluate the utility of pit-pattern analysis to differentiate neoplastic from non-neoplastic lesions. Generally speaking, positive predictive values (PPV) for neoplastic lesion range between 70 to 100% and negative predictive values (NPV) between 70 and 99%. Studies with the largest number of lesions show an overall accuracy of 80-95% [36-38]. One study focused in diminutive lesions, reported an overall accuracy of 95% [39]. There are also some randomized controlled trials comparing magnification plus chromoendoscopy to conventional chromoendoscopy. Konishi et al. [40] showed an accuracy of magnification colonoscopy in distinguishing non-neoplastic from neoplastic lesions < 10 mm in size of 92% vs 68% for conventional chromoendoscopy. Emura el al. [41] using a similar design showing an overall accuracy of 95% vs 84%. These figures were similar whenthe subgroup of lesions ≤ 5 mm was analyzed. Conventional colonoscopy, chromoendoscopy and magnification chromoendoscopy were compared in the study by Fu et al. [42], and the latter was found to have the highest accuracy (95.6%).

Magnification chromoendoscopy has also been evaluated in the prediction of malignant histology and invasive depth of cancer with variable results. Overall, it seems that its sensitivity and accuracy are lower. For instance, Bianco et al. [43] showed that endoscopic differentiation between invasive and noninvasive neoplasm had a PPV of 79% and a NPV of 95%. Hurlstone et al. reported an accuracy of 78% and a specificity of 50% [44]. Some authors use a modification of the Kudo classification with different subtypes of the type V pattern that may be quite cumbersome to use [45].

In conclusion, high-magnification chromoendoscopy allows the prediction of histology even in small and diminutive lesions, but is better differentiating nonneoplastic from neoplastic lesions than differentiating invasive from noninvasive neoplasms. Moreover, it must be kept in mind that overall accuracy is not 100%, despite the fact that a technology with a NPV of 95% for adenomatous histology fulfils the PIVI criteria for leaving suspected rectosigmoid hyperplastic polyps ≤ 5 mm in size in place [33].

2.2. Narrow-band imaging

2.2.1. Predicting histology by means of vascular features

Angiogenesis is a main step in the progression of neoplasms; therefore the diagnosis based on vascular morphological changes seems ideal for early detection and diagnosis of colon neoplasms. NBI enhances the visibility of the capillary network on the surface layer of the mucosa.

Normal mucosa displays a regular hexagonal or honeycomb-like pattern of capillary vessels around the crypt of the gland. This capillary meshwork, named meshed capillary (MC), is invisible or faintly visible (Figure 2a). In the neoplastic lesion, vessels grow thicker, with increasing diameter size, disruption and rise of vessel density as the lesion progresses. Therefore, recognizing the lesion becomes easier because it appears as a brownish area (Figure 2b).

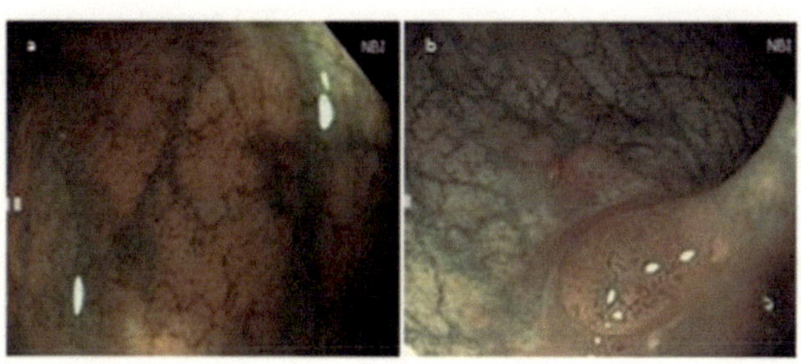

Figure 2. NBI image of normal mucosa (a) and a diminutive adenoma (b)

Several studies have evaluated the performance of NBI in characterizing colorectal lesions, focusing in the characteristics of the vascular capillary network. Generally speaking, NBI sensitivity and specificity for diagnosing neoplastic lesions ranges between 77% and 99% and 59 – 100% respectively (table 2). This heterogeneity may be explained by the use of different descriptions of vascular networks. Examples are, brown blob or dense vascular network to predict neoplasia [46-48]; fine capillary network, dark dots, light rounds, tubular or gyrus like [49]; microvessel thickness (invisible, thin, thick) and microvessel irregularity (invisible, regular, mildly irregular, severely irregular) [50]; vascular patter intensity (weaker, the same or darker than the surrounding mucosa) [51]; fine vascular network or dilated corkscrew type vessels and abnormal branching patterns [52]; and finally, capillary pattern (CP type I: invisible or faintly visible, CP type II: capillaries elongated and thicker and CP type III: capillaries of irregular sizes, thicker and branched) [53-55].Other causes of heterogeneity are the use of magnification or high-resolution endoscopes since the results with the latter are not as encouraging (see section 2.2.5) [46,49,56], and finally, better results are reported by experts.

2.2.2. Predicting histology by means of pit pattern evaluation

Most of the published studies, mainly from Japan, use optical magnification in combination with NBI, and the performance of pit pattern analysis with NBI ha salso been assessed (table 3). Sensitivity for neoplastic lesion ranges between 86 and 100%, while specificity ranges between 84 and 100%. Some studies have compared NBI with chromoendoscopy showing similar diagnostic accuracy, suggesting that NBI could replace chromoendoscopy in the diagnostic evaluation of colon lesions [46, 47, 52]. However, the original pit pattern classification was not designed for NBI, and has not been validated for this purpose. NBI fundamentals are different that those of chromoendoscopy. The latter uses dyes that lie inside the pits or stain their edges depending on the stain used while NBI highlights the capillary plexus that surrounds the opening of each pit. Machida et al. [57] described the use of NBI with magnification for pit pattern classification, showing that NBI was superior to conventional colonoscopy for pit pattern delineation but inferior to chromoendoscopy. The correlation between pit pattern analysis using chromoendoscopy and NBI is far from perfect especially for the pattern with the upmost clinical importance, type V. A study compared the pit pattern analysis obtained by NBI with stereoscopic examination and showed that the correlation was only 57% for type V_N[58]. East et al. [51] found a kappa score of only 0.23 between both types of pit pattern evaluation. Better results were obtained by Hirata et al. [48] (78% of agreement for pit pattern V_I and 100% for V_N).

Author	Mag	Patients/ Lesions	Sensitivity (%)	Specificity (%)	PPV (%)	NPV (%)	DA (%)
Su [47]	Yes	78/110	96	87	93	92	92
Tischendorf [52]	Yes	99/200	94	89	94	89	92
East [51] [a]	Yes	30/33	77-91	50-60	-	-	69-81

Author	Mag	Patients/ Lesions	Sensitivity (%)	Specificity (%)	PPV (%)	NPV (%)	DA (%)
Chiu [46][a]	Yes/No	133/180	87-95	88-72	96-92	67-80	87-90
Sano [53]	Yes	92/150	96	92	97	90	95
Hirata [50]	Yes	163/189	99	90	99	90	98
Hirata [48]	Yes	99/148	99	94	99	94	99
Rastogi [49]	No	40/123	96	86	90	95	92
Kanao [55]	Yes	223/289	95	100	100	20	99
Henry [54]	No	42/126	93	88	909	91	91
Ignjatovic [56]	Yes/No	48/80	93-74	59-56	-	-	76-85

Table 2. Vascular pattern analysis with NBI for prediction of adenomatous histology. Mag: use of optical magnification; PPV: positive predictive value; NPV: negative predictive value; DA: diagnostic accuracy. [a]Two observers. Values for each observer are shown.

Author	Mag	Patients/ Lesions	Sensitivity (%)	Specificity (%)	PPV (%)	NPV (%)	DA (%)
Machida [57]	Yes	34/43	100	75	91	100	93
East [51][a]	Yes	20/33	86-77	80-60	-	-	84-72
Tischendorf [52]	Yes	99/200	90	89	93	84	90
Van den Broek [59]	Yes	100/208	90	70	69	90	78

Table 3. Pit pattern analysis with NBI for prediction of adenomatous histology [a]Two observers. Values for each observer are shown. Mag: use of optical magnification; PPV: positive predictive value; NPV: negative predictive value; AC: diagnostic accuracy.

A systematic review which included 6 reports published until 2008 comparing NBI (pit pattern and vascular assessment) and chromoendoscopy showed a pooled sensitivity, specificity and overall accuracy of 92%, 86% and 89% respectively [60].

2.2.3. *Predicting submucosal invasion*

NBI has also been evaluated to diagnose early colorectal neoplasia and submucosal invasion. Katagiri et al. [61] used the capillary pattern classification in colon adenomas. Those showing CP type III harbored HGD or invasive cancer. In a recent report this group further developed this classification expanding CP type III in group IIIA (visible microvascular architecture and high microvessel density with lack of uniformity, branching and curtailed irregularity) and group IIIB (nearly avascular or loose microvascular area). This detailed classification allowed differentiation between lesions with Sm1 submucosal invasion from Sm2-Sm3 with a sensitivity, specificity and diagnostic accuracy of 84.8%, 88.7% and 87.7% respectively [62]. Hirata et al.[50] found that the accuracy of diagnosis of submucosal massive invasion on the basis of thick and severely irregular vascular pattern was 100%. Kanao et al. [55] used a combination of capillary pattern and pit pattern and showed that lesions with irregular microvessels with variable sizes and distribution, and pit absence with avascular areas harbored more often massive submucosal invasion.

2.2.4. NBI compared with other diagnostic modalities

NBI has been compared with other image enhancing technologies, most frequently with chromoendoscopy. Overall, the diagnostic accuracy of NBI is better than that of conventional colonoscopy and equivalent to that of chromoendoscopy (figure 3) [46,47,52], especially if vascular assessment rather than pit pattern is used [51].

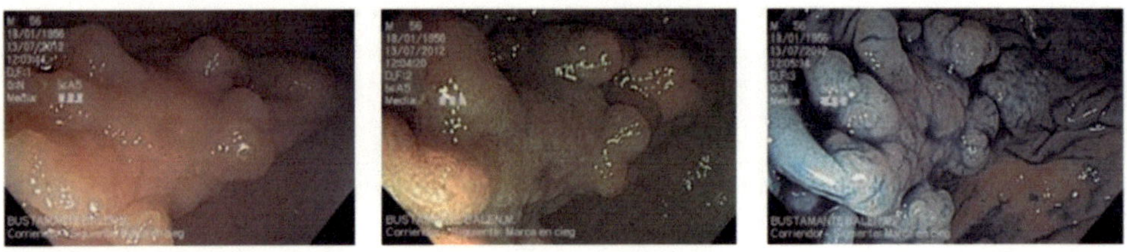

Figure 3. Invasive carcinoma in a depressed lesion observed with white light (a), NBI (b), and chromoendoscopy (c)

Four recent studies perform an evaluation of endoscopic trimodal imaging (high-resolution endoscopy, autofluorescence imaging and NBI) for colonic polyp characterization. Three studies from the same group show a poor diagnostic accuracy for NBI without magnification and autofluorescence with similar sensitivity but worse specificity [59,63,64]. Ignjatovic et al. [56] reported that NBI with magnification appeared to have the best accuracy, albeit modest and not adequate for in vivo diagnosis.

2.2.5. NBI without optical magnification

Most of the studies on prediction of histology using NBI have been carried out in Japan using Olympus equipments with optical magnification (Lucera), a feature not included in high-resolution systems (Exera) available in the USA and in continental Europe. Most of the capillary pattern descriptions or classifications have been designed using optical magnification, therefore are not directly applicable to high-resolution examinations. That is also the case for the Kudo´s pit pattern classification.

The results of NBI without optical magnification in predicting histology are variable with authors showing an accuracy similar to that of optical magnification NBI and authors obtaining worse results [56]. Again, different definitions for a vascular pattern typical of adenoma (table 4) may account for these discrepancies. None of these classifications have been appropriately validated and its reproducibility in different clinical settings is unknown.

http://dx.doi.org/10.5772/53205

Author	Predictive of adenoma	Predictive of hyperplastic
Rastogi [49, 65, 66]	Round/oval pattern (dark outer and a lighter central area) Tubulogyrus pattern	Fine capillary network alone but absent mucosal pattern Circular pattern with dots (central dark area surrounded by a lighter area)
Rex [67]	Overall brown color Short thick blood vessels Tubular or oval pits, variable size pits Central brown depression Straight blood vessels around pits forming rectangles, pentagons, etc.	Bland, featureless appearance Pattern of black dots surrounded by white Thin blood vessels coursing across polyp surface, and not surrounding pits
Rogart [68]	Modified Kudo´s classification	Vascular color intensity (light, medium, dark)
Sikka [69]	Neoplastic pit pattern (elongation of crypts, cerebriform pattern) Increased vascular markins	Non-neoplastic pit pattern (circular pit pattern) No vascular markins

Table 4. Prediction of histology using NBI without magnification

The group of the Indiana University has very recently designed a simple classification for determination of polyp histology (NICE classification) and has validated it for its use by experienced and non-experienced examinators (table 5) [70]. Further studies are needed to evaluate the reproducibility of this classification in real-time endoscopy.

2.2.6. Prediction of histology of diminutive polyps

Some authors have evaluated de diagnostic accuracy of NBI on diminutive polyps showing similar results to those on polyps of any size. In a study by Rex [67] the sensitivity of NBI in diagnosing adenomas was 92%, specificity 87%, PPV was 88%, NPV 91% and accuracy 89%. Grading the confidence on the endoscopic diagnosis in high and low, high confidence predictions of adenomas were correct in 92% of polyps and in 91% of ≤ 5 mm polyps. The equivalent figures for hyperplastic prediction were 95%. The same group evaluated the performance of NBI in real time for distal colorectal polyps, and showed a sensitivity of 96%, a specificity of 99.4%, and NPV and PPV of 99.4% and 96% respectively [71]. The authors concluded that NBI is sufficiently accurate to allow distal hyperplastic polyps to be left in place without resection and small, distal adenomas to be discarded without pathologic assessment. In the study of Henry et al. [54] the sensitivity for predicting histology was 87%, specificity was 93%, PPV was 89%, NPV was 91% and overall accuracy was 90%. Paggy et al. [72] found similar results both in the whole group of < 10 mm polyps and in diminutive polyps. Other authors have not showed as good results [56,73]. The most recent report using the NICE classification found an accuracy of 89%, sensitivity of 98% and a NPV of 95%. In conclusion, diagnostic accuracy of endoscopic prediction of histology of diminutive polyps seems equivalent to that of larger polyps, at least in expert hands.

NICE criterion	Type 1	Type 2
Color	Same or lighter than background	Browner relative to background
Vessels	None, or isolated lacy vessels coursing across the lesion	Brown vessels surrounding white structures
Surface pattern	Dark or white spots of uniform size, or homogeneous abscence of pattern	Oval, tubular, or branched white structures surrounded by brown vessels
Most likely pathology	Hyperplastic	Adenoma

Table 5. The NBI International colorectal endoscopic (NICE) classification

2.2.7. Learning NBI. Does expertise matters?

Most of the published studies have been performed by experts endoscopists, both in Japan and in Western countries. Reliable information about reproducibility of this results is lacking. Moreover, the overall accuracy in prediction of histology es markedly influenced by expertise in NBI interpretation, as has been shown in a study performed in a non academic setting in which sensitivity for high-confidence prediction was 77% and specificity 78% [73]. Experts have been shown to perform better than non-experts and with a higher interobserver agreement [74]. Fortunately, NBI interpretation of histology can be easily learned. Several studies have shown significant improvements in diagnostic accuracy and in interobserver agreement after following a computer-based training module [75] or a short teaching session [76].

2.3. Fujinon intelligent color enhancement system (FICE) and i-Scan

FICE also narrowes the bandwidth of light components using a computed spectral estimation technology that aritmetically processes the reflected photons to reconstitute virtual images for a choice of different wavelenghts [77]. Therefore, it no depends on optical filters to modify the image. There are less studies using FICE or i-Scan than NBI but its accuracy seems broadly similar.

In the study by Pohl et al. [77] FICE (with set 4 activated) was used to identify the pit pattern and the vascular pattern intensity in a similar way to NBI. The sensitivity and specificity of FICE for the prediction of adenoma was 93.2% and 61.2%, figures similar to those of chromoendoscopy. Parra et al. [78] showed that FICE performance in predicting histology was inferior to that of chromoendoscopy with magnification. Kim et al. [80] reported that FICE with magnification was better than without magnification especially for diminutive polyps [79]. Regarding i-Scan, a study compared this technology with NBI for histology prediction of diminutive polyps and showed a similar performance with good agreement between the two modalities (kappa index > 0.7).

http://dx.doi.org/10.5772/53205

3. Conclusion

New image-enhancing technologies may allow in vivo histological assessment of colorectal polyps, avoiding the need to pathological evaluation of all resected polyps. This would represent substantial savings and a more direct planning of surveillance intervals [81]. However, there are several steps to achieve before the resect and discard strategy is widely implemented. First a more simple, reproducible and validated way of characterize colon lesions is needed, especially in community practice. Learning the technique is also crucial because when learning curve is achieved NBI performs significantly better [68]. Moreover, implementing PIVI guidelines [33] implies accepting a 10% rate of false negative when in vivo assessing histology of rectal polyps. Endoscopists may feel more comfortable with a much lower rate before leaving polyps behind. Finally, if in vivo histology is applied in daily practice this represents a turning point in the management of colon polyps, which must be supported by Professional Societies.

In vivo histology seems here to stay, but we are still at the beginning of the way. Improvement in equipments and development of new technologies will help the medical community to take this step forward.

Author details

Marco Bustamante-Balén*

Address all correspondence to: mbustamantebalen@gmail.com

EndoscopyUnit. University Hospital La Fe.Valencia, Spain

References

[1] Siegel, R., Naishadham, D., & Jemal, A. (2012). Cancer Statistics . *CA Cancer J Clin*, 62, 10-29.

[2] Ferlay, J., Autier, P., Boniol, M., Heanue, M., Colombet, M., & Boyle, P. (2007). Estimates of the cancer incidence and mortality in Europe in 2006. *Ann Oncol*, 18, 581-92.

[3] Gellad, Z. F., & Provenzale, D. (2010). Colorectal cancer: national and international perspective on the burden of the disease and public health impact. *Gastroenterology*, 138, 2177-90.

[4] Oliva, J., Lobo, F., López-Bastida, J., Zozaya, N., & Romay, R. Pérdidas de productividad laboral ocasionadas por los tumores en España. http://docubib.uc3m.es/working-papers/DE/de050402.pdf.

[5] Markowitz, S. D., & Bertagnolli, M. M. (2009). Molecular bases of colorectal cancer. *N Engl J Med*, 361, 2449-60.

[6] Winawer, S. J., Zauber, A. G., Ho, N. M., O', Brien. M. J., Gottlieb, L. S., Sternberg, S. S., et al. (1993). Prevention of colorectal cancer by colonoscopic polypectomy. *N Engl J Med*, 329, 1977-81.

[7] Zauber, A. G., Winawer, S. J., O' Brien, MJ, Lansdorp-Vogelaar, I., van Ballegooijen, M., Hankey, B. F., et al. (2012). Colonoscopy polypectomy and long-term prevention of colorectal-cancer deaths. *N Engl J Med*, 366, 687-96.

[8] Pox, CP, Altenhofen, L., Brenner, H., Theilmeier, A., Von Stillfried, D., & Schmiegel, W. (2012). Efficacy of a nationwide screening colonoscopy program for colorectal cancer. *Gastroenterology*, 142, 1460-7.

[9] Lieberman, D. A., Rex, D. K., Winawer, S. J., Giardello, F. M., Johnson, D. A., & Levin, T. R. (2012). Guidelines for colonoscopy surveillance after screening and polypectomy: a consensus update by the US Multi-Society Task Force on colorectal cancer. *Gastroenterology*, 143, 844-57.

[10] Rex, D. K., Johnson, D. A., Anderson, J. C., Schoenfeld, P. S., Burke, C. A., & Inadomi, J. M. (2009). American College of Gastroenterology guidelines for colorectal cancer screening 2008. *Am J Gastroenterol*, 104, 739-50.

[11] European guidelines for quality assurance in colorectal cancer screening and diagnosis. (2012). First edition., http://screening.iarc.fr/doc/ND3210390ENC.pdf, Accesed: June.

[12] Winawer, S. J., Zauber, A. G., Fletcher, R. H., Stillman, J. S., O' Brien, M. J., Levin, B., et al. (2006). Guidelines for colonoscopic surveillance after polypectomy: a consensus update by the US Multi-Society Task Force on colorectal cancer and the American Cancer Society. *Gastroenterology*, 130, 1872-85.

[13] O' Brien, MJ, Winawer, S. J., Zauber, A. G., Gottlieb, L. S., Sternberg, S. S., Diaz, B., et al. (1990). The National Polyp Study. Patient and polyp characteristics associated with high-grade dysplasia in colorectal adenomas. *Gastroenterology*, 98, 371-9.

[14] Guía de práctica clínica sobre prevención del cáncer colorrectal. (2009). Actualización. *Asociación Española de Gastroenterología.*, http://www.guiasgastro.net/cgi-bin/wdbcgi.exe/gastro/guia_completa.portada?pident=4, Accessed: June.

[15] NCCN Clinical practice guidelines in oncology. (2012). Colorectal cancer screening. Version 2.2012. In: , http://www.nccn.org/professionals/physician_gls/pdf/colorectal_screening.pdf, Accessed: October.

[16] Rex, D. K., Cutler, C. S., Lemmel, G. T., Rahmani, E. Y., Clark, D. W., Helper, D. J., et al. (1997). Colonoscopic miss rates of adenomas determined by back-to-back colonoscopies. *Gastroenterology*, 112, 24-8.

[17] Sanaka, M. R., Deepinder, F., Thota, P., Lopez, R., & Burke, CA. (2009). Adenomas are detected more often in morning than in afternoon colonoscopy. *Am J Gastroenterol*, 104, 1659-64.

[18] Kaltenbach, T., Friedland, S., & Soetikno, R. (2008). A randomised tandem colonoscopy trial of narrow band imaging versus white light examination to compare neoplasia miss rates. *Gut*, 57, 1406-12.

[19] Bustamante-Balén, M., Bernet, L., Cano, R., Pertejo, V., & Ponce, J. (2010). Prevalence of nonpolypoid colorectal neoplasms in symptomatic patients scheduled for colonoscopy. A study with total colonic chromoscopy. *J Clin Gastroenterol*, 44, 280-5.

[20] Rex, D. K., & Helbig, C. C. (2007). High yields of small and flat adenomas with high-definition colonoscopes using either white light or narrow band imaging. *Gastroenterology*, 133, 42-7.

[21] Tsai, F. C., & Strum, W. B. (2011). Prevalence of advanced adenomas in small and diminutive colon polyps using direct measurement of size. *Dig Dis Sci*, 56, 2394-8.

[22] Unal, H., Selcuk, H., Gokcan, H., Tore, E., Sar, A., Korkmaz, M., et al. (2007). Malignancy risk of small polyps and related factors. *Dig Dis Sci*, 52, 2796-9.

[23] Gupta, N., Bansal, A., Rao, D., Early, DS, Jonnalagadda, S., Wani, S. B., et al. (2012). Prevalence of advanced histological features in diminutive and small colonic polyps. *Gastrointest Endosc*, 75, 1022-30.

[24] Chaput, U., Alberto, S. F., Terris, B., Beuvon, F., Audureau, E., Coriat, R., et al. (2011). Risk factors for advanced adenomas amongst small and diminutive colorectal polyps: a prospective monocenter study. *Dig Liv Dis*, 609-12.

[25] Bretagne, J. F., Manfredi, S., Piette, C., Hamonic, S., Durand, G., Riou, F., et al. (2010). Yield of high-grade dysplasia based on polyp size detected at colonoscopy: a series of 2295 examinations following a positive fecal occult blood test in a population-based study. *Dis Colon Rectum*, 53, 339-45.

[26] Lieberman, D., Moravec, M., Holub, J., Michaels, L., & Eisen, G. (2008). Polyp size and advanced histology in patients undergoing colonoscopy screening: implications for CT colonography. *Gastroenterology*, 135, 1100-5.

[27] Hassan, C., Pickhardt, P. J., Kim, D. H., Di Giulio, E., Laghi, A., Recipi, A., et al. (2010). Systematic review: distribution of advanced neoplasia according to polyp size at screening colonoscopy. *Aliment Pharmacol Ther*, 31, 210-7.

[28] Rex, D. K., Alikhan, M., Cummings, O., & Ulbright, T. M. (1999). Accuracy of pathological interpretation of colorectal polyps by general pathologists in community practice. *Gastrointest Endosc*, 50, 468-74.

[29] Terry, M. B., Neugut, A. I., Bostick, R. M., Potter, J. D., Haile, R. W., & Fenoglio-Preiser, C. M. (2002). Reliability in the classification of advanced colorectal adenomas. *Cancer Epidemiol Biomarkers Prev*, 11, 660-3.

[30] van Putten, P. G., Hol, L., van Dekken, H., Han van, Krieken. J., van Ballegooijen, M., Kuipers, E. J., et al. (2011). Inter-observer variation in the histological diagnosis of polyps in colorectal cancer screening. *Histopathology*, 58, 974-81.

[31] Lieberman, D. A., Rex, D. K., Winawer, S. J., Giardello, F. M., Johnson, D. A., & Levin, T. R. (2012). Guidelines for colonoscopy surveillance after screening and polypectomy: a consensus update by the US Multi-Society Task Force on colorectal cancer. *Gastroenterology*, 143, 844-57.

[32] Martinez, M. E., Baron, J. A., Lieberman, D. A., Schatzkin, A., Lanza, E., Winawer, S. J., et al. (2009). A pooled analysis of advanced colorectal neoplasia diagnosis following colonoscopicpolypectomy. *Gastroenterology*, 136, 832-41.

[33] Rex, D. K., Kahl, C., O′ Brien, M., Levin, T. R., Pohl, H., Rastogi, A., et al. (2011). The American Society for Gastrointestinal Endoscopy PIVI (Preservation and Incorporation of Valuable Endoscopic Innovations) on real-time endoscopic assessment of the histology of diminutive colorectal polyps. *Gastrointest Endosc*, 73, 419-22.

[34] Pellisé, M., Tasende, JD, Balaguer, F., Bustamante-Balén, M., Herraiz, M., Herreros de Tejada, A., et al. (2012). Technical review of advanced diagnostic endoscopy in patients at high risk of colorectal cancer. *Gastroenterol Hepatol*, 35, 278-92.

[35] Kudo, S., Hirota, S., Nakakima, T., Hosobe, S., Kusaka, H., Kobayashi, T., et al. (1994). Colorectal tumors and pit pattern. *J Clin Pathol*, 47, 880-5.

[36] Eisen, G. M., Kim, C. Y., Fleisher, D. E., Kozarek, R. A., Carr-Locke, D. L., Li, T. C. M., et al. (2002). High-resolution chromendoscopy for classifying colonic polyps: a multicenter study. *Gastrointest Endosc*, 55, 687-94.

[37] Hurlstone, D. P., Cross, S. S., Adam, I., Shorthouse, A. J., Brown, S., Sanders, DS, et al. (2004). Efficacy of high magnification chromoscopic colonoscopy for the diagnosis of neoplasia in flat and depressed lesions of the colorectum: a prospective analysis. *Gut*, 53, 284-90.

[38] Kiesslich, R., von Bergh, M., Hahn, M., Hermann, G., & Jung, M. (2001). Chromoendoscopy with indigocarmine improves the detection of adenomatous and nonadenomatous lesions in the colon. *Endoscopy*, 33, 1001-6.

[39] De Palma, G., Rega, M., Masone, S., Persico, M., Siciliano, S., Addeo, P., et al. (2006). Conventional colonoscopy and magnified chromoendoscopy for the endoscopic histological prediction of diminutive colorectal polyps: a single operator study. *World J Gastroenterol*, 12, 2402-5.

[40] Konishi, K., Kaneko, K., Kurahashi, T., Yamamoto, T., Kushima, M., Kanda, A., et al. (2003). A comparison of magnifying and nonmagnifiying colonoscopy for the diagnosis of colorectal polyps: a prospective study. *Gastrointest Endosc*, 57, 48-53.

[41] Emura, F., Saito, Y., Taniguchi, M., Fujii, T. K., Tagawa, K., & Yamakado, M. (2007). Further validation of magnifying chromocolonoscopy for differentiating colorectal neoplastic polyps in a health screening center. *J Gastroenterol Hepatol*, 22, 1722-7.

[42] Fu, K. I., Sano, Y., Kato, S., Fujii, T., Nagashima, F., Yoshino, T., Okuno, T., et al. (2004). Chromoendoscopy using indigo carmine dye sprying with magnifying observation is the most reliable method for differential diagnosis between non-neoplastic and neoplastic colorectal lesions: a prospective study. *Endoscopy*, 36, 1089-93.

[43] Bianco, MA, Rotondano, G., Marmo, R., Garofano, M. L., Piscopo, R., de Gregorio, A., et al. (2006). Predictive value of magnification chromoendoscopy for diagnosing invasive neoplasia in nonpolypoid colorectal lesions and stratifying patients for endoscopic resection or surgery. *Endoscopy*, 38, 470-6.

[44] Hurlstone, D. P., Cross, S. S., Adam, I., Shorthouse, A. J., Brown, S., Sanders, DS, et al. (2004). Endoscopic morphological anticipation of submucosal invasion in flat and depressed colorectal lesions: clinical implications and subtype analysis of the Kudo type V pit pattern using high-magnification-chromoscopic colonoscopy. *Colorectal Dis*, 6, 369-75.

[45] Nagata, S., Tanaka, S., Haruma, K., Yoshihara, M., Sumii, K., Kajiyama, G., et al. (2000). Pit pattern diagnosis of early colorectal carcinoma by magnifying colonoscopy: clinical and histological implications. *Int J Oncol*, 16, 927-34.

[46] Chiu, H. M., Chang, C. Y., Chen, C. C., Lee, Y. C., Wu, M. S., Lin, J. T., et al. (2007). A prospective comparative study of narrow-band imaging, chromoendoscopy, and conventional colonoscopy in the diagnosis of colorectal neoplasia. *Gut*, 56, 373-9.

[47] Su, M. Y., Hsu, C. M., Ho, Y. P., Chen, P. C., Lin, C. J., & Chiu, C. T. (2006). Comparative study of conventional colonoscopy, chromoendoscopy, and narrow-band imaging systems in differential diagnosis of neoplastic and nonneoplastic colonic polyps. *Am J Gastroenterol*, 101, 2711-6.

[48] Hirata, M., Tanaka, S., Oka, S., Kaneko, I., Yoshida, S., Yoshihara, M., et al. (2007). Magnifying endoscopy with narrow band imaging for diagnosis of colorectal tumors. *Gastrointest Endosc*, 65, 988-95.

[49] Rastogi, A., Bansal, A., Wani, S., Callahan, P., Mc Gregor, D. H., Cherian, R., et al. (2008). Narrow-band imaging colonoscopy- a pilot feasibility study for the detection of polyps and correlation of survface patterns with polyp histologic diagnosis. *Gastrointes Endosc*, 67, 280-6.

[50] Hirata, M., Tanaka, S., Oka, S., Kaneko, I., Yoshida, S., Yoshihara, M., et al. (2007). Evaluation of microvessels in colorectal tumors by narrow-band imaging magnification. *Gastrointest Endosc*, 66, 945-52.

[51] East, J. E., Suzuki, N., & Saunders, B. P. (2007). Comparison of magnified pit pattern interpretation with narrow band imaging versus chromendoscopy for diminutive colonic polyps: a pilot study. *Gastrointest Endosc*, 66, 310-6.

[52] Tischendorf, J. J. W., Wasmuth, H. E., Roch, A., Hecker, H., Trautwein, C., & Winograd, R. (2007). Value of magnifying chromendoscopy and narrow band imaging

(NBI) in classifying colorectal polyps: a prospective controlled study. *Endoscopy*, 39, 1092-6.

[53] Sano, Y., Ikematsu, H., Fu, K. I., Emura, F., Katagiri, A., Horimatsu, T., et al. (2009). Meshed capillary vessels by use of narrow-band imaging for differential diagnosis of small colorectal polyps. *Gastrointest Endosc*, 69, 278-83.

[54] Henry, Z. H., Yeaton, P., Shami, V. M., Kahaleh, M., Patrie, J. T., Cox, D. G., et al. (2010). Meshed capillary vessels found on narrow-band imaging without optical magnification effectively identifies colorectal neoplasia: a North American validation of the Japanese experience. *Gastrointest Endosc*, 72, 118-26.

[55] Kanao, H., Tanaka, S., Oka, S., Hirata, M., Yoshida, S., & Chayama, K. (2009). Narrow-band imaging magnification predicts the histology and invasion depth of colorectal tumors. *Gastrointest Endosc*, 69, 631-6.

[56] Ignjatovic, A., East, J. E., Guenther, T., Hoare, J., Morris, J., Ragunath, K., et al. (2011). What is the most reliable imaging modality for small colonic polyp characterization? Study of white-light, autofluorescence, and narrow-band imaging. *Endoscopy*, 43, 94-9.

[57] Machida, H., Sano, Y., Hamamoto, Y., Muto, M., Kozu, T., Tajin, H., et al. (2004). Narrow-band imaging in the diagnosis of colorectal mucosal lesions: a pilot study. *Endoscopy*, 36, 1094-8.

[58] Tanaka, S., Oka, S., Hirata, M., Yoshida, S., Kaneko, I., & Chayama, K. (2006). Pit pattern diagnosis for colorectal neoplasia using narrow band magnification. *Dig Endosc*, 18, S52-S56.

[59] Van den, Broek. F. J. C., Fockens, P., Van Eeden, S., Kara, MA, Hardwick, J. C. H., Reitsma, J. B., et al. (2009). Clinical evaluation of endoscopic trimodal imaging for the detection and differentiation of colonic polyps. *Clin Gastroenterol Hepatol*, 7, 288-95.

[60] Van den Broek, F. J. C., Reitsma, J. B., Curvers, W. L., Fockens, P., & Dekker, E. (2009). Systematic review of narrow-band imaging for the detection and differentiation of neoplastic and nonneoplastic lesions in the colon. *Gastrointest Endosc*, 69, 124-35.

[61] Katagiri, A., Fu, K. I., Sano, Y., Ikematsu, H., Horimatsu, T., Kaneko, K., et al. (2008). Narrow band imaging with magnifying colonoscopy as diagnostic tool for predicting histology of early colorectal neoplasia. *Aliment Pharmacol Ther*, 27, 1269-784.

[62] Ikematsu, H., Matsuda, T., Emura, F., Saito, Y., Uraoka, T., Fu, K. I., et al. (2010). Efficacy of capillary pattern type IIIA/IIIB by magnifying narrow band imaging for estimating depth of invasion of early colorectal neoplasms. *BMC Gastroenterol*, 10, 33.

[63] Kuiper, T., Van den Broek, F. J. C., Naber, A. H., Van Soest, E. J., Scholten, P., Mallant-Hent, R., et al. (2011). Endoscopic trimodal imaging detects colonic neoplasia as well as standard video endoscopy. *Gastroenterology*, 140, 1887-94.

[64] Van den Broek, F. J. C., van Soest, E. J., Naber, A. H., van Oijen, A., Mallant-Hent, R., et al. (2009). Combining autofluorescence imaging and narrow-band imaging for the differentiation of adenomas from non-neoplastic colonic polyps among experienced and non-experienced endoscopists. *Am J Gastroenterol*, 104, 1498-507.

[65] Rastogi, A., Pondugula, K., Bansal, A., Wani, S., Keighley, J., Sugar, J., et al. (2009). Recognition of surface mucosal and vascular patterns of colon polyps using narrow-band imaging: interobserver and intraobserver agreement and prediction of polyp histology. *Gastrointest Endosc*, 69, 716-22.

[66] Rastogi, A., Early, DS, Gupta, N., Bansal, A., Singh, V., Ansstas, M., et al. (2011). Randomized, controlled trial of standard-definition white-light, high-definition white light, and narrow-band imaging colonoscopy for the detection of colon polyps and prediction of polyp histology. *Gastrointest Endosc*, 74, 593-602.

[67] Rex, D. G. (2009). Narrow-band imaging without optical magnification for histologic analysis of colorectal polyps. *Gastroenterology*, 136, 1174-81.

[68] Rogart, J. N., Jain, D., Siddiqui, U. D., Oren, T., Lim, J., Jamidar, P., et al. (2008). Narrow-band imaging without high magnification to differentiate polyps during real-time endoscopy: improvement with experience. *Gastrointest Endosc*, 68, 1136-45.

[69] Sikka, S., Ringold, A., Jonnalagadda, S., & Banerjee, B. (2008). Comparison of white light and narrow band high definition images in predicting polyp histology, using standard colonoscopes without optical magnification. *Endoscopy*, 40, 818-22.

[70] Hewett, D. G., Kaltenbach, T., Sano, Y., Tanaka, S., Saunders, B. P., Ponchon, T., et al. (2012). Validation of a simple classification system for endoscopic diagnosis of small colorectal polyps using narrow-band imaging. *Gastroenterology*, 143, 599-607.

[71] Hewett, D. G., Huffman, M. E., & Rex, D. K. (2012). Leaving distal colorectal hyperplastic polyps in place can be achieved with high accuracy by using narrow-band imaging: an observational study. *Gastrointestinal Endosc*, 76, 374-80.

[72] Paggi, S., Rondonotti, E., Amato, A., Terruzi, V., Imperiali, G., Mandelli, G., et al. (2012). Resect and discard strategy in clinical practice: a prospective cohort study. *Endoscopy*, 10.1055/s-0032-1309891.

[73] Kuiper, T., Marsman, W. A., Jansen, J. M., Van Soest, E. J., Haan, Y., Bakker, G. J., et al. (2012). Accuracy for optical diagnosis of small colorectal polyps in nonacademic settings. *Clin Gastroenterol Hepatol*, 10, 1016-20.

[74] Gross, S., Tratuwein, C., Behreris, A., Winograd, R., Palm, S., Lutz, H. H., et al. (2011). Computer-based classification of small colorectal polyps by using narrow-band imaging with optical magnification. *Gastrointest Endosc*, 74, 1354-9.

[75] Ignjatovic, A., Thomas-Gibson, S., East, J. E., Haycock, A., Bassett, P., Bhandari, P., et al. (2011). Development and validation of a training module on the use of narrow-band imaging in differentiation of small adenomas from hyperplastic colorectal polyps. *Gastrointest Endos*, 73, 128-33.

[76] Raghavendra, M., Hewett, D. G., & Rex, D. K. (2010). Differentiating adenomas from hyperplastic colorectal polyps: narrow-band imaging can be learned in 20 minutes. *Gastrointest Endosc*, 72, 572-6.

[77] Pohl, J., Lotterer, E., Balzer, C., Sackmann, M., Schmidt, K. D., Gossner, L., et al. (2009). Computed virtual chromoendoscopy versus standard colonoscopy with targeted indigocarmin chromoendoscopy: a randomised multicentre trial. *Gut*, 58, 73-8.

[78] Parra-Blanco, A., Jimenez, A., Rembacken, B., González, N., Nicolás-Pérez, D., Gimeno-García, A. Z., et al. (2009). Validation of Fujinon intelligent chromoendoscopy with high definition endoscopes in colonoscopy. *World J Gastroenterol*, 15, 5266-73.

[79] Kim, Y. S., Kim, D., Chung, S. J., Park, M. J., Shin, C. S., Cho, S. H., et al. (2011). Differentiating small polyps histologies using real-time screening colonoscopy with Fuji Intelligent Color Enhancement. *Clin Gastroenterol Hepatol*, 9, 744-9.

[80] Lee, C. K., Lee, S. H., & Hwangho, Y. (2011). Narrow-band imaging versus I-Scan for the real-time histological prediction of diminutive colonic polyps: a prospective comparative study by using the simple unified endoscopic classification. *Gastrointest Endosc*, 74, 603-9.

[81] Hassan, C., Pickhardt, P. J., & Rex, D. K. (2010). A resect and discard strategy would improve cost-effectiveness of colorectal cancer screening. *Clin Gastroenterol Hepatol*, 8, 865-9.

Section 3

Complications of Colonoscopy: Minimizing the Risks of a Screening Tool

Chapter 9

The Major Complications of Colonoscopy: Sedation-Related, Hemorrhage Associated with Polypectomy and Colonic Perforation

Paul Miskovitz

Additional information is available at the end of the chapter

http://dx.doi.org/10.5772/51958

1. Introduction

"Complication, in medicine, is an unfavorable evolution of a disease, a health condition or a therapy. The disease can become worse in its severity or show a higher number of signs, symptoms, or new pathological changes, become widespread throughout the body or affect other organ systems. A new disease may also appear as a complication to a previous existing disease. A medical treatment, such as drugs or surgery may produce adverse effects and/or produce new health problem(s) by itself. Therefore, a complication may be iatrogenic, i.e., literally brought forth by the physician. Medical knowledge about a disease, procedure or treatment usually entails a list of the most common complications, so that they can be foreseen, prevented or recognized more easily and speedily.

Depending on the degree of vulnerability, susceptibility, age, health status, immune system condition, etc. complications may arise more easily. Complications affect adversely the prognosis of a disease. Non-invasive and minimally invasive medical procedures usually favor fewer complications in comparison to invasive ones." [1]

A currently popular focus in the gastroenterology and endoscopic literature is the quality of colonoscopy with regard to colorectal cancer screening [2]. This includes the collection of evidence regarding the use of colonoscopy as a tool for screening programs, defining and establishing quality indicators and minimum requirements that endoscopists involved in colorectal cancer screening programs should meet, and providing evidence about procedures that may improve the quality of colonoscopy. Those who have decades of experience performing colonoscopy will be quite familiar with the myriad of complications associated with the procedure, either through their reading of the gastrointestinal endoscopy literature, from personal experience or the experience of colleagues. That being said, three major categories of complications associated with colonoscopy are widely recognized. They are sedation-related complications, hemorrhage associated with colonic polypectomy and colonoscopy-related colonic perforation. Sedation-related complications are usually cardiovascular and/or pulmonary and include oxygen desaturation, respiratory arrest, alterations in heart rate (bradycardia and tachycardia), cardiac arrhythmias, myocardial infarction, stroke, seizures (at times attributed to the method of preparation) and shock. Hemorrhage is most often associated with snare electrocautery polypectomy but may also occur during the performance of diagnostic colonoscopy with or without biopsies. Two general subcategories of hemorrhage exist: hemorrhage immediately following the performance of polypectomy or delayed hemorrhage occurring up to several weeks after the therapeutic procedure. Colonic perforation resulting from colonoscopy may occur due to mechanical forces exerted against the colonic wall (colonoscope tip or shaft, biopsy forceps, dilatation of a stricture), barotrauma as a result of intraluminal air or carbon dioxide insufflation, or as a result of a therapeutic procedure such as polypectomy, foreign body extraction, or stent placement to name a few. A thorough understanding of these complications, their incidence and treatment, is part of the training of all those learning to perform colonoscopy and forms the basis for the physician obtaining informed consent (an explanation of the risks and benefits of the procedure) from the patient. This chapter will systematically review our current understanding of these complication categories and the methods of minimizing the likelihood of developing these complications. The latest treatments of specific complications will be reviewed with the intent of aiding the physician endoscopist's understanding of the principles of risk management as regards to performing colonoscopy.

"Primum non nocere" is the Latin phrase that means "First, do no harm". Non-maleficence, which is derived from this maxim, is one of the principal precepts of medical ethics taught to all medical students in medical school and is a fundamental principle for the provision of medical services world-wide. Another way to state it is that "given an existing problem, it may be better not to do something, or even to do nothing, than to risk causing more harm than good." It reminds the physician and other health care providers that they must consider the possible harm that any intervention might do. It is invoked when debating the use of an intervention that carries an obvious risk of harm but a less certain chance of benefit. This ancient principle should be kept in mind when contemplating colonoscopy and the possible complications of the procedure.

1.1. Informed consent for colonoscopy

The doctrine of informed consent (and its antithesis, informed refusal) for colonoscopy involves an assessment of the competence of the patient by the physician, disclosure of, in an understandable way, the information necessary to allow the patient to make an informed decision (risks and benefits considered) regarding the role of colonoscopy in his care, and the documentation of these proceedings in the medical record [3]. It is an intrinsic part of the doctor-patient relationship and an ethical obligation on the part of the physician in the clinical practice of medicine. In the United States, the doctrine of medical informed consent is most famously traced back to a 1914 New York court decision centered about the observa-

http://dx.doi.org/10.5772/51958

tion that since most surgical operations involve some use of force, there must be consent on the part of the patient. Because the nature of surgery is outside the experience of most patients, the consent must be granted only after the patient is properly informed of the risks and benefits. The most famous description of informed consent is a quote from New York Justice Benjamin Cardozo who, in 1914, stated that:

"Every human being of adult years and sound mind has a right to determine what shall be done with his own body; and a surgeon who performs an operation without his patient's consent commits an assault for which he is liable in damages" [4].

This advice is still applicable in the 21st century! Most important in considering the complications of colonoscopy is the need to meticulously document the obtaining of informed consent from the patient and the procedural technique, findings and outcome including any complications [5].

2. Sedation-related complications of colonoscopy

Sedation-related complications of colonoscopy are usually cardiovascular, pulmonary and occasionally neurological. The risk of these events occurring is associated with advancing age, higher American Society of Anesthesiologists Physical Status Classification System scores (ASA score—with category 6 not being applicable), and the patient's co-morbidities [6-8].

ASA Physical Status Classification System (I-VI)

ASA-I A normal healthy patient.

ASA-II A patient with mild systemic disease.

ASA-III A patient with severe systemic disease.

ASA-IV A patient with severe systemic disease that is a constant threat to life.

ASA-V A moribund patient who is not expected to survive without the operation.

ASA-VI A declared brain-dead patient whose organs are being removed for donor purposes.

ASA-E Emergency operation of any variety (used to modify one of the above classifications, i.e., ASA III-E)

In general, patients' inpatient status, trainee participation and the routine use of supplemental oxygen (the latter by possibly masking hypercapnea and hypoventilation) are associated with a higher risk of unplanned cardiopulmonary events [9]. The monitoring period for the "event rate" should likely include the 30 days post procedure [10].

2.1. Hypoxemia

Hypoxemia, which is usually transient but often anxiety provoking for the colonoscopist, is a common occurrence during sedation for colonoscopy and has lead to the often "routine" practice by colonoscopists and attending anesthesiologists and nurse anesthetists of providing patients with supplemental oxygen [9] delivered by nasal cannula and on occasion by a venturi air-entrapment mask (the latter providing a fixed and predictable oxygen concentration despite a variable respiration pattern). Prolonged hypoxemia associated with colonoscopy is rare. The etiology of hypoxemia is often multifactorial but not to be overlooked is the amount of air (or carbon dioxide) insufflated into the colon for adequate luminal distention and in some cases the passing of this gas into the small bowel through an incompetent ileocecal valve thereby affecting diaphragmatic function. This has lead most endoscopists to periodically monitor the degree of abdominal distention ("softness") by direct palpation of the abdomen either routinely during the procedure or when there are drops in the monitored oxygen saturation.

2.2. Hypercapnea

Capnography monitor use is widespread in hospitals but these devices are less commonly used in the gastrointestinal endoscopy suite and other ambulatory settings where propofol is often used. In 2012 the American Society of Anesthesiologists (ASA) advised its member to use such carbon dioxide monitoring devices that detect changes in the amount of carbon dioxide the patient is exhaling during monitored anesthesia care for upper gastrointestinal endoscopies [11]. The new policy states:

"Monitoring for exhaled carbon dioxide should be considered during endoscopic procedures in which sedation is provided with propofol alone or in combination with opioids and/or benzodiazepines, and especially during these procedures on the upper gastrointestinal tract. Careful attention to airway management must be provided during endoscopic retrograde cholangiopancreatography (ERCP) procedures performed in the prone position where ventilatory monitoring, airway maintenance and resuscitation may be especially difficult."

It has only been a matter of time since this recommendation has found application in the monitoring of sedated patients undergoing colonoscopy. The new policy has met with mixed reviews in the gastrointestinal endoscopy and anesthesiology communities but most have agreed that there is little downside to such monitoring.

It is important to emphasize that at least one individual with training in advanced cardiac life support (tracheal intubation, defibrillation, use of resuscitation medications, ACLS certification) that is capable of establishing an airway and providing positive-pressure ventilation should be present during colonoscopy sedation. Ability for communication with "back up" local paramedics or life support personnel should be confirmed.

2.3. Hypotension

The etiology of hypotension during colonoscopy is also multifactorial (pre-procedure antihypertensive medications, sedatives and analgesics used during the performance of the procedure, arrhythmias, pre-procedure cardiac performance status, etc.) but the state of hydration of the patient after (usually a polyethylene glycol containing) bowel preparation may reign supreme among the factors to consider. Intravenous replacement with crystalloid solutions should be considered during such events and in anticipation of such events in appropriately screened patients.

2.4. Arrhythmia

Cardiac arrhythmias including bradycardia, less often tachycardia, atrial premature contractions, paroxysms of atrial fibrillation, and ventricular premature contractions have been documented during procedural sedation. Most resolve with the intravenous administration of fluids or increased sedation. With regard to bradycardia there is asymptomatic bradycardia (heart rate less than 60 bpm) and symptomatic bradycardia defined as a heart rate less than 60/min that elicits signs and symptoms. In symptomatic bradycardia the heart rate will usually be less than 50/min. Symptomatic bradycardia exists when the following 3 criteria are present: 1.) The heart rate is slow; 2.) The patient has symptoms; and 3.) The symptoms are due to the slow heart rate. Atropine is the first drug of choice for symptomatic bradycardia [12]. The dose in the bradycardia ACLS algorithm is 0.5 mg IV push which may be repeated up to a total dose of 3 mg. (Anesthesiologists often choose glycopyrrolate [Robinul®] as an alternative to atropine.) Dopamine is a second line drug for symptomatic bradycardia when atropine is not effective. The dosage is 2-10 micrograms/kg/min infusion. Epinephrine can be used as an equal alternative to dopamine when atropine is not effective. The dosage is 2-10 micrograms/min. Rare cases of ventricular tachycardia and cardiac arrest during ventricular fibrillation have been reported necessitating the need for continuous EKG monitoring, the availability of ACLS trained personnel, as well as obtaining a history of cardiac or pulmonary disease prior to initiating the procedure.

2.5. Pulmonary embolism

Although the prevalence of coexistent pulmonary embolism at the time of colon cancer detection has been estimated to be as high as 2% (with the concurrent prevalence of deep venous thrombosis being as high as 8%) there are no accepted statistics for the incidence of pulmonary embolism complicating diagnostic or therapeutic colonoscopy [13].

2.6. TIA/stroke

The risk of stroke in patients with AF whose anticoagulation is adjusted for endoscopies is low, but almost tenfold higher in patients with complex clinical situations [14]. Age, history of stroke, hypertension, hyperlipidemia, and family history of vascular disease may increase the risk of suffering a stroke during or immediately after undergoing a gastrointestinal endoscopic procedure. Comprehensive guidelines for the management of anticoagulation and antiplatelet therapy in patients undergoing gastrointestinal endoscopic procedures including colonoscopy have recently been published [15] and should serve as a reference and guide when dealing with such patients.

2.7. Myocardial infarction

Recent myocardial infarction has traditionally precluded the performance of elective colonoscopy for at least several months but recently this issue has been closely addressed in the literature [16]. Colonoscopy performed in patients who have experienced a recent myocardial infarction is associated with a higher rate of minor, transient, and primarily cardiovascular complications when compared with control patients but is relatively infrequently associated with major complications. In certain circumstances, despite the higher risk, colonoscopy may be beneficial in this setting, particularly given the higher frequency of ischemic colitis in this patient population. The occurrence of cardiac ischemia (and concomitant cardiac rhythm disturbances) in patients undergoing colonoscopy who have known cardiac disease or cardiac risk factors has recently been quantified [17]. Holter EKG recordings and measurement of cTnI troponin I levels showed a high incidence of new but silent ischemic and arrhythmic EKG changes during colonoscopy and do a lesser extent those patients with one or more risk factors for heart disease. Two patients with known heart disease died within 30 days of colonoscopy.

3. Colonic hemorrhage associated with polypectomy

Although hemorrhage can occur during diagnostic colonoscopy (particularly when "cold" or "hot" forceps biopsy techniques are used) it most often complicates polypectomy occurring immediately or being delayed for several weeks after the procedure [18]. The overall incidence of hemorrhage has been reported to be in the range of 1 to 6 per 1,000 colonoscopies [19,6] (this being a useful figure to quote when obtaining informed consent from the patient) with the number of polyps [20], polyp size [19] recent anticoagulant use [22,23] and even polyp histology(!) [6,24,25] being modifying factors! The effects of aspirin, nonsteroidal anti-inflammatory drugs and clopidogrel both alone and in combination on this complication of colonoscopy have also been addressed [26,27].

Patients requiring colonoscopy with or without biopsy and/or polypectomy are often taking antithrombotic agents including anticoagulants such as warfarin, heparin, and low molecular weight heparin, and antiplatelet agents such as aspirin, non-steroidal anti-inflammatory drugs, thienopyridines such as clopidrogel and ticlopidine, and glycoprotein IIb/IIIa receptor inhibitors. The indications for the use of these medications include atrial fibrillation, acute coronary syndrome, deep venous thrombosis, hypercoagulable states and indwelling endoprostheses such as coronary artery stents. When hemorrhage does occur in patients taking these agents it is most commonly from the gastrointestinal tract [28]. Risk stratification for these patients can generally be relegated to two categories. Low risk procedures include diagnostic colonoscopy including mucosal biopsy [29,30] and high-risk procedures include colonoscopy with polypectomy and the dilatation of either benign or malignant colonic strictures (guidelines extrapolated in part from experience reported in the upper gastrointestinal endoscopy literature) [31-33]. A comprehensive review of the types of antithrombotic therapies, their implications for patients undergoing colonoscopy, and recommendations and a management algorithm for such patients using these agents has recently been published [34]. Newer anticoagulants, for which current guidelines regarding their being held for endoscopic procedures, are lacking and these agents are reaching the market at an increasing rate. They include danaparoid, a low molecular weight heparinoid consisting of a mixture of heparin sulfate, dermatan sulfate, and chondroitin sulfate [35,36] which was recently removed from the US market due to shortages; the direct thrombin inhibitors recombinant hirudin (lepirudin), argatroban, desirudin and bivalirudin [37-39]; the recently available orally active direct thrombin inhibitor dabigatran etexlate [40]; and the factor Xa inhibitors idraparinux, rivaroxaban, and apixaban [41]. There is no doubt that as these agents are used they will affect practice standards with regard to colonoscopy and polypectomy.

Acute postpolypectomy bleeding is often immediately localizable by or apparent on colonoscopy and amenable to endoscopic therapy using clips, ligatures, cautery or argon plasma coagulation [42,43] or nonendoscopic techniques such as angiographic embolizaton or surgery [44]. Recent endoscopic clip application devices have undergone redesign and improvements to optimize their clinical effectiveness [45]. The site of delayed postpolypectomy colonic hemorrhage can be identified by colonoscopy, by red cell nuclear scintigraphy and/or by selective angiography [46] and dealt with in a similar fashion.

A variety of procedural techniques have been proposed to minimize the risk of hemorrhage complicating polypectomy. These include the avoidance of the use of the "hot biopsy" technique [47], the use of clips or detachable snares [48,49] and possibly the use of epinephrine injections to the base of the polyp prior to initiating the polypectomy [50,51]. Proper technique for the removal of pendunculated polyps includes planning for the application of pressure by regrasping the pedicle with the snare if immediate bleeding occurs, the injection of epinephrine 1:10,000 to 1:20,000 dilution into the bleeding site, the application of cautery (with thermal probes, bipolar cautery [BICAP], the argon plasma coagulator, or the tip of the polypectomy snare), the use of hemoclips, and/or the use of loops and band ligators on the pedicle. Similar techniques may be used in those with delayed bleeding who seem to be actively bleeding. Up to 50 percent of patients with delayed hemorrhage may require blood transfusion [23].

4. Colonic perforation associated with polypectomy

Perforation of the colon is the most dreaded complication of colonoscopy and polypectomy and this risk, albeit small, should be cited in the process of obtaining informed consent form the patient for the procedure.

Abdominal pain, abdominal distention, +/- abdominal tenderness, hiccoughs, loss of bowel sounds indicative of ileus, and late developing peritoneal signs are the hallmarks of perforation following colonoscopy. As physical examination, chest x-ray and abdominal flat and upright x-ray alone or in combination may not be diagnostic of colonic perforation patients suspected of having this complication should undergo CT scanning of the abdomen and pelvis [52]. The rate of perforation after colonoscopy ranges from 0.1-0.3% [19] and may be increased (along with the risk of hemorrhage) in those physicians who have a low procedure volume [53]. It has been suggested that physicians who have a high perforation rate should be evaluated for inappropriate colonoscopy practice technique [54].

Perforation risk for polypectomy may be minimized by proper technique. One should avoid ensnaring colonic folds, particularly when the anatomy is obscured by large penduculated or sessile lesions. By not properly lifting an ensnare polyp into the lumen of the colon before applying current, there may be spread of thermal injury to the deeper layers of the bowel wall increasing the risk of delayed perforation. Likewise, a pedunculated polyp should not be resected close to the bowel wall. Care should be taken to leave some residual stalk. The polypectomy snare should be tightly closed before applying coagulation in order to avoid the tip of the snare behind the polyp from touching the bowel wall.

Endoscopic mucosal resection for the piecemeal removal of benign appearing sessile colonic adenomas has become routine. Endoscopic submucosal dissection is a resection technique applied to early gastrointestinal cancers. Complications rates are higher with endoscopic submucosal dissection than with endoscopic mucosal resection with perforations occurring in up to 10 percent of patients. Often these perforations can be managed by endoscopic clipping and conservative therapy, however surgery is still required in some cases and prolonged hospital stays are common. [55-57].

All patients found to have evidence of colonic perforation following colonoscopy should be seen in surgical consultation because perforation often requires surgical repair which in some cases may be accomplished using a laparoscopic technique with avoidance of diverting colostomy formation [58,59]. It has been reported that nonsurgical management may be appropriate for some individuals [60,61] but these patients should still undergo surgical consultation and close monitoring for signs of deterioration. Successful endoscopic repair of an iatrogenic colonic perforation occurring during *diagnostic* colonoscopy has been reported [62] and the efficacy of a new Over-the Scope-Clip (OTSC-Ovesco Endoscopy AG, Tübingen, Germany) device (a bear trap-like, large clip with a wingspan of 12 mms. that grasps much more tissue than the small endoscopic clips used previously and can create a full-thickness closure of perforations up to 3 cms. in diameter) in treating acute perforation of the gastrointestinal tract has been reported [63].

5. Miscellaneous complications of colonoscopy with and without polypectomy

5.1. Abdominal discomfort

Commonly reported but minor complications of colonoscopy include bloating and abdominal discomfort and or pain [64-66]. The incidence of these complications may be reduced by avoiding "looping" of the colonoscope, avoiding excess traction applied to the bowel mesentery, adequately removing insufflated gas, using carbon dioxide instead of insufflated air [67] and by using a water insufflation technique instead of the insufflation of gas [68].

5.2. Postpolypectomy electrocoagulation syndrome

Postpolypectomy electrocagulation syndrome refers to a transmural burn and localized peritonitis occurring up to a few days after the removal of a polyp without clinical or radiographic evidence of perforation of the viscus. Patients may present with localized abdominal pain, fever, and leukocytosis. Inpatient [69] and outpatient [70] therapy have both proven to be successful in treatment of this complication.

5.3. Infection

Transient bacteremia after colonoscopy with polypectomy is rare and signs and symptoms of infection are even rarer [71,72]. Current guidelines exist generally advocating against antibiotic prophylaxis for those undergoing colonoscopy with or without polypectomy [73]. As these represent only guidelines it is best for the endoscopist to consult with the patient and the referring physician before deciding to forego the use of antibiotic prophylaxis in certain clinical situations (prosthetic heart valve, history of endocarditis, newly placed prosthetic joint, etc.). Both diverticulitis [74] and appendicitis [75] the latter possibly due to barotrauma have been reported complicating colonoscopy done with and without polypectomy. These clinical possibilities must be kept in mind in patients with post-procedure abdominal pain.

5.4. Rare complications

Rare complications of colonoscopy with and without polypectomy have been reported and include infections related to instrument cleanliness [76] incarceration of the colonoscope in an inguinal hernia [77], splenic injury during colonoscopy [78], and intracolonic gas explosion during colonoscopic polypectomy [79,80]. CT colonography, the alternative to colonoscopy in many patients, however, is not without its own complications and adverse events [81].

6. Conclusion

It is incumbent upon physicians performing colonoscopy to stay current in their field, keep abreast of the medical literature and the ongoing technological advances associated with endoscopic equipment and technique, and to be meticulous in their approach to detail in caring for their patients, particularly when gastrointestinal endoscopic diagnostic and therapeutic procedures are involved.

GENERAL
♥Obtain informed consent from the patient prior to the colonoscopy procedure with emphasis on the risks of, benefits of and alternatives to the proposed procedure
♥Be cognizant of your limitations as an endoscopist
♥Be certain that all necessary equipment to perform the colonoscopy procedure (diagnostic and therapeutic) is available and in working order
SEDATION RELATED COMPLICATIONS
♥Perform and document a medical history and physical examination prior to the initiation of the procedure. Include a review of the patient's current medications, known allergies, past experiences with anesthesia, Mallampati score and ASA Physical Status Classification
♥Ensure that the patient is properly monitored during the procedure including blood pressure, pulse, oximetry, capnography monitoring if available, cardiac rhythm monitoring, and airway management. If working with an anesthesiologist thoroughly discuss with your colleague the patient's medical history and the goals of the procedure. Maintain a dialogue with the anesthesiologist throughout the procedure
♥Ensure that tracheal intubation and cardiac defibrillation equipment as well as resuscitation medications are available and have up to date certification in Advanced Cardiac Life Support
COLONIC HEMORRHAGE ASSOCIATED WITH POLYPECTOMY
♥Take a history of the patient's anticoagulant use, antiplatelet agent use, and past history of bleeding diathesis if any
♥Be thoroughly familiar with proper snare electrocautery polypectomy technique including the use of saline or epinephrine injection into the base of the polyp before initiating electrocautery
♥Avoid the use of the "hot biopsy" technique for small (several millimeter) polyps
♥Have available for use if necessary clips, ligatures, epinephrine, a bipolar electrocautery device and/or an argon plasma coagulation device or heater probe
♥Give specific written post-procedure instructions to the patient regarding the use of anticoagulants and antiplatelet agents
COLONIC PERFORATION ASSOCIATED WITH POLYPECTOMY
♥Cite the risk of colonic perforation when obtaining informed consent
♥Avoid ensnaring colonic folds
♥Do not perform polypectomy when the anatomy is obscured by the size or shape of the lesion or the adequacy of the preparation
♥Have training and familiarity with endoscopic clipping techniques
♥Have a predetermined "game plan" to expeditiously evaluate a patient suspected of having a perforation
MISCELLANEOUS COMPLICATIONS OF COLONOSCOPY WITH AND WITHOUT POLYPECTOMY
♥If available, use carbon dioxide for colonic insufflation
♥Monitor the degree of abdominal distension by palpation throughout the procedure
♥Examine the patient in the recovery area post procedure to ensure that there has been adequate evacuation of colonic gas
♥Be cognizant of and practice infection control measures routinely
♥Keep abreast of the medical literature and ongoing technological advances associated with endoscopic equipment and technique

Table 1. Recommendations to prevent specific colonoscopy complications

http://dx.doi.org/10.5772/51958

Author details

Paul Miskovitz

Division of Gastroenterology and Hepatology, Department of Medicine, Weill Cornell Medical College, New York-Presbyterian Hospital, New York, USA

References

[1] http://en.wikipedia.org/wiki/Complication_%28medicine%29 accessed 7/24/2012

[2] Jover, R., Herrálz, M., Alarcón, O., Brullet, E., Bujanda, L., Bustamante, M., Campo, R., Carreño, R., Castells, A., Cubiella, J., Garcia-Iglesias, P., Hervás, A.J., Menchén, P., Ono, A., Panadés, A., Parra-Blanco, A., Pellisé, M., Ponce, M., Quintero, E., Reñé, J.M., Sánchez del Rio, A., Seoane, A., Serradesanferm, A., Soriano Izquierdo, A., Vázquez Sequeiros, E., Spanish Society of Gastroenterology (AEG) and Spanish Society of Gastrointestinal Endoscopy (SEED) Working Group. (2012) Clinical practice guidelines: quality of colonoscopy in colorectal cancer screening. Endoscopy. Vol.44, No.4, (April 2012) pp. 444-451. ISSN 0013-726X

[3] Stunkel, L., Benson, M., McLellan, L., Sinaii, N., Bedarida, G., Emanuel, E., Grady, C. (2010) Comprehension and informed consent: assessing the effect of a short consent form. IRB. Vol.32, No.4, (July-August 2010) pp. 1-9. ISSN 0193-7758

[4] Schloendorff v Society of New York Hospital, 105 N.E. 92, N. Y., (1914)

[5] Miskovitz, P. Gibofsky, A. (1995) Risk management in endoscopic practice. Gastrointest Endosc Clin North Am. Vol.5, No.2, (April 1995) pp. 391-401. ISSN 1052-5157

[6] Warren, J.L., Klabunde, C.N., Mariotto, A.B., Meekins, A., Topor, M., Brown, M.L., Ransohoff, D.F. (2009) Adverse events after outpatient colonoscopy in the Medicare population. Ann Intern Med. Vol.150, No.12., (June 2009) pp. 849-57. W152 ISSN 1539-3704

[7] Baudet, J.S., Diaz-Bethencourt, D., Avilès, J., Aguirre-Jaime, A. (2009) Minor adverse events of colonoscopy on ambulatory patients: the impact of moderate sedation. Eur J Gastroenterol Hepatol. Vol.21, Issue.6, (June 2009) pp. 656-61. ISSN 1473-5687

[8] Vargo, J.J., Holub, J.L., Faigel, D.O., Lieberman, D.A., Eisen, G.M. (2006) Risk factors for cardiopulmonary events during propofol mediated upper endoscopy and colonoscopy. Aliment Pharmacol Ther. Vol.24, No.6., (September 2006) pp. 955-63. ISSN 1365-2036

[9] Sharma, V.K., Nguyen, C.C., Crowell, M.D., Lieberman, D.A., de Garmo, P., Fleischer, D. (2007) A national study of cardiopulmonary unplanned events after GI endoscopy. Gastrointest Endosc. Vol.66, No.1., (July 2007) pp. 27-34. ISSN 1097-6779

[10] Ko, C.W., Riffle, S., Michaels, L., Morris, C., Holub, J., Shapiro, J.A., Ciol, M.A., Kimmey, M.B., Seef, L.C., Lieberman, D. (2010) Serious complications within 30 days of screening and surveillance colonoscopy are uncommon. Clin Gastroenterol Hepatol. Vol.8, No.2., (February 2010) pp. 166-73. ISSN 1452-3565

[11] Marcus, A. and Gordon, C.J. (2010) ASA recommends capnography for propofol sedation in upper endoscopy procedures. Gastroenterol and Endosc News. Vol.61., No. 2., (February 2010) pp 1. ISSN 0883-8348

[12] Advanced Cardiac Life Support (ACLS) Provider Manual 2012 American Heart Association, Dallas, TX. ISBN 978-1-61669-010-6

[13] Stender, M.T., Nielsen, T.S., Frøkjaer, J.B., Larsen, T.B., Lundbye-Christensen, S., Thorlacius-Ussing, O. (2007) High preoperative prevalence of deep venous thrombosis in patients with colorectal cancer. Br J Surg. Vol.94., No.9., (September 2007) pp. 1100-3. ISSN 1365-2168

[14] Blacker, D.J., Wijdicks, E.F., McClelland, R.L. (2003) Stroke risk in anticoagulated patients with atrial fibrillation undergoing endoscopy. Neurology. Vol.61., No.7. (October 2003) pp. 964-8. ISSN 0028-3879

[15] Veitch, A.M., Baglin, T.P., Gershlick, A.H., Harnden, S.M., Tighe, R., Cairns, S. (2008) Guidelines for the management of anticoagulant and antiplatelet therapy in patients undergoing endoscopic procedures. Gut. Vol.5., No.9., (September 2008) pp. 1322-9. ISSN 1468-3288

[16] Cappell, M.S. (2004) Safety and efficacy of colonoscopy after myocardial infarction: an analysis of 100 study patients and 100 control patients at two tertiary cardiac referral hospitals. Gastrointest Endosc. Vol.60., No.6., (December 2004) pp. 901-9. ISSN 1097-6779

[17] George, A.T., Davis, C., Rangaraj, A., Edwards, C., Chamary, V.L., Khan, H., Javed, M., Campbell, P.G., Allison, M.C., Swarnkar, K.J. (2010) Cardiac ischaemia and rhythm disturbances during elective colonoscopy. Frontline Gastroenterol. Vol.1., No.3., (October 2010) pp. 131-7. ISSN 2041-4145

[18] Singaram, C., Torbey, D.F., Jacoby, R.F. (1995) Delayed postpolypectomy bleeding. Am J Gastroenterol. Vol.90., No.1., (January 1990) pp. 146-7. ISSN 0002-9270

[19] Ko, C.W., Dominitz, J.A. (2010) Complications of colonoscopy: magnitude and management. Gastrointest Endosc Clin N Am. Vol.20., No.4., (October 2010) pp. 659-71. ISSN 1052-5157

[20] Witt, D.M., Delate, T., McCool, K.H., Dowd, M.B., Clark, N.P., Crowther, M.A., Garcia, D.A., Ageno, W., Dentali, F., Hylek, E.M., Rector, W.G., WARPED Consortium. (2009) Incidence and predictors of bleeding or thrombosis after polypectomy in patients receiving and not receiving anticoagulation therapy. J Thromb Haemost. Vol. 7., No.12, (December 2009) pp. 1982-89. ISSN 1538-7836

[21] Watabe, H., Yamaji, Y., Okamoto, M., Kondo, S., Ohta, M., Ikenoue, T., Kata, J., Togo, G., Matsumura, M., Yoshida, H., Kawabe, T., Omata, M. (2006) Risk assessment for delayed hemorrhagic complication of colonic polypectomy: polyp-related factors and patient-related factors. Gastrointest Endosc. Vol.64., No.1., (July 2006) pp.73-78. ISSN 1097-6779

[22] Hui, A.J., Wong, R.M., Ching, J.Y., Hung, L.C., Chung, S.C., Sung, J.J. (2004) Risk of colonoscopic polypectomy bleeding with anticoagulants and antiplatelet agents: analysis of 1657 cases. Gastrointest Endosc. Vol.59., No.1., (January 2004) pp. 44-8. ISSN 1097-6779

[23] Sawhney, M.S., Salfiti, N., Nelson, D.B., Lederle, F.A., Bond, J.H. (2008) Risk factors for severe delayed postpolypectomy bleeding. Endoscopy. Vol.40., No.2., (February 2008) pp. 115-9. ISSN 0013-726X

[24] Consolo, P., Luigiano, C., Stranio, G., Scaffidi, M.G., Giacobbe, G., DiGiuseppe, G., Zirilli, A., Familiari, L. (2008) Efficacy, risk factors and complications of endoscopic polypectomy: ten year experience at a single center. World J Gastroenterol. Vol.14., No.15., (April 2008) pp. 2364-9. ISSN 1007-9327

[25] Kim, H.S., Kim, T.I., Kim, W.H., Kim, Y.H., Kim, H.J., Yang, S.K., Myung, S.J., Byeon, J.S., Lee, M.S., Chung, J.K., Jung, S.A., Jeen, Y.T., Choi, J.H., Choi, K.Y., Choi, H., Han, D.S., Song J.S. (2006) Risk factors for immediate postpolypecotmy bleeding of the colon: a multicenter study. Am J Gastroenterol. Vol.101, No.6., (June 2006) pp.1333-41. ISSN 0002-9270

[26] Shiffman, M.L., Farrel, M.T., Yee, Y.S. (1994) Risk of bleeding after endoscopic biopsy or polypectomy in patients taking aspirin or other NSAIDS. Gastrointest Endosc. Vol.40., No.4., (July-August 1994) pp. 458-62. ISSN 1097-6779

[27] Singh, M., Mehta, N., Murth, U.K., Kaul, V., Arif, A., Newman, N. (2010) Postpolypectomy bleeding in patients undergoing colonoscopy on uninterrupted clopidogrel therapy. Gastrointest Endosc. Vol.71., No.6., (May 2010) pp. 998-1005. ISSN 1097-6779

[28] Choudari, C.P., Rajgopal, C., Palmer, K.R. (1994) Acute gastrointestinal haemorrhage in anticoagulated patients: diagnoses and response to endoscopic treatment. Gut. Vol.35, No.4, (April 1994) pp. 464-6. ISSN 0017-5749

[29] Sieg, A., Hachmoeller-Eisenbach, U., Eisenbach, T. (2001) Prospective evaluation of complications in outpatient GI endoscopy: a survey among German gastroenterologists. Gastrointest Endosc. Vol.53, No.6, (May 2001) pp. 620-7. ISSN 1097-6779

[30] Parra-Blanco, A., Kaminaga, N., Kojima, T., Endo, Y., Uragami, N., Okawa, N., Hattori, T., Takahashi, H., Fujita, R. (2000) Hemoclipping for postpolypectomy and postbiopsy colonic bleeding. Gastrointest Endosc. Vol.51, No.1, (January 2000) pp. 37-41. ISSN 1097-6779

[31] Singh, V.V., Draganov, P., Valentine, J. (2005) Efficacy and safety of endoscopic balloon dilation of symptomatic upper and lower gastrointestinal Crohn's disease strictures. J Clin Gastroenterol. Vol.39, No.4, (April 2005) pp. 284-90. ISSN 0192-0790

[32] Solt, J., Bajor, J., Szabó, M., Horváth, O.P. (2003) Long-term results of balloon catheter dilation for benign gastric outlet stenosis. Endoscopy. Vol.35, No.6, (June 2003) pp. 490-5. ISSN 0013-726X

[33] DiSario, J.A., Fennerty, M.B., Tietze, C.C., Hutson, W.R., Burt, R.W. (1994) Endoscopic balloon dilation for ulcer-induced gastric outlet obstruction. Am J Gastroenterol. Vol.89, No.6, (June 1994) pp. 868-71. ISSN 0002-9270

[34] ASGE Standards of Practice Committee, Anderson, M.A., Ben-Menachem, T., Gan, S.I., Appalaneni, V., Banerjee, S., Cash, B.D., Fisher, L., Harrison, M.E., Fanelli, R.D., Fukami, N., Ikenberry, S.O., Jain, R., Khan, K., Krinsky, M.L., Lichtenstein, D.R., Maple, J.T., Shen, B., Strohmeyer, L., Baron, T., Dominitz, J.A. (2009) Management of antithrombotic agents for endoscopic procedures. Gastrointest Endosc. Vol.70, No.6, (December 2009) pp. 1060-70. ISSN 1097-6779

[35] Danhof, M., de Boer, A., Magnani, H.N., Stiekema, J.C. (1992) Pharmacokinetic considerations on Orgaran (Org 10172) therapy. Haemostasis Vol.22, No.2, (February 1992) pp. 73-84. ISSN 0340-5338

[36] Nurmohamed, M.T., Fareed, J., Hoppensteadt, D., Walenga, J.M., ten Cate, J.W. (1991) Pharmacological and clinical studies with Lomoparan, a low molecular weight glycosaminoglycan. Semin Thromb Hemost. Vol.17 Suppl.2, pp. 205-13. ISSN 0094-6176

[37] Greinacher, A., Warkentin, E. (2008) The direct thrombin inhibitor hirudin. Thromb Haemost. Vol.99, No.5, (May 2008) pp. 819-29. ISSN 0340-6245

[38] Clarke, R.J., Mayo, G., FitzGerald, G.A., Fitzgerald, D.J. (1991) Combined administration of aspirin and a specific thrombin inhibitor in man. Circulation. Vol.83, No.5. (May 1991) pp. 1510-8. ISSN 0009-7322

[39] Warkentin T.E., Greinacher, A., Koster, A. (2008) Bivalirudin. Thromb Haemost. Vol. 99, No.5. (May 2008) pp. 830-9. ISSN 0340-624

[40] Schulman, S., Kearon, C., Kakkar, A.K., Mismetti, P., Schellong, S., Eriksson, H., Baanstra, D., Schnee, J., Goldhaber, S.Z.; RE-COVER Study Group. (2009) Dabigatran versus warfarin in the treatment of acute venous thromboembolism. N Engl J Med. Vol.361, No.24, (December 2009) pp. 2342-52. ISSN 0028-4793

[41] Turpie, A.G. (2008) New oral anticoagulants in atrial fibrillation. Eur Heart J. Vol.29, No.2. (December 2008) pp. 155-65. ISSN 0195-668X

[42] Carpenter, S., Petersen, B.T., Chuttani, R., Croffie, J., DiSario, J., Liu, J., Mishkin, D., Shar, R., Somogyi, L., Tierney, W., Song, L.M. (2007) Polypectomy devices. Gastrointest Endosc. Vol.65., No.6., May 2007) pp741-9. ISSN 1097-6779

[43] ASGE Technology Committee, Conway, J.D., Adler, D.G., Diehl, D.L., Farraye, F.A., Kantsevoy, S.V., Kaul, V., Kethu, S.R., Kwon, R.S., Mamula, P., Rodriguez, S.A., Tierney, W.M. (2009) Endoscopic hemostatic devices. Gastrointest Endosc. Vol.69, No.6, (May 2009) pp. 987-96. ISSN 1097-6779

[44] Sorbi, D., Norton, I., Conio, M., Balm, R., Zinsmeister, A., Gostout, C.J. (2000) Postpolypectomy lower GI bleeding: descriptive analysis. Gastrointest Endosc. Vol.51, No. 6., (June 2000) pp. 690-6. ISSN 1097-6779

[45] Kato, M., Jung, Y, Gromski, M.A., Chuttani, R., Matthes, K. (2012) Prospective, randomized comparison of 3 different hemoclips for the treatment of acute upper GI hemorrhage in an established experimental setting. Gastrointest Endosc. Vol.75, No. 1., (January 2012) pp. 3-10. ISSN 1097-6779

[46] Gibbs, D.H., Opelka, F.G., Beck, D.E., Hicks, T.C., Timmcke, A.E., Gathright, J.B., Jr., (1996) Postpolypectomy colonic hemorrhage. Dis Colon Rectum. Vol.39, No.7., (July 1996) pp. 806-10. ISSN 1530-0358

[47] Tappero, G., Gaia, E., De Giuli, P., Martini, S., Gubetta, L., Emanuelli, G. (1992) Cold snare excision of small colorectal polyps. Gastrointest Endosc. Vol.38, No.3, (June 1992) pp. 310-13. ISSN 1097-6779

[48] Iishi, H., Tatsuta, M., Narahara, H., Iseki, K., Sakai, N. (1996) Endoscopic resection of large pedunculated colorectal polyps using a detachable snare. Gastrointest Endosc. Vol.44., No.5., (November 1996) pp. 594-7. ISSN 1097-6779

[49] Shioji, K., Suzuki, Y., Kobayashi, M., Nakamura, A., Azumaya, M., Takeuchi, M., Baba, Y., Honma, T., Narisawa, R. (2003) Prophylactic clip application does not decrease delayed bleeding after colonoscopic polypectomy. Gastrointest Endosc. Vol. 57., No. 6., (May 2003) pp. 691-4. ISSN 1097-6779.

[50] Hsieh, Y.H., Lin, H.J., Tseng, G.Y., Perng, C.L., Li, A.F., Chang, F.Y., Lee, S.D. (2001) Is submucosal epinephrine injection necessary before polypectomy? A prospective, comparative study. Hepato-Gastroenterology. Vol.48, No.41., (September-October 2001) pp. 1379-82. ISSN 0172-6390

[51] Di Giorgio, P., De Luca, L., Calcagno, G., Rivellini, G., Mandato, M., De Luca, B. (2004) Detachable snare versus epinephrine injection in the prevention of postpolypectomy bleeding: a randomized and controlled study. Endoscopy. Vol.36, No.10., (October 2004) pp. 860-3. ISSN 0013-726X

[52] Stapakis, J.C., Thickman, D. (1992) Diagnosis of pneumoperitoneum: abdominal CT vs. upright chest film. J Comput Assist Tomogr. Vol.16., No.5., (September-October 1992) pp. 713-6. ISSN 1532-3145

[53] Rabeneck, L., Paszat, L.F., Hilsden, R.J., Saskin, R., Leddin, D., Grunfield, E., Wai, E., Godwasser, M., Sutradhar, R., Stukel, T.A. (2008) Bleeding and perforation after outpatient colonoscopy and their risk factors in usual clinical practice. Gastroenterology. Vol.135., No.6., (December 2008) pp.1899-1906. ISSN 0016-5085

[54] Rex, D.K., Petrini, J.L., Baron, T.H., Chak, A., Cohen, J., Deal, S.E., Hoffman, B., Jacobson, B.C., Mergener, K., Petersen, B.T., Safdi, M.A., Faigel, D.O., Pike, I.M. (2006) Quality indicators for colonoscopy. Gastrointest Endosc. Vol.63., Suppl.4., (April 2006) pp. S 16-28. ISSN 1097-6779

[55] Tamegai, Y., Saito, Y., Masaki, N., Hinohara, C., Oshima, T., Kogure, E., Liu, Y., Uemura, N., Saito, K. (2007) Endoscopic submucosal dissection: a safe technique for colorectal tumors.. Endoscopy. Vol.39., No.5., (May 2007) pp. 418-22. ISSN 0013-726X

[56] Kakushima, N., Fujishiro, M., Kodashima, S., Muraki, Y., Tateishi, A., Yahagi, N., Omata, M. (2007) Technical feasibility of endoscopic submucosal dissection for gastric neoplasm in the elderly Japanese population. J Gastroenterol Hepatol. Vol.22., No.3., (March 2007) pp. 311-4. ISSN 1440-1746

[57] Yoshida, N., Wakabayashi, N., Kanemasa, K., Sumida, Y., Hasegawa, D., Inoue, K., Morimoto, Y., Kashiwa, A., Konishi, H., Yagi, N., Naito, Y., Yanagisawa, A., Yoshikawa, T. (2009) Endoscopic submucosal dissection for colorectal tumors: technical difficulties and rate of perforation. Endoscopy. Vol.41., No.9. (September 2009) pp. 758-61. ISSN 0013-726X

[58] Putcha, R.V., Burdick, J.S. (2003) Management of iatrogenic perforation. Gastroenterol Clin North Am. Vol.32, No.4, (December 2003) pp. 1289-309. ISSN 0889-8553

[59] Mattel, P., Alonso, M., Justinich, C. (2005) Laparoscopic repair of colon perforation after colonoscopy in children: report of two cases and review of the literature. J. Pediat Surg. Vol.40, No.10., (October 2005) pp. 1651-3. ISSN 0022-3468

[60] Orsoni, P., Berdah, S., Verrier, C., Caamano, A., Sastre, B., Boutboul, R., Grimaud, J.C., Picaud, R. (1997) Colonic perforation due to colonoscopy: a retrospective study of 48 cases. Endoscopy. Vol.28., No.3., (March 1997) pp. 160-4. ISSN 0013-726X

[61] Won, D.Y., Lee, I.K., Lee, Y.S., Cheung, D.Y., Choi, S.B., Jung, H., Oh, S.T. (2012) The indications for nonsurgical management in patients with colorectal perforation after colonoscopy. Am Surg. Vol.78., No.5., (May 2012) pp. 550-4. ISSN 0003-1348

[62] Lee, S.H. and Cheong, Y.S. (2012) Successful endoscopic repair of an iatrogenic colonic perforation during diagnostic colonoscopy. J Am Board Fam Med. Vol.25., No.3, (May-June 2012) pp. 383-9. ISSN 1544-8770

[63] Voermans, R.P., Le Moine, O., von Rentein, D., Ponchon, T., Giovannini, M., Bruno, M., Weusten, B., Seewald, S., Costamagna, G., Deprez, P., Fockens, P., CLIPPER Study Group. (2012) Efficacy of endoscopic closure of acute perforations of the gastrointestinal tract. Clin Gastroenterol Hepatol. Vol.10., No.6., (June 2012) pp. 603-8. ISSN 1542-3565

[64] Zubarik, R., Fleischer, D.E., Mastropietro, C., Lopez, J., Carroll, J., Benjamin, S., Eisen, G. (1999) Prospective analysis of complications 30 days after outpatient colonoscopy. Gastrointest Endosc. Vol.50., No.3., (September 1999) pp. 322-8. ISSN 1097-6779

[65] Bini, E.J., Firoozi, B., Choung, R.J., Ali, E.M., Osman, M., Weinshel, E.H. (2003) Systematic evaluation of complications related to endoscopy in a training setting: A prospective 30-day outcomes study. Gastrointest Endosc. Vol.57., No.1., (January 2003) pp. 8-16. ISSN 1097-6779

[66] Ko, C.W., Riffle, S., Shapiro, J.A., Saunders, M.D., Lee, S.D., Tung, B.Y., Kuver, R., Larson, A.M., Kowdley, K.V., Kimmey, M.B. (2007) Incidence of minor complications and time lost from normal activities after screening or surveillance colonoscopy. Gastrointest Endosc. Vol.65., No.4., (April 2007) pp. 648-56. ISSN 1097-6779

[67] Wong, J.C., Yau, K.K., Cheung, H.Y., Wong, D.C., Chung, C.C., Li, M.K. (2008) Towards painless colonoscopy: a randomized controlled trial on carbon dioxide-insufflating colonoscopy. ANZ J Surg. Vol.78., No.10., (October 2008) pp. 871-4. ISSN 1445-2197

[68] Leung, J.W., Mann, S.K., Siao-Salera, R., Ransibrahmanakui, K., Lim, B., Cabrera, H., Canete, W., Barredo, P., Gutierrez, R., Leung, F.W. (2009) A randomized, controlled comparison of warm water infusion in lieu of air insufflation versus air insufflation for aiding colonoscopy insertion in sedated patients undergoing colorectal cancer screening and surveillance. Gastrointest Endosc. Vol.70., No.3., (September 2009) pp. 505-10. ISSN 1097-6779

[69] Nivatvongs, S. (1986) Complications in colonoscopic polypectomy, an experience with 1,555 polypectomies. Dis Colon Rectum. Vol.29., No.12., (December 1986) pp. 825-30. ISSN 1530-0358

[70] Waye, J.D., Lewis, B.S., Yessayan, S. (1992) Colonoscopy: a prospective report of complications. J Clin Gastroenterol. Vol.15., No.4., (December 1992) pp. 347-51. ISSN 1539-2031

[71] Nelson, D.B. (2003) Infectious disease complications of GI endoscopy: part I, endogenous infections. Gastrointest Endosc. Vol.57., No.4., (April 2003) pp. 546-56. ISSN 1097-6779

[72] Nelson, D.B. (2003) Infectious disease complications of GI endoscopy: part II, exogenous infections. Gastrointest Endosc.Vol.57., No.6., (May 2003) pp. 695-711. ISSN 1097-6779

[73] ASGE Standards of Practice Committee, Banerjee, S., Shen, B., Baron, T.H., Nelson, D.B., Anderson, M.A., Cash, B.D., Dominitz, J.A., Gan, S.I., Harrison, M.E., Ikenberry, S.O., Jagannath, S.B., Lichtenstein, D., Fanelli, R.D., Lee, K., van Guilder, T., Stewart, L.E. (2008) Antibiotic prophylaxis for GI endoscopy. Gastrointest Endosc. Vol.67., No.6., (May 2008) pp. 791-8. ISSN 1097-6779

[74] Rutter, C.M., Johnson, E., Miglioretti, D.L., Mandelson, M.T., Inadomi, J. Buist, D.S. (2012) Adverse events after screening and follow-up colonoscopy. Cancer Causes Control. Vol. 23., No.2., (February 2012) pp. 289-96. ISSN 1573-7225

[75] Izzedine, H., Thauvin, H., Maisel, A., Bourry, E., Deschamps, A. (2005) Post-colonoscopy appendicitis: case report and review of the literature. Am J Gastroenterol. Vol. 100., No.12., (December 2005) pp. 2815-7. ISSN 0002-9270

[76] ASGE Quality Assurance in Endoscopy Committee, Petersen, B.T., Chennat, J., Cohen, J., Cotton, P.B., Greenwald, D.A., Kowalski, T.E., Krinsky, M.L., Park, W.G., Pike, I.M., Romagnuolo, J.: Society for Health care Epidemiology of America, Rutala, WA. (2011) Multisociety guideline on reprocessing flexible gastrointestinal endoscopes: 2011. Gastrointest Endosc. Vol.73., No.6., (June 2011) pp. 1075-84. ISSN 1097-6779

[77] Kume, K., Yoshikawa, I., Harada, M. (2009) A rare complication: incarceration of a colonoscope in an inguinal hernia. Endoscopy. Vol.41., Supplement 2. (2009) pp. E172 ISSN 0013-726X

[78] Shankar, S., and Rowe, S. (2011) Splenic injury after colonoscopy: a case report and review of the literature. Ochsner J. Vol.11., No.3., (Fall 2011) pp. 276-81. ISSN 1524-5012

[79] Avgerinos, A., Kalantzis, N., Rekoumis, G., Pallikaris, G., Arapakis, G., Kanaghinis, T. (1984) Bowel preparation and the risk of explosion during colonoscopic polypectomy. Gut. Vol.15., No.4., (April 1984) pp. 361-4. ISSN 1468-3288

[80] La Brooy, S.J., Avgerinos, A., Fendick, C.L., Williams, C.B., Misiewicz, J.J. (1981) Potentially explosive colonic concentrations of hydrogen after bowel preparation with mannitol. Lancet. Vol.21., No.1.(8221), (March 1981) pp. 634-6. ISSN 0140-6736

[81] Pendsé, D.A., and Taylor, S.A. (2012) Complications of CT colonography: a review. Eur J Radiol. (May 15, 2012) [Epub ahead of print] ISSN 0720-048X

Chapter 10

Complications of Colonoscopy

Muhammed Sherid, Salih Samo and
Samian Sulaiman

Additional information is available at the end of the chapter

http://dx.doi.org/10.5772/53202

1. Introduction

Colonoscopy is a common procedure in medical practice for a variety of gastrointestinal indications. It is widely used in the United Stated, especially since 2001, when Medicare expanded its coverage for screening for colorectal cancer to include colonoscopy. An estimated 14.2 million colonoscopies were performed in 2002 in the United States, with screening indications representing half of cases [1]. Although generally considered a safe procedure, complications of colonoscopy as an invasive procedure should be noted. Complications vary from minor symptoms such as minor abdominal discomfort to more serious complications such as colonic perforation, cardiopulmonary arrest, or even death (Table). Although most studies have focused on serious complications, the less serious complications are important because they are more frequent than reported and may have an impact on willingness of patients and their peers to undergo future colonoscopy. Colonoscopy complications are categorized as immediate; occurring during the procedure or before discharge from endoscopy unit, or delayed; occurring within 30 days of the procedure. We will present in this chapter these potential complications in detail.

2. Complications of colonoscopy

2.1. Death

Death has been reported as a complication of colonoscopy in 30 days from the procedure. Its rate varies between studies from 0 to 83.3 per 10,000 colonoscopies [2-15]. In 3 studies with a total of 16,747 patients of mean age 59 years, there was no single death within 30 days of colonoscopy [6-8]. In a study in outpatient colonoscopy in the Medicare population by using Surveillance,

Epidemiology and End Result (SEER) database, there were 53 deaths within 30 days of 53,220 patients (9.9 deaths per 10,000 colonoscopies) [2]. The main focus in that study was not the death rate but the serious gastrointestinal and cardiopulmonary events which increased with advance age, history of stroke, congestive heart failure (CHF), chronic obstructive pulmonary disease (COPD), atrial fibrillation, diabetes mellitus (DM), and use of polypectomy.

Most deaths are not related directly to the procedure itself, rather to severe underlying comorbidities such as CHF, severe underlying coronary artery disease, COPD, cirrhosis, stroke, and pneumonia [3,4,11]. In a study of 9,223 patients from the UK, there were 10 deaths within 30 days of procedure (10.8 deaths per 10,000 colonoscopies); however, four cases were considered to be due to severe comorbidities rather than the procedure itself [4]. The mean age of study population was 58 years (range: 16-95 years) with 14.1% were 75 years or older. The reported causes of death were pneumonia, CHF, myocardial infarction, stroke and cirrhosis [4]. In a study of 13,580 patients, one single death occurred during colonoscopy in patient with massive GI bleeding (0.7 deaths per 10,000 colonoscopies) [5]. One single death occurred in 26,162 colonoscopies in another study done by Tran (0.38 deaths per 10,000 colonoscopies) which occurred in a patient with underlying coronary artery disease and COPD who developed perforation and died postoperatively from myocardiac ischemia [11].

Polypectomy has been shown to be an independent risk factor for death. In a study from Germany with 82,416 colonoscopies, death rate was 0.1 per 10,000 colonoscopies, which was 7-fold higher if polypectomy was performed [9].

However, the mortality rate was as high as 83.3 deaths per 10,000 colonoscopies in an Australian study of 23,508 outpatients with 196 deaths within 30 days of the procedure, although only 3 deaths were attributed to the colonoscopy itself (1.2 deaths per 10,000 colonoscopies) [13]. In a 2010 review of complications of colonoscopy from large studies, there were 128 deaths attributed to colonoscopy among 371,099 colonoscopies (3.4 deaths per 10,000 colonoscopies) [14,15].

2.2. Cardiopulmonary complications

Cardiopulmonary complications may be related to the preparation, conscious sedation, or the procedure itself. It might occur during or immediately after the procedure, including respiratory depression, hypoxia, dyspnea, hypotension, hypertension, bradycardia, tachycardia, vasovagal reactions, cardiac arrhythmias, and chest pain. Most of these events occur at endoscopy unit; however, they may occur days after the procedure. Fortunately, most of these complications are self-limited and resolve with minor interventions. In a study of 21,375 patients by Ko,et al. there were 160 cases of respiratory depression (74.8 per 10,000 colonoscopies) [3]. Also in this study, there were 105 cases of immediate cardiovascular complications (49.1 per 10,000 colonoscopies), with the vast majority being hypotension (65 cases; 30.4 per 10,000 colonoscopies) and bradycardia (32 cases; 14.9 per 10,000 colonoscopies). Vasovagal reaction occurred in 14 cases (6.5 per 10,000 colonoscopies), tachycardia in 2 cases (0.9 per 10,000 colonoscopies), and hypertension in one case (0.4 per 10,000 colonoscopies). One hundred and thirty four cases required supplemental oxygen (62.6 per 10,000 colonoscopies), 48 cases intravenous fluids (22.4 per 10,000 colonoscopies), 29 cases naloxone (13.5 per 10,000 colonoscopies), 20 cases atropine (9.3 per 10,000 colonoscopies), and 16 cases required flumazenil (7.4 per 10,000 colonoscopies).

Complications	Rate of complications (cases per 10,000 colonoscopies)
Death	0-83.3
Cardiopulmonary events	
Hypotension	0.2-48
Hypertension	0.4-2.1
Vasovagal reaction	6.5-19
Arrhythmia	1.9-102
Bradycardia	0.3-28
Tachycardia	0.7-0.9
Chest pain	0.7-45.2
Pulmonary edema	0.2-57.3
Transient hypoxia	0.8-23
Respiratory depression	0.7-74.8
Perforation	0.4-19
Bleeding	8.5-63.8
Postpolypectomy electrocoagulation syndrome	0.3-9.3
Gas explosion	Case reports in the literature
Infections	
Bacterial endocarditis	Case reports in the literature
Acute diverticulitis	0.8-8.4
Pneumonia	0.4-0.9
Per-perineum infections	0.9-3.1
Minor GI symptoms	133.1-4100
Cerebrovascular events	0.8-6.5

Table 1. Rate of complications of colonoscopy

In a retrospective study of 174,255 colonoscopies in the Clinical Outcomes Research Initiative (CORI) database, there were 1995 unplanned cardiopulmonary events (114.4 per 10,000 colonoscopies) which were significantly higher than in EGD [16]. Hypotension occurred in 867 cases (48 per 10,000 colonoscopies), bradycardia in 507 cases (28 per 10,000 colonoscopies), vasovagal reaction in 341 cases (19 per 10,000 colonoscopies), transient hypoxia in 410 (23 per 10,000 colonoscopies), low oxygen saturation in 128 (7 per 10,000 colonoscopies), prolonged hypoxia in 14 cases (0.7 per 10,000 colonoscopies), hypertension in 38 cases(2.1 per 10,000 colonoscopies), arrhythmia in 34 cases (1.9 per 10,000 colonoscopies), chest pain in 14 cases (0.7 per 10,000 colonoscopies), respiratory distress in 13 cases(0.7 per 10,000 colonoscopies), tachycardia in 13 cases (0.7 per 10,000 colonoscopies), pulmonary edema in 4 case (0.2 per 10,000 colonoscopies), wheezing in 3 cases (0.1 per 10,000 colonoscopies), and tracheal compression in one case (0.05 per 10,000 colonoscopies) [16]. The risk factors were advanced age, high *American Society of Anesthesiologists* (ASA) class, inpatient status, trainee participation, and non-university and veterans hospitals [16].

Higher doses of meperidine required for colonoscopy were associated with higher cardiopulmonary events, whereas there was an inverse association with doses of fentanyl and midazolam in the study by Sharma [16]. The association between lower dose of benzodiazepines use in endoscopy and cardiopulmonary events was suggested first in a small earlier study [17]. Droperidol has been used effectively for conscious sedation in difficult endoscopy, but has notable potential complications including QT prolongation and torsade de pointes. In one study, the use of droperidol for conscious sedation was not associated with increased cardiopulmonary events [16].

In a study of 53,220 outpatient colonoscopies in the Medicare population using the SEER database and diagnosis coding system, there were total of 1030 cardiovascular events (193.5 per 10,000 colonoscopies) with arrhythmias compromised more than half events which were statistically significant than matched group [2]. There were 241 cases of acute coronary syndrome and 115 cases of cardiopulmonary arrest in 30 days which was not statistically significant from matched group. Advanced age, polypectomy during procedure, CHF, atrial fibrillation, DM, COPD, and stroke were the independent risk factors for adverse cardiovascular events [2]. It has been shown that life expectancy decreases significantly for patients with 3 or more chronic conditions at the time of colon cancer diagnosis, illustrating importance of considering chronic comorbidities in elderly patients when evaluating for screening colonoscopy [18].

In a study of 82,416 colonoscopies from Germany, there were 12 cases of cardiopulmonary complications during the procedure (1.4 per 10,000 colonoscopies); oxygen desaturation in 7 cases (0.8 per 10,000 colonoscopies) which were treated by oxygen supplement or flumazenil, bradycardia in 3 cases (0.3 per 10,000 colonoscopies) which were treated by atropine, and hypotension in 2 cases (0.2 per 10,000 colonoscopies) which were treated by intravenous fluids [9]. Most of these complications occurred in patients received the combination of benzodiazepines with opioids, whereas no cardiopulmonary event was recorded when use propofol [9].

Appropriate evaluation for anesthesia risk, identifying high-risk patients, consulting other specialties based on their comorbidities, and appropriate monitoring before, during and after the procedure may reduce the rate of cardiopulmonary complications.

2.3. Perforation

Colonic perforation may occur due to therapeutic endoscopic interventions, barotrauma due to air insufflation during colonoscopy, mechanical forces against colon wall, or during maneuvering of the scope. Persistent abdominal pain after colonoscopy and abdominal distension may present initially, however a late presentation with abdominal abscess is possible. Although plain X-Rays may reveal sub-diaphragmatic free air, CT scan is more sensitive to detect any free air in the abdomen and pelvis which should be considered in cases with high suspicion of perforation. The rate of perforation varies between studies from 0.4-19 cases per 10,000 colonoscopies.

There were 4 cases of perforation in a study of 82,416 colonoscopies without poypectomy (0.4 per 10,000 colonoscopies), but it was 14 times higher if polypectomy was performed during the procedure (6.3 per 10,000 colonoscopies) [9]. Although the majority of polypectomy was done in the left colon, half of the perforations after polypectomy occurred in the right colon [9].

In another study of 21,375 patients, there were 4 cases of perforation (1.8 per 10,000 colonoscopies); all of them female, two occurred without biopsy or polypectomy [3]. The risk of serious complications including perforation, GI bleeding, post-polypectomy syndrome and diverticulitis (all combined) increased with pre-procedure warfarin use and performance of polypectomy with cautery [3].

In a population-based cohort study of 67,632 colonoscopies performed in persons between 50-75 years of age, there were 37 cases of perforation (5.4 per 10,000 colonoscopies); 57% were detected on the day of procedure, 92% within 2 days, and all within 5 days [19]. In 62% of these cases snare polypectomy was performed. The median length of stay was 6 days (0-18), comparing to 2 days (0-15) when GI bleeding occurred as a complication of colonoscopy. Although 68% of them underwent surgery; one of them died after hemicolectomy, 32% were treated conservatively without mortality [19].

In a study of 53,220 Medicare beneficiaries (age 66-95 years) who had outpatient colonoscopy, there were 33 cases of perforation (6.2 per 10,000 colonoscopies) with 21 cases of them (63.6%) underwent polypectomy [2]. The independent risk factors for serious gastrointestinal complications including perforation and GI bleeding were advanced age, DM, CHF, COPD, atrial fibrillation, stroke, and performing polypectomy [2].

A study from the UK with 9,223 pediatric and adult patients, there were 12 cases of perforation (13 per 10,000 colonoscopies); half of them diagnosed at the time of colonoscopy, another two before discharge from the unit, and the rest presented 1, 7, 16, and 24 days after the procedure [4]. Four of the perforations followed biopsy or polypectomy from 1841 patients underwent any kind of therapeutic or diagnostic interventions (21.7 per 10,000 colonoscopies).

There were 15 cases of perforation in a study of 16,318 patients (9.1 per 10,000 colonoscopies); 12 cases either had biopsy or polypectomy (80%) [12]. The rate of serious complications (including perforation, bleeding, diverticulitis, postpolypectomy syndrome; all combined) after removal of polyps larger than 10 mm was significantly higher than in those with removal of smaller polyps. All perforations were detected in 7 days of the procedure. The risk factors were increasing age, female gender, and polypectomy.

In a large retrospective cohort study of 277,434 patients, 228 cases of perforation occurred (8.2 per 10,000 colonoscopies) [20]. The predictors for perforation were advanced age, obstruction as an indication for the colonoscopy, significant comorbidities, and performance of invasive interventions during the procedure.

In an Australian study of 23,508 patients over 10 years, there were 23 perforations (9.7 per 10,000 colonoscopies), 78% occurred with a mucosal intervention (hot snare polypectomy) [13]. The rectosigmoid was the most common site of perforation, followed by the cecum. Surgical intervention was performed in 83%, and one death occurred. Median time to diagnosis was 1 day (0-5 days) with length of hospitalization stay 8 days (3-26 days).

The sigmoid colon is probably susceptible to perforation due to the mechanical forces on the sigmoid during colonoscopy, the common occurrence of diverticular disease in sigmoid, and frequency of colonic polyps in this area. The relatively thin-walled right colon is more predisposed to barotrauma and thermal injury during polypectomy.

Twenty cases of perforation occurred in a study of 10,486 patients (19 per 10,000 colonoscopies); 65% in sigmoid colon and 25% in cecum [10]. Comparing to flexible sigmoidoscopy, there were only two cases of perforation in 49,501 sigmoidoscopies (0.4 per 10,000 sigmoidoscopies). Although most of perforations (91%) detected in 2 days of colonoscopy, 9% presented after 2 weeks with abdominal abscess. All patients except an 87 year old who died underwent surgery with 37% required only simple closure without any resection. The average length of stay was 7.7 ± 2.8 days. Female gender was an independent risk factor for perforation. Transmural electrocautery burns (36%), mechanical injury (32%) from the tip and shaft of scope, and barotrauma (5%) were the main mechanisms of perforation [10]. Defects caused by diagnostic intervention tend to be larger than those caused by electrocautery injury.

Perforations occurring more often in female which may be due to frequency of pelvic surgery in females, diverticular disease, or the higher likelihood of looping because of longer colonic lengths [3,10,21].

In a large study of 116,000 patients underwent colonoscopy at ambulatory centers, 37 cases of perforation occurred (3.1 per 10,000 colonoscopies); most of them female (73%), 49% had diverticular disease, 54% had history of pelvic or colon surgery [21]. Sigmoid colon was the most common site of perforation (62%) then ascending colon (16%). The time to diagnosis ranged from immediate (29 patients) to 3 days (8 patients). Surgery was performed in 95%, and conservative treatment in the rest. No mortality occurred.

Although surgery consultation should be obtained in any case of perforation, conservative treatment with bowel rest, hydration, and intravenous antibiotics has been increasingly used in selected cases [5,19,21]. There are also case reports revealing successful closure with endoscopic clips to repair perforations [22].

In a study of 97,091 outpatient colonoscopies, the rate of perforation was 8.5 per 10,000 colonoscopies. The risk factors for colonoscopy-related perforation were older age, increased comorbidity score, polypectomy, and low-volume endoscopists (when perforation combined with bleeding) [23]. However, this finding was different from a study by Wexner which showed neither an absolute number of prior colonoscopies, nor any ongoing annual experience affected the serious complication rates [5]. Also Ko and colleagues did not find any relation between complication rate and annual colonoscopy volume, trainee participation, or practice setting [3].

Preventative measures to avoid perforation have been suggested, including decreasing the risk of barotrauma by minimal air insufflation, minimizing loop formation, encouraging the use of cold techniques in the removal of small polyps, and injection of saline into the submucosa for removal of flat or sessile polyps [14,15].

2.4. Bleeding

Colonic bleeding is the most common serious complication following colonoscopy. Although it may occur after diagnostic procedure, it mostly follows therapeutic colonoscopy from either biopsy or polypectomy, and can be immediate or delayed up to several weeks after colonoscopy.

In a population-based study of 97,091 patients aged 50-75 years, bleeding rate within 30 days was 16.4 per 10,000 outpatient colonoscopies. The independent risk factors for colonoscopy-related bleeding were older age, male gender, polypectomy, and low-volume endoscopists [23].

In another population-based, matched cohort study of 53,220 Medicare patients of age 66-95 years, there were 340 cases of GI bleeding (63.8 per 10,000 outpatient colonoscopies) which was significantly higher than matched group [2]. The risk of bleeding was 4 times higher when polypectomy was performed (21 bleeding episodes per 10,000 colonoscopies without polypectomy compared to 87 per 10,000 colonoscopies with polypectomy). Older age, history of COPD, CHF, atrial fibrillation, and stroke were other independent risk factors for serious GI events (bleeding and perforation) [2].

In a study of 23,508 patients, 49 cases of GI bleeding occurred (20.8 cases per 10,000 colonoscopies); all cases associated with biopsy or polypectomy, median time to presentation with bleeding was 6 days (0-14 days), and length of stay was 2 days (1-18 days) [13]. No death was contributed to bleeding, none required surgery, colonoscopic interventions was performed in 4 cases (8%), and blood transfusion in 7 cases (14%) [13].

Use of aspirin or any other non-steroidal anti-inflammatory drugs (NSAIDs) alone does not increase risk of postpolypectomy bleeding. Thus, the American Society for Gastrointestinal Endoscopy (ASGE) recommends continuing aspirin and NSAIDs if one of them is used alone and if its use is necessary [24-27]. However, there is some evidence that combination of aspirin with one or more NSAIDs may increase the risk of bleeding after polypectomy; therefore discontinuation of NSIADs 2-3 days before polypectomy is recommended in patients receiving aspirin [24-27]. Also, use of clopidogrel alone does not increase risk of post-polypectomy bleeding; however, concomitant use of aspirin or any other NSAIDs increases the risk of bleeding [3,24,25,28].

Pre-procedure warfarin use increases risk of bleeding after colonoscopy, thus discontinuation of warfarin is recommended 3-5 days before colonoscopy, however bridging with heparin or its equivalents is important in high risk patients for thrombosis such as a mechanical cardiac valve [3,14,24,25,29].

A prospective cohort study of 21,375 patients of age over 40 years using CORI database, there were 34 cases of GI bleeding requiring hospitalization within 30 days following colonoscopy (15.9 per 10,000 colonoscopies), and half of them required blood transfusion [3]. Pre-procedure warfarin use and snare polypectomy with cautery had an increased risk of serious complications. Risk increased even further if more than one polypectomy with cautery was done.

Size of resected polyps, number of polyps removed, and histology type of polyps have been reported as increased risk factors for postpolypectomy bleeding [3,28-30].

Management of bleeding detected during colonoscopy can be performed with endoscopic approach; however, delayed bleeding is managed conservatively with bowel rest, intravenous hydration and blood transfusion if required. Repeat colonoscopy is often required for hemostasis. Angiographic embolization and surgery are preserved for selected cases with massive, severe, persistent bleeding [3,15,31]. However, many cases of bleeding are minimal and self-limited.

Twenty one cases of bleeding occurred within 30 days in a study of 24,509 patients aged 16 years or older who underwent lower GI endoscopy including colonoscopy and sigmoidoscopy (8.5 per 10,000 colonoscopies) [31]. Seven of them required blood transfusion, 15 required repeat endoscopy and 2 required laparotomy. The average time to present was 6 days (0-16 days).

Some measures suggested to decrease the bleeding rate after polypectomy including use of cold snare instead of hot biopsy forceps, prophylactic use of mechanical methods such as clips and detachable snare loops, and injection of epinephrine into submucosa of large sessile polyps [14,15,32].

2.5. Postpolypectomy electrocoagulation syndrome

Postpolypectomy syndrome results from electrocoagulation injury to the bowel wall when electrocautery is used which causes transmural burn and focal peritoneal inflammation without radiologic evidence of frank colonic perforation. It is characterized by severe localized abdominal pain, fever, localized peritonitis signs, and leukocytosis without any radiologic evidence of perforation. Patients usually present within 1-5 days after colonoscopy performed with electrocautery polypectomy. The rate of this syndrome varies from 0.3 to 9.3 cases per 10,000 colonoscopies, depending on differences in defining this syndrome [12,14,15,31].

In a study of 16,318 patients aged 40 years or older, 6 cases of postpolypectomy syndrome occurred in 11,083 colonoscopies with biopsy performed (5.4 cases per 10,000 colonoscopies) [12].

The recognition of postpolypectomy syndrome is of importance because it does not require surgical treatment as frank perforation. The diagnosis can be made by CT scan in the appropriate clinical scenario which shows focal thickening of the colonic wall at a polypectomy site with peri-colonic fat stranding [33]. The treatment is conservative, including bowel rest, intravenous hydration and antibiotics [15,33]. Outpatient management with oral antibiotics also has been reported [12].

Postpolypectomy syndrome occurs more often with resection of large sessile polyps when prolonged, high thermal energy is applied. Therefore saline injection into the sub mucosa of large sessile polyps before polypectomy may decrease the rate of this complication [33].

2.6. Gas explosion

Gas explosion during colonoscopy is rare but has potential life-threatening consequences including death. It triggers when three elements are available in the colon lumen: high level of combustible gases such as hydrogen and methane produced by fermentation of non-absorbable carbohydrates by colonic flora, high level of oxygen, and electrical energy that produces heat such as electrocautery and argon plasma coagulation [15,34,35]. High levels of hydrogen and methane are produced in the colonic lumen by fermentation of non-absorbable carbohydrates (lactulose, mannitol) or incompletely absorbed carbohydrates (lactose, fructose, sorbitol) by the colonic bacteria, or the presence of stool in the colonic lumen due to poor cleansing preparation or using enema for sigmoidoscopy [15,34-38]. In a review in 2007 searching from 1952-2006, there were only ten cases reported in the literature including one case from the reviewer [15,34]. Most of cases caused colonic perforation with one death. Bowel preparation using manitol which is rarely used in current practice for colonic cleansing, using cleansing solutions containing sorbitol, or using enemas containing no fermentable agents were participating factors for gas explosions [34]. Newer bowel preparation solutions such as polyethylene glycol (PEG) and sodium phosphate are safer for electrocautery and argon plasma coagulation by not producing inflammable levels of hydrogen and methane. Using argon plasma coagulation during sigmoidoscopy following enemas carries risk for gas explosion which should only be performed after complete colonic preparation with new solutions not containing manitol or sorbitol. It has been suggested using frequent air insufflation and suction before performing these procedures, using carbon dioxide during colonoscopy, and using oral antibiotics to decrease combustible levels of hydrogen and methane in colonic lumen when using manitol or sorbitol [15,35-37].

2.7. Acute diverticulitis

Acute diverticulitis is another potential complication of colonoscopy. It is caused by microscopic perforation of the colon which may develops following colonoscopy in persons with pre-existing diverticulosis due to barotrauma or mechanical forces from the endoscope. Acute diverticulitis following colonoscopy has been poorly investigated and infrequently mentioned in studies reporting other complications of colonoscopy. The rate of diverticulitis as a complication of colonoscopy has been reported from 0.8 to 8.4 cases per 10,000 colonoscopies [3,12,14,31].

In a study of 16,318 patients aged 40 years or older, there were 6 cases of diverticulitis within 30 days of colonoscopy (3.6 cases per 10,000 colonoscopies); 2 cases required surgery and the rest were treated conservatively, 5 of them developed in colonoscopy with biopsy performed [12].

In another study of 21,375 patients aged 40 or older, there were 18 cases of diverticulitis within 30 days of colonoscopy (8.4 per 10,000 colonoscopies) with majority did not require hospitalization [3]. The risk factors for serious GI complications (perforation, bleeding, postpolypectomy syndrome, and diverticulitis) were prior warfarin use, and polypectomy with cautery; however, these risks were not individualized to each complication but all combined [3].

In third study of 24,509 outpatients who underwent colonoscopy or sigmoidoscopy, there 2 cases of acute diverticulitis within 30 days of colonoscopy (0.8 per 10,000 colonoscopies) [31].

2.8. Infection

Transient bacteremia can occur during and after colonoscopy due to bacterial translocation of normal colonic flora to blood stream. Then these bacteria may potentially adhere to distant tissue such as endocardium and artificial devices, however clinical infections are rare. Transient bacteremia associated with colonoscopy occurs in average of 4.4% ranging from 0-25% [24,39,40]. However, harmless transient bacteremia occurs in some daily activities such as tooth brushing in 23-68% [24,39,41]. These isolated bacteria during colonoscopy are generally believed to have little potential to cause endocarditis. The most common isolated organisms are normal skin flora which could contamination during blood draw [24,42,43]. Despite more than 14 million colonoscopies are performed each year in the United States, there have been only 15 reported cases of infectious endocarditis with temporal relation with colonoscopy; thus, potential side effects of prophylactic antibiotic outweigh their possible benefit of preventing endocarditis [24,39,44]. Due to the lack of convincing evidence of risk of endocarditis, both the American Heart Association (AHA) and ASGE have revised their recommendations against prophylactic antibiotics before colonoscopy [39,44].

In cirrhotic patients with or without ascites in the absence of acute GI bleeding who undergo colonoscopy, the risk of bacteremia is low. In a study of 58 cirrhotic patients who underwent colonoscopy, there were 4 cases of positive blood culture (6.9%) without in development of infections [42].

Patients on peritoneal dialysis may be at risk for infectious complications after colonoscopy. There are several reported cases of peritonitis in patients on peritoneal dialysis after colonoscopy especially postpolypectomy [45,46]. The International Society for Peritoneal Dialysis (ISPD) in 2005 recommended prophylactic antibiotics and emptying the peritoneal fluid before colonoscopy; however 2010 ISPD recommendations did not address these prevention strategies [47,48].

Infections in prosthetic joints has been reported after colonoscopy, however the risk is too low which led ASGE to recommend against using prophylactic antibiotics for patients who have prosthetic orthopedic devices undergoing colonoscopy [39,49,50].

http://dx.doi.org/10.5772/53202

Acute appendicitis following colonoscopy has been described in the literature. In a review in 2008, there were only 12 cases reported in literature from 1985 to 2007 [51]. Pre-existing subclinical disease of the appendix, barotrauma, impaction of stool into the appendix, direct intubation of appendiceal lumen, and focal edema in appendiceal orifice from trauma leading to obstruction are proposed mechanisms of acute appendicitis after colonoscopy [51].

Pneumonia within 30 days of colonoscopy has been reported. In a study of 21,375 patients, there were 2 cases of pneumonia within 30 days of colonoscopy (0.9 cases per 10.000 colonoscopies) [3]. Another study of 24,509 patients, 1 case of pneumonia developed in 30 days of colonoscopy (0.4 per 10,000 colonoscopies) [31]. The mechanism is mostly aspiration secondary to sedation and anesthesia more than related to the procedure itself.

Local infections in perineum including perianal abscess and Fournier's gangrene have been described following colonoscopy. In a study of 3,196 patients, there was one case of Fournier's gangrene occurring 2 days after colonoscopy (3.1 cases per 10,000 colonoscopies) [6]. In another study of 21,375 patients, 2 cases of perirectal abscess occurred during 30 days of colonoscopy (0.9 per 10,000 colonoscopies) [3]. The mechanism is local mechanical trauma to the perineum area during the procedure.

2.9. Abdominal pain and other minor GI symptoms

Although abdominal pain can be the symptom of above mentioned serious complications, less severe abdominal discomfort is more common following colonoscopy. The mechanism is multifactorial including mechanical trauma, barotrauma, gaseous distension secondary to air insufflation. It is usually self-limited and rarely required hospitalization; however it is of importance because it may affect the adherence for any future surveillance colonoscopy. In a study by Ko et al. there were 5 cases of abdominal pain requiring hospitalization (2.3 cases per 10,000 colonoscopies) [3]. In a study of 53,220 patients, abdominal pain occurred in 176 patients (33 cases per 10,000 colonoscopies), paralytic ileus in 172 patients (32.3 cases per 10,000 colonoscopies), and nausea and vomiting in 361 patients (67.8 cases per 10,000 colonoscopies) which all were significantly higher compared to the matched group [2]. The risk of these symptoms was higher if polypectomy was performed.

Minor adverse events that defined as any health problem that patient experienced in 30 days of colonoscopy not requiring a hospital visit were reported in telephone interview in 466 patients of a study of 1,528 patients (41%) with majority were GI symptoms including 195 cases of abdominal discomfort, 64 cases of self-limited rectal bleeding which lasted 1-3 days, 6 cases of nausea, and 62 cases of change in bowel habits including diarrhea (n=20), constipation (n=11), flatulence (n=8), fecal incontinence(n=3), fecal urgency (n=3), and mucus discharge (n=2) [8]. There were also 2 cases of severe abdominal pain that required hospitalization. Among the patients who were not retired and reported minor adverse events, 26.1% missed one extra day of work after the day of procedure, 5.9% missed 2 days beside the day of colonoscopy, and 8.8% missed 3 days or more [8].

Minor complications occurred in 162 subjects (34%) in a prospective cohort study by Ko et al. most commonly bloating (25%) and abdominal pain (11%) [52]. Minor adverse events were more common in women, and when the procedure lasted 20 minutes or longer. Colonic preparation was reported by patients as the most difficult part of the procedure in 77%. Most patients (94%) missed 2 or fewer days from normal activities for the preparation, procedure itself, or recovery [52].

These minor adverse events have 3 aspects of effect; they are inconvenience to patients, have indirect cost by missing work, and can affect the willingness of patients to undergo any further colonoscopy in future if need it.

Reducing looping of the endoscope and minimizing air insufflation may decrease some of these symptoms [53]. It has been also suggested using carbon dioxide, which is rapidly absorbed and excreted through lungs, as an insufflating gas for colonoscopy to reduce these symptoms [54,55]. Also water immersion technique instead of air insufflation has been proposed to reduce these minor events especially in cases of minimal sedation [56] (Leung 2010).

2.10. Miscellaneous

The most serious miscellaneous complications have reported within 30 days of colonoscopy are cerebrovascular accident (CVA), transient ischemic attack (TIA), and pulmonary embolisms which most likely related to temporary cessation of anticoagulation agents and antiplatelet medications peri-procedure period [3,6-8,13].

Stroke or TIA occurred within 30 days of colonoscopy in 3.3 cases per 10,000 colonoscopies in study of 21,375 patients [3]. In a study of 1,528 patients, there was one case of TIA, and one case of pulmonary embolism within 30 days of colonoscopy (6.5 cases of each per 10,000 colonoscopies) [8]. A third study of 23,508 patients, there were two cases of TIA and reversible ischemic neurologic deficit lasting 24 hours and 72 hours, occurring in recovery period following the procedure (0.8 per 10,000 colonoscopies) [13]. However, these rates are comparable with the expected annual adjusted rate of stroke in general population [3].

Splenic hematoma and rupture, intramural hematoma, subcutaneous emphysema in the absence of frank colonic perforation, tearing of mesenteric vessels with intra-abdominal bleeding, thrombosis in carotid-subclavian artery bypass graft, thrombophlebitis in the intravenous site, intestinal obstruction, and ischemic and chemical colitis secondary to glutaraldehyde or air insufflation have been reported following colonoscopy in literature [3,14,15,23,31,57,58].

2.11. Polyp and cancer miss rates

Although it is not a true complication of colonoscopy, missing colorectal polyps and cancer is of importance because it affects patient's safety, malpractice, and determining the surveillance interval for repeat colonoscopy. In a study of 235 patients, the miss rate for advanced adenomas which defined as polyps ≥10 mm with or without a villous component or high-grade dysplasia was 2.5% and 3.3% for patients who had complete colonoscopy and satisfactory colon preparation on second and third repeat colonoscopy, respectively [59]. There was no cancer missed [59].

In another prospective study with repeated colonoscopy performed within 2 months of first colonoscopy, the miss rate of colorectal polyps was 21.2%; however, as number of polyps found on first colonoscopy increased, the miss rate increased to reach 77.8% when 4 polyps found [60]. The miss rate decreased inversely with polyps' size from 23.9% with polyps of 1-4 mm to 10% for polyps of size ≥10 mm [60].

However, the overall miss rate for adenomas was as high as 24% in a study of 183 patients who underwent 2 consecutive colonoscopies on the same day. The miss rate increased with number of polyps detected on first colonoscopy, inversely with polyps' size, and right colon [61].

In a systematic review of 6 studies of a total of 465 patients, the pooled polyps miss rate was 22% which increased inversely with polyps' size to reach 26% for polyps of 1-5 mm [62].

Also withdrawal time of endoscope is an important factor for detecting adenomas with minimal recommended time of 6 minutes. The detection rates for adenomas ≥ 10 mm were only 2.6% for endoscopists with mean withdrawal time less than 6 minutes, compared to 6.4% for those with withdrawal time greater than 6 minutes [63]. Therefore, polyp miss rate increases with short withdrawal time.

3. Complications associated with specific colonoscopic interventions

3.1. Colonoscopic tattooing

Colonic tattooing is an injection of permanent dye into the submucosal layer of colon wall that adjacent to the lesion for easier future localization either for surgical resection or colonoscopic follow-up. Although three studies with a total of 264 patients who underwent colonoscopic tattooing reported no fever, abdominal pain, or any major complications [64-66], a systematic review of 447 patients with colonoscopic tattooing described 5 cases of complications with only one was an overt clinical complication (22.3 per 10,000 tattooing) [67].

It has been reported cases of intramural hematoma, colonic abscess, rectus muscle abscess following colonoscopic tattooing, bowel obstruction, retroperitoneal colonic perforation due to localized necrosis, adhesion ileus, and spread of the dye following colonoscopic tattooing [68-75].

3.2. Colonic balloon dilation

Colonic dilation has been used as a non-surgical treatment for benign strictures that associated with Crohn's disease and those at surgical anastomoses [76].

In a systematic review in 2007 of 13 studies with 347 patients with Crohn's disease with colonic strictures who underwent 695 sessions of colonic dilation, there were 14 cases of major complications (201.4 cases per 10,000 colonic dilations); 13 cases being bowel perforation (92.8%) [77].

Two prospective studies with a total of 42 patients with benign colorectal anastomotic stenosis, not associated with Crohn's disease, who underwent 81 sessions of colonic dilation reported no procedure-related complications [78,79].

3.3. Colonic stent placement

Self-expandable metal stents (SEMS) have been used in the management of colorectal obstruction as a bridge to surgery or as a palliative treatment especially malignant obstruction. In a pooled analysis of 54 studies with 1,198 patients who underwent colonic stent placement, the major complications related to stent placement included stent migration (11.81%), reobstruction (7.34%), perforation (3.76%), and mortality (0.58%) [80]. The risk factors for stent migration which may occur proximally or distally were using covered stent, laser treatment, dilation prior stent insertion, and the use of chemotherapy and radiotherapy. The causes for reobstruction were tumor ingrowth (73.2%), fecal impaction, mucosal prolapse, stent migration, tumor overgrowth, and peritoneal seeding. The reobstruction was significantly higher in uncovered stents. The perforation was related to stent wires, balloon dilation, guide wires, or related to laser recanalization prior stent placement. The death was related to colonic perforation and its consequences in majority of cases [80].

In another systematic review of 1,785 patients with 1,845 stent placements, colonic reobstruction in 12%, migration of the stent occurred in 11%, perforation in 4.5%. Other reported complications of stent placement included GI bleeding, anal pain, abdominal pain, and tenesmus which were relatively rare and generally well tolerated by patients [81]. It is not recommended to perform dilation around the time of stent placement due to increased perforation risk [76,80].

Despite of the early termination of 3 randomized controlled trials comparing SEMS to surgery because of high rate of complications in SEMS groups, a recent systematic review in 2012 with 234 patients including these 3 trials showed that the clinical perforation rate was 6 9% and the silent perforation rate 14%. There was no difference between SEMS arm and emergent surgery in primary anastomosis, permanent stoma, in-hospital mortality, anastomotic leak, 30-day reoperation and surgical-site infection rates [82-85].

3.4. Colonic decompression tube placements

Transanal endoscopic decompression tube placement has been used in acute colorectal obstruction or pseudo-obstruction before surgery or stenting.

In 5 series consisting of 153 patients with acute colonic obstruction treated with transanal decompression tube placement, two cases of bowel perforation occurred (1.3%) [86-90].

In a series of 50 patients with acute colonic pseudo-obstruction who underwent 54 decompression tube placements, one case of bowel perforation occurred (2%), and overall in-hospital mortality was 30% reflecting severe underlying comorbidities [91].

3.5. Percutaneous endoscopic colostomy

Percutaneous endoscopic colostomy (PEC) is considered a minimally invasive endoscopic procedure that has been used as an alternative modality to surgery in poor surgical candidates who have recurrent sigmoid volvulus, recurrent colonic pseudo-obstruction, neurogenic bowel or severe slow-transit constipation [76,92-94].

The complications of PEC that has been reported are fecal peritonitis (8.5%), fecal leakage, recurrent infections (77%), buried internal bolster, abdominal wall bleeding and pain [92-94]. All-cause mortality has been reported as high as 26% reflecting the often frail patients who undergo PEC [92-94].

3.6. Colonic hemostasis

Colonic hemostasis devices are used to treat GI bleeding including diverticular bleeding, postpolypectomy bleeding, angiodysplasia, and radiation-induced angioectasias. Colonic hemostasis devices include contact thermal devices (eg, heater probe [HP], multipolar electrocautery [MPEC] probes, and hemostatic graspers), noncontact thermal devices (eg, argon plasma coagulator [APC]), mechanical devices (eg, band ligators, clips, and loops) and injection needles [95].

Initial worsening of bleeding may occur when applying any of these devices which can be successfully treated by an additional application of the same or different device [15]. Colonic perforation especially right colon has been reported as high as 2.5% with thermal devices [15,95,96]. Distention of the GI tract with argon gas, submucosal emphysema, pneumomediastinum, pneumoperitoneum, and gas explosion has been reported as complications of ACP [95,97,98].

There are multiple reports of premature deployment of the clip, and the failure to separate the clip from the catheter after deployment [95]. Colonic perforation, initial worsening bleeding, clip retention, immediate or delayed bleeding secondary to slippage of loop when using detachable loop ligating devices have been described [95,99].

The complications of injection needles are usually related to injected substances such as cardiac arrhythmias and hypertension due to epinephrine, however, there are reports of needles separating from the catheter in the patient and requiring retrieval, and of needles failing to extend from their sheaths [95].

3.7. Foreign body removal

Colorectal foreign bodies may result from the insertion in the rectum for sexual pleasure, non-sexual purposes such as body packing of illicit drugs for transportation purposes, accidentally, by swallowing solid objects such as bones and toothpicks, or migration into the colon from the adjacent organs such as intrauterine contraceptive devices and inguinal hernia mesh [15,100-103]. Numerous kinds of objects have been described in the literature including fruits, vegetables, cans, bottles, bull horn, batteries, light bulbs, cosmetic containers, and children or sex toys [100,104]. The presenting symptoms of colorectal foreign bodies are pelvic pain, abdominal pain, the peritoneal signs if perforation occurs, rectal bleeding, rectal mucous drainage, fecal incontinence, bowel obstruction, or drug overdose if bag ruptures during removal attempts in body pocking of illicit drugs [15,100,101,104].

These symptoms and the management varies considerably based on the type of inserted objects (sharp versus blunt), traumatic or not, and illicit drug involved or not [15,101]. Management of colorectal foreign bodies can be challenging and a systematic approach should be employed including abdominal plain film and CT scan to evaluate for free intra-abdominal air, shape and size of object, and its location and relations to the pelvis [15,100,101]. The majority of cases can be successfully managed conservatively, but occasionally such as large objects or tightly wedged in the pelvis surgical intervention is warranted [15,100]. It not recommended removing drug-containing bags endoscopically because of potential rupture of bags that can lead to systemic absorption of the drug which may cause death from rapid drug overdose [15,105].

3.8. Advanced techniques for colonoscopic tissue removal

These advanced techniques include endoscopic mucosal resection (EMR) and endoscopic submucosal dissection (ESD) that have been used to remove benign and early malignant lesions that confined to superficial layers (mucosa and submucosa) [15,106]. Perforation and bleeding are the most common complications for EMR and ESD which are more frequent than with standard polypectomy [15]. The size of lesion, location, histology, the type of device used, and operator experience are the factors that affects complication rates [15,107-109].

Intraprocedural bleeding rate has been reported over 10% in several large studies with delayed bleeding to up to 14% [15,101,102]. Bleeding usually is managed endoscopically, although it may require blood transfusion [15,110].

Perforation may occur in 0-5% and 5-10% in EMR and ESD respectively which is usually recognized during the procedure and managed endoscopically, although delayed perforation has been reported in 0.4% [15,107-111].

4. Conclusion

Despite these varieties of potential complications of colonoscopy and colonoscopic interventions, they occur in low rate. It is important for both patients and physicians to know these potential complications. Informing patients regarding the symptoms of these complications is of importance to seek medical attention in timely manner without delay. Also knowledge of these potential complications their frequency, risk factors, and appropriate interventions is essential for endoscopists to minimize their incidence, detect and treat them without delay.

Acknowledgements

Special thanks to Dr. Eugene F Yen who took his time to review the chapter.

Author details

Muhammed Sherid, Salih Samo and Samian Sulaiman

Saint Francis hospital, University of Illinois at Chicago, Evanston, Illinois, USA

References

[1] Seeff LC, Richards TB, Shapiro JA, Nadel MR, Manninen DL, Given LS, Dong FB, Winges LD, McKenna MT. How many endoscopies are performed for colorectal cancer screening? Results from CDC's survey of endoscopic capacity. Gastroenterology. 2004 Dec;127(6):1670-7.

[2] Warren JL, Klabunde CN, Mariotto AB, Meekins A, Topor M, Brown ML, Ransohoff DF. Adverse events after outpatient colonoscopy in the Medicare population. Ann Intern Med. 2009 Jun 16;150(12):849-57, W152.

[3] Ko CW, Riffle S, Michaels L, Morris C, Holub J, Shapiro JA, Ciol MA, Kimmey MB, Seeff LC, Lieberman D. Serious complications within 30 days of screening and surveillance colonoscopy are uncommon. Clin Gastroenterol Hepatol. 2010 Feb;8(2): 166-73.

[4] Bowles CJ, Leicester R, Romaya C, Swarbrick E, Williams CB, Epstein O. A prospective study of colonoscopy practice in the UK today: are we adequately prepared for national colorectal cancer screening tomorrow? Gut. 2004 Feb;53(2):277-83.

[5] Wexner SD, Garbus JE, Singh JJ; SAGES Colonoscopy Study Outcomes Group. A prospective analysis of 13,580 colonoscopies. Reevaluation of credentialing guidelines. Surg Endosc. 2001 Mar;15(3):251-61.

[6] Nelson DB, McQuaid KR, Bond JH, Lieberman DA, Weiss DG, Johnston TK. Procedural success and complications of large-scale screening colonoscopy. Gastrointest Endosc. 2002 Mar;55(3):307-14.

[7] Rathgaber SW, Wick TM. Colonoscopy completion and complication rates in a community gastroenterology practice. Gastrointest Endosc. 2006 Oct;64(4):556-62.

[8] De Jonge V, Nicolaas JS, van Baalen O, Brouwer JT, Stolk MF, Tang TJ, van Tilburg AJ, van Leerdam ME, Kuipers EJ. The incidence of 30-day adverse events after colonoscopy among outpatients in the Netherlands. Am J Gastroenterol. 2012 Jun;107(6): 878-84. doi: 10.1038/ajg.2012.40.

[9] Sieg A, Hachmoeller-Eisenbach U, Eisenbach T. Prospective evaluation of complications in outpatient GI endoscopy: a survey among German gastroenterologists. Gastrointest Endosc. 2001 May;53(6):620-7.

[10] Anderson ML, Pasha TM, Leighton JA. Endoscopic perforation of the colon: lessons from a 10-year study. Am J Gastroenterol. 2000 Dec;95(12):3418-22.

[11] Tran DQ, Rosen L, Kim R, Riether RD, Stasik JJ, Khubchandani IT. Actual colonoscopy: what are the risks of perforation? Am Surg. 2001 Sep;67(9):845-7; discussion 847-8.

[12] Levin TR, Zhao W, Conell C, Seeff LC, Manninen DL, Shapiro JA, Schulman J. Complications of colonoscopy in an integrated health care delivery system. Ann Intern Med. 2006 Dec 19;145(12):880-6.

[13] Viiala CH, Zimmerman M, Cullen DJ, Hoffman NE. Complication rates of colonoscopy in an Australian teaching hospital environment. Intern Med J. 2003 Aug;33(8): 355-9.

[14] Ko CW, Dominitz JA. Complications of colonoscopy: magnitude and management. Gastrointest Endosc Clin N Am. 2010 Oct;20(4):659-71.

[15] Fisher DA, Maple JT, Ben-Menachem T, Cash BD, Decker GA, Early DS, Evans JA, Fanelli RD, Fukami N, Hwang JH, Jain R, Jue TL, Khan KM, Malpas PM, Sharaf RN, Shergill AK, Dominitz JA; ASGE Standards of Practice Committee. Complications of colonoscopy. Gastrointest Endosc. 2011 Oct;74(4):745-52.

[16] Sharma VK, Nguyen CC, Crowell MD, Lieberman DA, de Garmo P, Fleischer DE. A national study of cardiopulmonary unplanned events after GI endoscopy. Gastrointest Endosc. 2007 Jul;66(1):27-34.

[17] Arrowsmith JB, Gerstman BB, Fleischer DE, Benjamin SB. Results from the American Society for Gastrointestinal Endoscopy/U.S. Food and Drug Administration collaborative study on complication rates and drug use during gastrointestinal endoscopy. Gastrointest Endosc. 1991 Jul-Aug;37(4):421-7.

[18] Gross CP, McAvay GJ, Krumholz HM, Paltiel AD, Bhasin D, Tinetti ME. The effect of age and chronic illness on life expectancy after a diagnosis of colorectal cancer: implications for screening. Ann Intern Med. 2006 Nov 7;145(9):646-53.

[19] Rabeneck L, Saskin R, Paszat LF. Onset and clinical course of bleeding and perforation after outpatient colonoscopy: a population-based study. Gastrointest Endosc. 2011 Mar;73(3):520-3.

[20] Arora G, Mannalithara A, Singh G, Gerson LB, Triadafilopoulos G. Risk of perforation from a colonoscopy in adults: a large population-based study. Gastrointest Endosc. 2009 Mar;69(3 Pt 2):654-64.

[21] Korman LY, Overholt BF, Box T, Winker CK. Perforation during colonoscopy in endoscopic ambulatory surgical centers. Gastrointest Endosc. 2003 Oct;58(4):554-7.

[22] Trecca A, Gaj F, Gagliardi G. Our experience with endoscopic repair of large colonoscopic perforations and review of the literature. Tech Coloproctol. 2008 Dec;12(4): 315-21; discussion 322.

[23] Rabeneck L, Paszat LF, Hilsden RJ, Saskin R, Leddin D, Grunfeld E, Wai E, Goldwasser M, Sutradhar R, Stukel TA. Bleeding and perforation after outpatient colonoscopy and their risk factors in usual clinical practice. Gastroenterology. 2008 Dec; 135(6):1899-1906, 1906.e1.

[24] Deepak P, Sifuentes H, Sherid M, Ehrenpreis ED. (2011). Preparing for Colonoscopy. In Jose Josquim Ribeiro da Rocha (Ed.), Endoscopic Procedures in Colon and Rectum (pp. 1-26).

[25] Anderson MA, Ben-Menachem T, Gan SI, Appalaneni V, Banerjee S, Cash BD, Fisher L, Harrison ME, Fanelli RD, Fukami N, Ikenberry SO, Jain R, Khan K, Krinsky ML, Lichtenstein DR, Maple JT, Shen B, Strohmeyer L, Baron T, Dominitz JA. ASGE Standards of Practice Committee. Management of antithrombotic agents for endoscopic procedures. Gastrointest Endosc. 2009 Dec;70(6):1060-70.

[26] Hui AJ, Wong RM, Ching JY, Hung LC, Chung SC, Sung JJ. Risk of colonoscopic polypectomy bleeding with anticoagulants and antiplatelet agents: analysis of 1657 cases. Gastrointest Endosc. 2004 Jan;59(1):44-8.

[27] Grossman, E.B; Maranino, A.N; Zamora, D.C; et al (2010). Antiplatelet medications increase the risk of post-polypectomy bleeding. Gastrointest Endosc, Vol.71, (2010), pp.AB138, ISSN: 0016-5107.

[28] Singh M, Mehta N, Murthy UK, Kaul V, Arif A, Newman N. Postpolypectomy bleeding in patients undergoing colonoscopy on uninterrupted clopidogrel therapy. Gastrointest Endosc. 2010 May;71(6):998-1005.

[29] Witt DM, Delate T, McCool KH, Dowd MB, Clark NP, Crowther MA, Garcia DA, Ageno W, Dentali F, Hylek EM, Rector WG; WARPED Consortium. Incidence and predictors of bleeding or thrombosis after polypectomy in patients receiving and not receiving anticoagulation therapy. J Thromb Haemost. 2009 Dec;7(12):1982-9. Epub 2009 Aug 28.

[30] Consolo P, Luigiano C, Strangio G, Scaffidi MG, Giacobbe G, Di Giuseppe G, Zirilli A, Familiari L. Efficacy, risk factors and complications of endoscopic polypectomy: ten year experience at a single center. World J Gastroenterol. 2008 Apr 21;14(15): 2364-9.

[31] Singh H, Penfold RB, DeCoster C, Kaita L, Proulx C, Taylor G, Bernstein CN, Moffatt M. Colonoscopy and its complications across a Canadian regional health authority. Gastrointest Endosc. 2009 Mar;69(3 Pt 2):665-71.

[32] Di Giorgio P, De Luca L, Calcagno G, Rivellini G, Mandato M, De Luca B. Detachable snare versus epinephrine injection in the prevention of postpolypectomy bleeding: a randomized and controlled study. Endoscopy. 2004 Oct;36(10):860-3.

[33] Christie JP, Marrazzo J 3rd. "Mini-perforation" of the colon--not all postpolypectomy perforations require laparotomy. Dis Colon Rectum. 1991 Feb;34(2):132-5.

[34] Ladas SD, Karamanolis G, Ben-Soussan E. Colonic gas explosion during therapeutic colonoscopy with electrocautery. World J Gastroenterol. 2007 Oct 28;13(40):5295-8.

[35] Avgerinos A, Kalantzis N, Rekoumis G, Pallikaris G, Arapakis G, Kanaghinis T. Bowel preparation and the risk of explosion during colonoscopic polypectomy. Gut. 1984 Apr;25(4):361-4.

[36] Hofstad B. Explosion in rectum. [Article in Norwegian with English abstract]. Tidsskr Nor Laegeforen. 2007 Jun 28;127(13):1789-90.

[37] Taylor EW, Bentley S, Youngs D, Keighley MR. Bowel preparation and the safety of colonoscopic polypectomy. Gastroenterology. 1981 Jul;81(1):1-4.

[38] Monahan DW, Peluso FE, Goldner F. Combustible colonic gas levels during flexible sigmoidoscopy and colonoscopy. Gastrointest Endosc. 1992 Jan-Feb;38(1):40-3.

[39] Banerjee, S; Shen, B; Baron, T.H; Nelson, D.B; Anderson, M.A; Cash, B.D; Dominitz, J.A; Gan, S.I; Harrison, M.E; Ikenberry, S.O; Jagannath, S.B; Lichtenstein, D; Fanelli, R.D; Lee, K; van Guilder, T & Stewart, L.E (2008). ASGE STANDARDS OF PRACTICE COMMITTEE. Antibiotic prophylaxis for GI endoscopy. Gastrointest Endosc, Vol. 67, No. 6, (May 2008), pp. 791-8, ISSN: 0016-5107.

[40] Nelson, D.B (2003). Infectious disease complications of GI endoscopy: part I, endogenous infections. Gastrointest Endosc, Vol.57, (2003), pp.546-56, ISSN: 0016-5107.

[41] Lockhart, P.B; Brennan, M.T; Sasser, H.C; Fox, P.C; Paster, B.J & Bahrani-Mougeot, F.K (2008). Bacteremia associated with tooth brushing and dental extraction. Circulation. Vol.117, No.24, (Jun 2008), pp.3118-25, ISSN: 0009-7322.

[42] Llach, J; Elizalde, J.I; Bordas, J.M; et al (1999). Prospective assessment of the risk of bacteremia in cirrhotic patients undergoing lower intestinal endoscopy. Gastrointest Endosc, Vol.49, (1999), pp.214-7, ISSN: 0016-5107.

[43] Levy, M.J; Norton, I.D; Clain, J.E; et al (2007). Prospective study of bacteremia and complications with EUS FNA of rectal and perirectal lesions. Clin Gastroenterol Hepatol, Vol.5, (2007), pp.684-9, ISSN: 1542-3565.

[44] Wilson, W; Taubert, K.A; Gewitz, M; Lockhart, P.B; Baddour, L.M; Levison, M; Bolger, A; Cabell, C.H; Takahashi, M; Baltimore, R.S; Newburger, J.W; Strom, B.L; Tani, L.Y; Gerber, M; Bonow, R.O; Pallasch, T; Shulman, S.T; Rowley, A.H; Burns, J.C; Ferrieri, P; Gardner, T; Goff, D & Durack, D.T (2007); American Heart Association Rheumatic Fever, Endocarditis, and Kawasaki Disease Committee; American Heart Association Council on Cardiovascular Disease in the Young; American Heart Association Council on Clinical Cardiology; American Heart Association Council on Cardiovascular Surgery and Anesthesia; Quality of Care and Outcomes Research Interdisciplinary Working Group. Prevention of infective endocarditis: guidelines from the American Heart Association: a guideline from the American Heart Association Rheumatic Fever, Endocarditis, and Kawasaki Disease Committee, Council on Cardiovascular Disease in the Young, and the Council on Clinical Cardiology, Coun-

cil on Cardiovascular Surgery and Anesthesia, and the Quality of Care and Outcomes Research Interdisciplinary Working Group. Circulation, Vol.116, No.15, (Oct 2007), pp.1736-54, ISSN: 0009-7322.

[45] Bac, D.J; van Blankenstein, M; de Marie, S & Fieren, M.W (1994). Peritonitis following endoscopic polypectomy in a peritoneal dialysis patient: the need for antibiotic prophylaxis. Infection, Vol.22, No.3, (May-Jun 1994), pp.220-1, ISSN: 0163-4453.

[46] Ray, S.M; Piraino, B & Holley, J (1990). Peritonitis following colonoscopy in a peritoneal dialysis patient. Perit Dial Int, Vol.10, No.1, (1990), pp.97-8, ISSN: 0896-8608; 1718-4304 (online).

[47] Piraino, B; Bailie, G.R; Bernardini, J; Boeschoten, E; Gupta, A; Holmes, C; Kuijper, E.J; Li, P.K; Lye, W.C; Mujais, S; Paterson, D.L; Fontan, M.P; Ramos, A; Schaefer, F &Uttley, L; ISPD Ad Hoc Advisory Committee (2005). Peritoneal dialysis-related infections recommendations: 2005 update. Perit Dial Int, Vol.25, No.2, (Mar-Apr 2005), pp. 107-31, ISSN: 0896-8608 (print); 1718-4304 (online).

[48] Li, P.K; Szeto, C.C; Piraino, B; Bernardini, J; Figueiredo, A.E; Gupta, A; Johnson, D.W; Kuijper, E.J; Lye, W.C; Salzer, W; Schaefer, F & Struijk, D.G (2010). Peritoneal dialysis-related infections recommendations: 2010 update. Perit Dial Int, Vol.30, No. 4, (Jul-Aug 2010), pp.393-423, ISSN: 0896 8608 (print); 1718-4304 (online).

[49] Vanderhooft, J.E & Robinson, R.P (1994). Late infection of a bipolar prosthesis following endoscopy. A case report. J Bone Joint Surg Am, Vol.76, (1994), pp.744-6, ISSN: 0021-9355.

[50] Cornelius, L.K; Reddix, R.N & Jr, Carpenter, J.L (2003). Periprosthetic knee joint infection following colonoscopy. A case report. J Bone Joint Surg Am, Vol.85-A, No.12, (Dec 2003), pp.2434-6, ISSN: 0021-9355.

[51] Johnston P, Maa J. Perforated appendicitis after colonoscopy. JSLS. 2008 Jul-Sep; 12(3):335-7.

[52] Ko CW, Riffle S, Shapiro JA, Saunders MD, Lee SD, Tung BY, Kuver R, Larson AM, Kowdley KV, Kimmey MB. Incidence of minor complications and time lost from normal activities after screening or surveillance colonoscopy. Gastrointest Endosc. 2007 Apr;65(4):648-56. Epub 2006 Dec 14.

[53] Waye JD. The most important maneuver during colonoscopy. Am J Gastroenterol. 2004 Nov;99(11):2086-7.

[54] Church J, Delaney C. Randomized, controlled trial of carbon dioxide insufflation during colonoscopy. Dis Colon Rectum. 2003 Mar;46(3):322-6.

[55] Wong JC, Yau KK, Cheung HY, Wong DC, Chung CC, Li MK. Towards painless colonoscopy: a randomized controlled trial on carbon dioxide-insufflating colonoscopy. ANZ J Surg. 2008 Oct;78(10):871-4.

[56] Leung CW, Kaltenbach T, Soetikno R, Wu KK, Leung FW, Friedland S. Water immersion versus standard colonoscopy insertion technique: randomized trial shows promise for minimal sedation. Endoscopy. 2010 Jul;42(7):557-63. Epub 2010 Jun 30.

[57] Ahishali E, Uygur-Bayramiçli O, Dolapçioğlu C, Dabak R, Mengi A, Işik A, Ermiş E. Chemical colitis due to glutaraldehyde: case series and review of the literature. Dig Dis Sci. 2009 Dec;54(12):2541-5.

[58] Sherid M, Ehrenpreis ED. Types of colitis based on histology. Dis Mon. 2011 Sep; 57(9):457-89.

[59] Shehadeh I, Rebala S, Kumar R, Markert RJ, Barde C, Gopalswamy N. Retrospective analysis of missed advanced adenomas on surveillance colonoscopy. Am J Gastroenterol. 2002 May;97(5):1143-7.

[60] Ji JS, Choi KY, Lee WC, Lee BI, Park SH, Choi H, Kim BW, Chae HS, Park YM, Park YJ. Endoscopic and histopathologic predictors of recurrence of colorectal adenoma on lowering the miss rate. Korean J Intern Med. 2009 Sep; 24(3):196-202.

[61] Rex DK, Cutler CS, Lemmel GT, Rahmani EY, Clark DW, Helper DJ, Lehman GA, Mark DG. Colonoscopic miss rates of adenomas determined by back-to-back colonoscopies. Gastroenterology. 1997 Jan; 112(1):24-8.

[62] van Rijn JC, Reitsma JB, Stoker J, Bossuyt PM, van Deventer SJ, Dekker E. Polyp miss rate determined by tandem colonoscopy: a systematic review. Am J Gastroenterol. 2006 Feb;101(2):343-50.

[63] Barclay RL, Vicari JJ, Doughty AS, Johanson JF, Greenlaw RL. Colonoscopic withdrawal times and adenoma detection during screening colonoscopy. N Engl J Med. 2006 Dec 14;355(24):2533-41.

[64] Aboosy N, Mulder CJ, Berends FJ, Meijer JW, Sorge AA. Endoscopic tattoo of the colon might be standardized to locate tumors intraoperatively. Rom J Gastroenterol. 2005 Sep;14(3):245-8.

[65] Feingold DL, Addona T, Forde KA, Arnell TD, Carter JJ, Huang EH, Whelan RL. Safety and reliability of tattooing colorectal neoplasms prior to laparoscopic resection. J Gastrointest Surg. 2004 Jul-Aug;8(5):543-6.

[66] McArthur CS, Roayaie S, Waye JD. Safety of preoperation endoscopic tattoo with india ink for identification of colonic lesions. Surg Endosc. 1999 Apr;13(4):397-400.

[67] Nizam R, Siddiqi N, Landas SK, Kaplan DS, Holtzapple PG. Colonic tattooing with India ink: benefits, risks, and alternatives. Am J Gastroenterol. 1996 Sep;91(9):1804-8.

[68] Yagnik V. Re: Bowel obstruction associated with endoscopic tattooing of the colon with India ink (Asian J Endosc Surg 3 (2010) 150-152). Asian J Endosc Surg. 2011 Feb; 4(1):43. doi: 10.1111/j.1758-5910.2010.00063.x.

[69] Marques I, Lagos AC, Pinto A, Neves BC. Rectal intramural hematoma: a rare complication of endoscopic tattooing. Gastrointest Endosc. 2011 Feb;73(2):366-7.

[70] Gianom D, Hollinger A, Wirth HP. [Intestinal perforation after preoperative colonic tattooing with India ink]. [Article in German with English abstract] Swiss Surg. 2003;9(6):307-10.

[71] Yano H, Okada K, Monden T. Adhesion ileus caused by tattoo-marking: unusual complication after laparoscopic surgery for early colorectal cancer. Dis Colon Rectum. 2003 Jul;46(7):987.

[72] Hellmig S, Stüber E, Kiehne K, Fölsch UR. Unusual course of colonic tattooing with India ink. Surg Endosc. 2003 Mar;17(3):521. Epub 2002 Dec 20.

[73] Alba LM, Pandya PK, Clarkston WK. Rectus muscle abscess associated with endoscopic tattooing of the colon with India ink. Gastrointest Endosc. 2000 Oct;52(4): 557-8.

[74] Dell'Abate P, Iosca A, Galimberti A, Piccolo P, Soliani P, Foggi E. Endoscopic preoperative colonic tattooing: a clinical and surgical complication. Endoscopy. 1999 Mar; 31(3):271-3.

[75] Cappell MS, Courtney JT, Amin M. Black macular patches on parietal peritoneum and other extraintestinal sites from intraperitoneal spillage and spread of India ink from preoperative endoscopic tattooing: an endoscopic, surgical, gross pathologic, and microscopic study. Dig Dis Sci. 2010 Sep;55(9):2599-605. Epub 2009 Dec 3.

[76] Harrison ME, Anderson MA, Appalaneni V, Banerjee S, Ben-Menachem T, Cash BD, Fanelli RD, Fisher L, Fukami N, Gan SI, Ikenberry SO, Jain R, Khan K, Krinsky ML, Maple JT, Shen B, Van Guilder T, Baron TH, Dominitz JA, ASGE Standards of Practice Committee. The role of endoscopy in the management of patients with known and suspected colonic obstruction and pseudo-obstruction. Gastrointest Endosc. 2010 Apr;71(4):669-79.

[77] Hassan C, Zullo A, De Francesco V, Ierardi E, Giustini M, Pitidis A, Taggi F, Winn S, Morini S. Systematic review: Endoscopic dilatation in Crohn's disease. Aliment Pharmacol Ther. 2007 Dec;26(11-12):1457-64. Epub 2007 Sep 28.

[78] Di Giorgio P, De Luca L, Rivellini G, Sorrentino E, D'amore E, De Luca B. Endoscopic dilation of benign colorectal anastomotic stricture after low anterior resection: A prospective comparison study of two balloon types. Gastrointest Endosc. 2004 Sep;60(3): 347-50.

[79] Ambrosetti P, Francis K, De Peyer R, Frossard JL. Colorectal anastomotic stenosis after elective laparoscopic sigmoidectomy for diverticular disease: a prospective evaluation of 68 patients. Dis Colon Rectum. 2008 Sep;51(9):1345-9.

[80] Sebastian S, Johnston S, Geoghegan T, Torreggiani W, Buckley M. Pooled analysis of the efficacy and safety of self-expanding metal stenting in malignant colorectal obstruction. Am J Gastroenterol. 2004 Oct;99(10):2051-7.

[81] Watt AM, Faragher IG, Griffin TT, Rieger NA, Maddern GJ. Self-expanding metallic stents for relieving malignant colorectal obstruction: a systematic review. Ann Surg. 2007 Jul;246(1):24-30.

[82] Tan CJ, Dasari BV, Gardiner K. Systematic review and meta-analysis of randomized clinical trials of self-expanding metallic stents as a bridge to surgery versus emergency surgery for malignant left-sided large bowel obstruction. Br J Surg. 2012 Apr;99(4): 469-76. doi: 10.1002/bjs.8689. Epub 2012 Jan 19.

[83] Van Hooft JE, Fockens P, Marinelli AW, Timmer R, van Berkel AM, Bossuyt PM, Bemelman WA; Dutch Colorectal Stent Group. Early closure of a multicenter randomized clinical trial of endoscopic stenting versus surgery for stage IV left-sided colorectal cancer. Endoscopy. 2008 Mar;40(3):184-91.

[84] Van Hooft JE, Bemelman WA, Oldenburg B, Marinelli AW, Holzik MF, Grubben MJ, Sprangers MA, Dijkgraaf MG, Fockens P; collaborative Dutch Stent-In study group. Colonic stenting versus emergency surgery for acute left-sided malignant colonic obstruction: a multicentre randomised trial. Lancet Oncol. 2011 Apr;12(4):344-52.

[85] Pirlet IA, Slim K, Kwiatkowski F, Michot F, Millat BL. Emergency preoperative stenting versus surgery for acute left-sided malignant colonic obstruction: a multicenter randomized controlled trial. Surg Endosc. 2011 Jun;25(6):1814-21.

[86] Fischer A, Schrag HJ, Goos M, Obermaier R, Hopt UT, Baier PK. Transanal endoscopic tube decompression of acute colonic obstruction: experience with 51 cases. Surg Endosc. 2008 Mar;22(3):683-8.

[87] Horiuchi A, Nakayama Y, Tanaka N, Kajiyama M, Fujii H, Yokoyama T, Hayashi K. Acute colorectal obstruction treated by means of transanal drainage tube: effectiveness before surgery and stenting. Am J Gastroenterol. 2005 Dec;100(12):2765-70.

[88] Tanaka T, Furukawa A, Murata K, Sakamoto T. Endoscopic transanal decompression with a drainage tube for acute colonic obstruction: clinical aspects of preoperative treatment. Dis Colon Rectum. 2001 Mar;44(3):418-22.

[89] Horiuchi A, Nakayama Y, Kajiyama M, Kamijima T, Kato N, Ichise Y, Tanaka N. Endoscopic decompression of benign large bowel obstruction using a transanal drainage tube. Colorectal Dis. 2012 May;14(5):623-7.

[90] Horiuchi A, Maeyama H, Ochi Y, Morikawa A, Miyazawa K. Usefulness of Dennis Colorectal Tube in endoscopic decompression of acute, malignant colonic obstruction. Gastrointest Endosc. 2001 Aug;54(2):229-32.

[91] Geller A, Petersen BT, Gostout CJ. Endoscopic decompression for acute colonic pseudo-obstruction. Gastrointest Endosc. 1996 Aug;44(2):144-50.

[92] Baraza W, Brown S, McAlindon M, Hurlstone P. Prospective analysis of percutaneous endoscopic colostomy at a tertiary referral centre. Br J Surg. 2007 Nov;94(11): 1415-20.

[93] Cowlam S, Watson C, Elltringham M, Bain I, Barrett P, Green S, Yiannakou Y. Percutaneous endoscopic colostomy of the left side of the colon. Gastrointest Endosc. 2007 Jun;65(7):1007-14.

[94] Bertolini D, De Saussure P, Chilcott M, Girardin M, Dumonceau JM. Severe delayed complication after percutaneous endoscopic colostomy for chronic intestinal pseudo-obstruction: a case report and review of the literature. World J Gastroenterol. 2007 Apr 21;13(15):2255-7.

[95] Conway JD, Adler DG, Diehl DL, Farraye FA, Kantsevoy SV, Kaul V, Kethu SR, Kwon RS, Mamula P, Rodriguez SA, Tierney WM; ASGE Technology Committee. Endoscopic hemostatic devices. Gastrointest Endosc. 2009 May;69(6):987-96.

[96] Foutch PG. Angiodysplasia of the gastrointestinal tract. Am J Gastroenterol 1993;88:807-18.

[97] Johanns W, Luis W, Janssen J, et al. Argon plasma coagulation (APC) in gastroenterology: experimental and clinical experiences. Eur J Gastroenterol Hepatol 1997;9:581-7.

[98] Wahab PJ, Mulder CJ, den Hartog G, Thies JE. Argon plasma coagulation in flexible gastrointestinal endoscopy: pilot experiences. Endoscopy. 1997 Mar;29(3):176-81.

[99] Katsinelos P, Kountouras J, Paroutoglou G, et al. Endoloop-assisted polypectomy for large pedunculated colorectal polyps. Surg Endosc 2006;20:1257-61.

[100] Kasotakis G, Roediger L, Mittal S. Rectal foreign bodies: A case report and review of the literature. Int J Surg Case Rep. 2012;3(3):111-5. Epub 2011 Dec 8.

[101] Goldberg JE, Steele SR. Rectal foreign bodies. Surg Clin North Am. 2010 Feb;90(1): 173-84, Table of Contents.

[102] Assarian A, Raja MA. Colonoscopic retrieval of a lost intrauterine contraceptive device: a case report and review of articles. Eur J Contracept Reprod Health Care. 2005 Dec;10(4):261-5.

[103] Celik A, Kutun S, Kockar C, Mengi N, Ulucanlar H, Cetin A. Colonoscopic removal of inguinal hernia mesh: report of a case and literature review. J Laparoendosc Adv Surg Tech A. 2005 Aug;15(4):408-10.

[104] Aggarwal G, Satsangi B, Raikwar R, Shukla S, Mathur R. Unusual rectal foreign body presenting as intestinal obstruction: a case report. Ulus Travma Acil Cerrahi Derg. 2011 Jul;17(4):374-6.

[105] Ikenberry SO, Jue TL, Anderson MA, Appalaneni V, Banerjee S, Ben-Menachem T, Decker GA, Fanelli RD, Fisher LR, Fukami N, Harrison ME, Jain R, Khan KM, Krinsky ML, Maple JT, Sharaf R, Strohmeyer L, Dominitz JA; ASGE Standards of Practice Committee. Management of ingested foreign bodies and food impactions. Gastrointest Endosc. 2011 Jun;73(6):1085-91.

[106] Kantsevoy SV, Adler DG, Conway JD, Diehl DL, Farraye FA, Kwon R, Mamula P, Rodriguez S, Shah RJ, Wong Kee Song LM, Tierney WM; ASGE TECHNOLOGY COMMITTEE. Endoscopic mucosal resection and endoscopic submucosal dissection. Gastrointest Endosc. 2008 Jul;68(1):11-8.

[107] Saito Y, Uraoka T, Yamaguchi Y, Hotta K, Sakamoto N, Ikematsu H, Fukuzawa M, Kobayashi N, Nasu J, Michida T, Yoshida S, Ikehara H, Otake Y, Nakajima T, Matsuda T, Saito D. A prospective, multicenter study of 1111 colorectal endoscopic submucosal dissections (with video). Gastrointest Endosc. 2010 Dec;72(6):1217-25. Epub 2010 Oct 27.

[108] Tanaka S, Oka S, Kaneko I, Hirata M, Mouri R, Kanao H, Yoshida S, Chayama K. Endoscopic submucosal dissection for colorectal neoplasia: possibility of standardization. Gastrointest Endosc. 2007 Jul;66(1):100-7.

[109] Toyonaga T, Man-i M, Fujita T, East JE, Nishino E, Ono W, Morita Y, Sanuki T, Yoshida M, Kutsumi H, Inokuchi H, Azuma T. Retrospective study of technical aspects and complications of endoscopic submucosal dissection for laterally spreading tumors of the colorectum. Endoscopy. 2010 Sep;42(9):714-22. Epub 2010 Aug 30.

[110] Niimi K, Fujishiro M, Kodashima S, Goto O, Ono S, Hirano K, Minatsuki C, Yamamichi N, Koike K. Long-term outcomes of endoscopic submucosal dissection for colorectal epithelial neoplasms. Endoscopy. 2010 Sep;42(9):723-9.

[111] Repici A, Pellicano R, Strangio G, Danese S, Fagoonee S, Malesci A. Endoscopic mucosal resection for early colorectal neoplasia: pathologic basis, procedures, and outcomes. Dis Colon Rectum. 2009 Aug;52(8):1502-15.

Section 4

Colonoscopy Is Not the End of the Way: Other Screening Technologies

Chapter 11

Colon Capsule Endoscopy: Quo Vadis?

Samuel N. Adler and Cesare Hassan

Additional information is available at the end of the chapter

http://dx.doi.org/10.5772/53055

1. Introduction

Capsule endoscopy was independently invented in the last decade of the 20th century by Gabriel Iddan and Paul Swain. They both were committed to develop a wireless camera that would transmit images for the insides of the digestive tract to an extracorporeal receiver. They faced many significant challenges. The last hurdle to be taken was made possible by the miniaturization of the photosensitive chip (CMOS). This device transmits images in digital format and is very economical with modest energy consumption. In this capsule the following elements were implanted: a light source (LED), a lens, the photosensitive chip, a power source (batteries) and a transmitter with and antenna (see Figure 1).

In the year1996 the stomach of a pig was visualized by this method. The importance of this discovery remained as yet elusive to the medical community at large. Yet Paul Swain and Gabriel Iddan pursued their invention. Internal Review Board approval was obtained and the first human ingestion of a wireless capsule endoscope was performed by Paul Swain in Israel on October 17th 1999. In the year 2000 the scientific journal Nature realized that something of importance was taking place and devoted an article to wireless capsule endoscopy[1]. The question had to be addressed whether capsule endoscopy was a cute high tech toy or whether this device had clinical importance for the medical community. The results of a double blind controlled study comparing capsule endoscopy to push enteroscopy (the best available method at that time) in patients with occult gastrointestinal bleeding were presented at the Digestive Disease Week meeting in Atlanta in the year 2001. Capsule endoscopy was superior to push enteroscopy at a rate of two to one[2]. A few months later the US Food and Drug Administration approved the use of capsule endoscopy. From there on capsule endoscopy has captured the field of small bowel endoscopy. Capsule endoscopy of the small bowel was superior to conventional methods in diagnosing NSAID induced enteropathy, Crohn's disease of the small bowel, tumors of the small bowel and other diseases. Direct visualization of the gastrointestinal mucosa was superior to barium studies. For this reason the gastroscope had replaced upper gastrointestinal series, the colonoscope had replaced barium enemas and it was now the capsule endoscopy's turn to replace the small bowel follow through examinations.

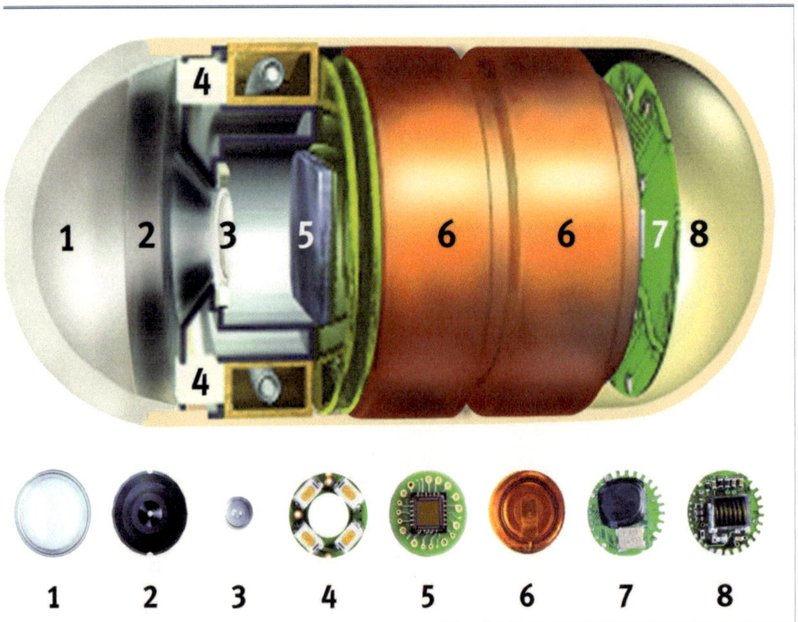

Figure 1. Optical dome, 2 Lens holder, 3. Lens, 4.Illuminating LEDs (light emitting diodes), 5. CMOS (Complementary Metal Oxide Semiconductor) image, 6. Battery, 7.ASIC (Application Specific Integrated Circuit) transmitter, 8. Antenna

Once capsule endoscopy had proven itself as a very useful and important diagnostic tool in the work up of small bowel disease, the concept of non invasive endoscopy sought expansion to other areas of the gastrointestinal tract as well. This chapter deals with capsule endoscopy of the colon.

2. History of capsule endoscopy of the colon

In contrast to capsule endoscopy of the small bowel, capsule endoscopy of the colon faces serious challenges for the following reasons.

1. Problem:

The small bowel is narrow (hence its name). As the capsule camera enters the small bowel it remains by and large fixed in its orientation and facing the same direction, either camera first or transmitter first. The capsule as a rule does not flip around its own axis. The capsule travels along its journey through the small bowel in the same orientation as it enters the small bowel. For this reason the single camera of the capsule will screen the entire small bowel mucosa either in forward view if the capsule enters the small bowel with the camera end first or in backward view if the capsule enters with the transmitter end first. This is not true for the colon. In the large bowel with its wide diameter the capsule can tumble around its axis. A capsule with a single camera would screen certain areas twice and other areas not at all.

Solution:

The engineers solved this challenge by offering a colon capsule that has two cameras, one camera at each end. The colonic mucosa is visualized from both directions simultaneously. This guarantees complete visual coverage of the entire colonic surface.

2. Problem:

The capsule transit time to reach the end of the colon is significantly longer than the time required for the capsule to reach the cecum and the colon capsule consumes more energy than the small bowel capsule since it transmits images from two cameras. Yet the energy supply is limited to two watch batteries.

Solution:

To reduce energy requirements the colon capsule was put to sleep for an hour and a half, five minutes after ingestion. This hour and a half of transmit time became now available for transmission from the colon.

3. Problem:

The third hurdle is bowel cleansing. In standard colonoscopy some minimal amount of liquid debris can be aspirated, yet minimal amount of debris may compromise the capsule's ability to identify pathological findings.

Solution:

A more vigorous bowel preparation had to be offered to patients to assure proper cleansing for colon capsule examinations.

The first colon capsule was tested in the year 2005 and 2006[3]. The results of three studies were encouraging. Firstly the bowels could be adequately cleansed in 72 to 84% of patients. Secondly the capsule passed through the entire gastrointestinal tract while transmitting images from the entire colon in 81% of patients within 8 hours. Finally the capsule did indentify pathologies such as polyps, tumors, colitis, diverticulosis and internal hemorrhoids. Proof of principle had been obtained. However the sensitivity of 58 to 64% to identify patients with polyps equal to or larger than 6 mm as compared to standard colonoscopy was suboptimal and fell short of expectations [4].

3. New features of colon capsule 2

The shortcomings of this first colon capsule were analyzed and the capsule underwent a thorough overhaul. The second generation colon capsule has the following improvements.

The angle of view of this new colon capsule camera was extended from 154 to 172 degrees for each camera. This change provides a near full panorama view (see Figure 2).

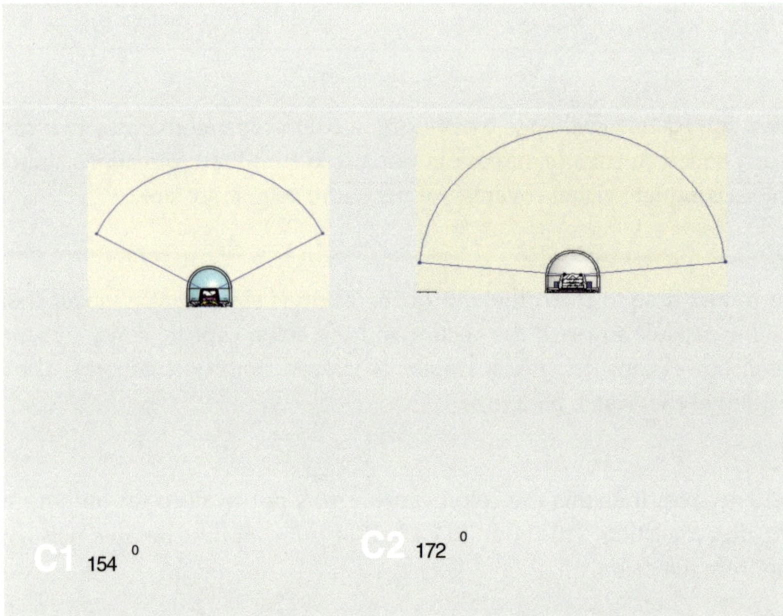

Figure 2. The left side image demonstrates the angle of view of the out dated C1 colon capsule. The right hand image demonstrates the angle of view of the C2 colon capsule with a near panoramic view.

The Data Recorder 3 (DR3), the device that collects the transmitted digital information from the capsule, is a true revolution in capsule endoscopy. Smart features have been imbedded in this device. Bidirectional communication between capsule and DR3 takes place. The DR3 receives information from the capsule and accordingly directs the capsule with corresponding instructions. The capsule receives online orders by the DR3. The capsule transmits its images at four images per second when in stationary condition. When DR3 recognizes that the incoming images indicate that the capsule is in motion it orders the capsule to raise the transmission rate to 35 images per second. This entire circle of receiving optical information from the capsule, online analysis by the DR3 and execution of the DR3 orders by the capsule takes place within a split second. Furthermore, DR3 also communicates with the patient undergoing the colon capsule examination and instructs the patient if and when to take a prokinetic agent, which shortens gastric transit time and moves the capsule more expediently form stomach into small bowel. The DR3 notifies the patient

a. when to ingest the first booster laxative which accelerates small bowel transit time of the capsule and keeps the colon clean,

b. if and when to ingest a second booster laxative

c. if and when to insert a bisacodyl suppository

http://dx.doi.org/10.5772/53055

d. and finally notifies that the patient may eat and that the procedure is over.

This is how the second generation colon capsule system works. Three minutes after swallowing the capsule the rate of transmission is reduced to 16 images per minute to conserve energy. The received images are constantly analyzed by DR3. If after one hour DR3 notices that the colon capsule has not left the stomach it will instruct the subject by ringing an alarm tone and activating a vibrating device attached to the antenna to look at the LCD screen where the digit 0 is displayed. The patient's instruction sheet indicates that the appearance of digit 0 requires the subject to take a prokinetic agent such domperidone or metoclopramide. However if the capsule has left the stomach and entered the small bowel, the smart features of DR3 recognize that the capsule is now in the small bowel. DR3 orders the capsule to raise its transmission rate from 16 images per minute to 4 images per second and the patient to ingest the booster laxative. The purpose of this booster laxative is to shorten small bowel transit time of the colon capsule and to maintain adequate cleanliness of the bowel. Furthermore, all incoming images from the colon capsule are analyzed online by this "intelligent" DR3 that recognizes if the capsule is stationary or in motion. Once DR3 recognizes that the capsule is in motion it orders the capsule to raise its transmission rate of images to a staggering 35 frames per second. As mentioned, the process of recognition to execution takes place in a fraction of a second. This rapid transmission rate (35 frames per second) provides adequate number of colonic images while the capsule is in motion especially while flying through the transverse colon.

Polyp size is of course clinically very relevant. The larger the size of a polyp the greater the chances that the polyp has advanced neoplastic changes. The software program for colon capsule 2 is equipped with a polyp size assessor. The cursor is drawn from one side of the polyp to the other and the algorithm spits out the size of the polyp in mm. The same polyp seen from distance or from close up will have the same size measurement.

These technological achievements are very impressive (a data recorder communicating with capsule and patient, a data recorder that analyzes images, determines location, position –stationary versus motion, and accordingly alters transmission rate of frames per second by the capsule). Yet the gnawing question remains. Is this device medically relevant?

4. Results of clinical trials with colon capsule 2

We engaged in a five center prospective double blind feasibility study in Israel in which this second generation colon capsule was compared to standard colonoscopy for the identification of patients with colonic polyps. 104 patients were enrolled. Whereas in the European multicenter trial published in 2009 the sensitivity to identify patients with polyps was only 58% the sensitivity in the multicenter Israel trial with the second generation colon capsule rose to 89% [5]. This marked improved diagnostic sensitivity was reproduced by a recent European study with the second generation colon capsule [6]. This improvement (raise in diagnostic sensitivity from 58% to 89%) has to be attributed to the revolutionary new capsule platform of this second generation colon capsule for the following reasons. Firstly, the three previous studies with the first generation colon capsule had a very similar design as the present studies with colon capsule 2 and are thus comparable. Secondly, good bowel cleansing is a determining factor for a successful study. Good bowel cleansing was obtained at similar rates in the studies with colon capsule 1 as in the new studies with colon capsule 2. Thirdly, capsule exrection of a capsule still transmitting images is a prerequisite for a successful colon capsule study. Capsule excretion rates of the studies with colon capsule 1 and the studies with colon capsule 2 were the same. The only factor which set this second generation colon capsule study apart from the previous studies is the new technological platform. It is for this reason that we credit the improvement in technology for the improved diagnostic sensitivity of 30%.

Colon capsule 2's negative predictive value of 97% is very high and is clinically very meaningful. The physician discussing the results of a negative colon capsule 2 study with his patient can reassure her/him that that a negative colon capsule 2 study has a 97% accuracy that there are no polyps.

The fact that the smart features of DR3 enable communication with the patient has opened the door to offer colon capsule examination as an out of clinic procedure [7].

5. Colon capsule endoscopy, Quo Vadis?

In the year 2011 the European Society of Gastrointestinal Endoscopy(ESGE) recognized the potential that colon capsule endoscopy offers and ordered the establishment of evidence based guidelines for colon capsule endoscopy[8]. This initiative was endorsed by the governing board of ESGE.

Technical concerns in relation to colon capsule endoscopy were addressed. Will the colon be adequately cleansed for high quality inspection? Will the power of the batteries within the capsule supply adequate energy to transmit images from the colon until excretion of the capsule? The experts therefore formulated precise guidelines and devoted an entire section on how to perform capsule endoscopy. To achieve high quality colon capsule endoscopy (good bowel preparation, high rate of capsule passage rate through entire colon and proper reading) strict implementation of all guidelines must be followed (diet, laxatives, booster ingestion, controlled frame rate during reading).

Here are some of the attractive features of colon capsule endoscopy that are mentioned in the published guidelines.

- "CCE (Colon capsule endoscopy) has consistently been shown to be a very safe procedure: no major complication has been reported in over 1500 procedures, of which around 40% were in asymptomatic individuals. CCE also appears to be a feasible procedure, with a very low rate of technical failures (i. e. 3%) and a high capsule excretion rate of about 90%".
- "A previous cost–effectiveness analysis has compared first-generation CCE with colonoscopy in a screening setting. Although CCE was not a cost-effective alternative when

equal uptake (adherence to participate in colon cancer screening) was assumed, it became an efficient option when it was assumed that uptake of CCE would be higher than that of colonoscopy for CRC screening, a premise that has not been demonstrated yet."

- "CCE is a feasible and safe tool for visualization of the colonic mucosa in patients with incomplete colonoscopy and without stenosis."
- "Small-bowel capsule endoscopy provides a very high diagnostic yield for small-bowel mucosal lesions and its use is recommended in specific scenarios of IBD (Inflammatory Bowel Disease). Similarly, CCE could be used to identify mucosal changes in the colorectal mucosa. ..."

We will dwell on two mentioned issues raised in the European Guidelines, namely the use of capsule colonoscopy in screening for colonic polyps and the use of capsule endoscopy in incomplete colonoscopy.

6. Can colon capsule endoscopy play a role in clinical medicine today?

a. Screening patients for presence of colonic polyps as primary colon cancer prevention.

Colonoscopy is the accepted gold standard and the most sensitive method to investigate patients for the presence of colonic polyps. While colon cancer screening programs are available the participation rate of the general population has been disappointingly low. The reasons for the low adherence rate are multifactorial. Colonoscopy is associated with discomfort/pain, so there is a need for sedation, there are complications, albeit small, the procedure leads to loss of work and there is the issue of the invasion of one's privacy. Recently it has been reported that post procedural pain necessitating visits to the emergency room following colonoscopy has been underestimated. While these reservations may appear trivial to gastroenterologists, this is perceived differently in the general public. Inadomi et al published the results of a prospective randomized trial [9]. In the office setting eligible patients were offered either colonoscopy or fecal occult blood testing (FOBT). 12 months thereafter 38% of patients offered colonoscopy had completed the procedure, while 31% more, a total of 69% of patients offered FOBT had done the test.

They concluded that our common practice of universally recommending only colonoscopy may actually reduce adherence to colorectal cancer screening.

In a prospective study performed in Germany to examine whether colon capsule endoscopy could increase adherence to screening colonoscopy in a healthy population Groth et al found that offering capsule endoscopy led to a fourfold increase of screening uptake compared to standard colonoscopy [10].

Rex and Lieberman published a survey study that colon capsule endoscopy could raise colorectal cancer screening adherence rates among patients who decline screening colonoscopy. This was especially apparent when the participants in this survey were offered colon capsule endoscopy as an out of clinic test with no loss of work. We published a cohort study of 41 patients who underwent colon capsule endoscopy as an out of clinic study. Successfully completed colon capsule endoscopy examinations in this out-of-clinic trial, including capsule excretion rates and colon cleansing levels were similar to those of the two published in-clinic trials. This study concluded that second generation colon capsule endoscopy may be offered as an out-of-clinic medically supervised procedure [11].

To summarize the above: offering colonoscopy only in colon cancer screening programs reduces adherence. Loss of work and the need to have a person accompany the subject to be screened by colonoscopy are significant reasons for decreased adherence to undergo colonoscopy screening. Reduced adherence compromises the effectiveness of colonoscopy even if colonoscopy admittedly is the gold standard. Colon capsule endoscopy can offer itself as a non invasive test to identify patients with colonic polyps. In the future colon capsule endoscopy could be offered as an out of clinic test which potentially could further increase adherence rates for colon cancer screening programs. Modern technology has set the tone. Invasive diagnostic tests will be replaced with less or non invasive tests. Colon capsule endoscopy may fit this paradigm.

b. Incomplete Colonoscopy.

For colonoscopy to reduce colon cancer rates certain criteria have to be met. Colonoscopy has to be carried out by competent endoscopists (operator dependent). Bowel cleansing has to be optimal. Cecal intubation has to be achieved (complete colonoscopy). Incomplete colonoscopy, ie the failure to intubate the cecum with the colonoscope, in general practice is higher than expected [12]. Complete colonoscopy rates have been reported from 60% to over 90% [13],[14],[15]. If for whatever reason complete colonoscopy cannot be achieved then ingestion of the colon capsule endoscope for visualization of the uninspected part of the colon is feasible. Colon capsule endoscopy in this setting may be especially attractive since it is the right colon which is usually not visualized in incomplete conventional colonoscopy whereas the right colon is routinely visualized by capsule endoscopy. A prospective multicenter European study demonstrated that colon capsule endoscopy in case of incomplete colonoscopy (74 cases) or contraindicated colonoscopy (26 cases) yields a high number of relevant diagnostic findings (36 %) including one right sided colonic cancer. Furthermore, the authors report that during a one year follow up of this study no adenocarcinoma of the colon was missed by the colon capsule[16]. It should be emphasized that this study was performed with the inferior (today outdated) first generation colon capsule.

7. Conclusion

Colon capsule endoscopy has come a long way in a very short time. Technological developments are so rapid that studies performed in the years 2006 and 2007 with the first generation of colon capsules are already outdated. Second generation colon capsule endoscopy has a diagnostic sensitivity of 89% or higher to identify patients with polyps equal to or larger than 5 mm. In addition to this high sensitivity colon capsule endoscopy is non invasive, painless, protects one's privacy, may be offered in the future as an out of clinic (or possibly home procedure) and for all these reasons may increase adherence rates to participate in colon cancer screening. Therefore colon capsule endoscopy may become clinically important to practicing gastroenterologists.

Author details

Samuel N. Adler[1] and Cesare Hassan[2]

1 Division of Gastroenterology, BikurHolim Hospital, Jerusalem, Israel

2 Ospedale Nuovo Regina Margherita, Via Morosini, Roma, Italia

References

[1] Iddan G, Meron G, Glukhovsky A, Swain P. Wireless capsule endoscopy. NATURE 2000;405. 417

[2] Lewis BS, Swain P. Capsule endoscopy in the evaluation of patients with suspected small intestinal bleeding: Results of a pilot study. Gastrointest Endosc. 2002;56(3): 349-53.

[3] Eliakim R, Fireman Z, Gralnek IM, Yassin K, Waterman M, Kopelman Y, Lachter J, Koslowsky B, Adler SN. Evaluation of the PillCam Colon capsule in the detection of colonic pathology: results of the first multicenter, prospective, comparative study. Endoscopy 2006; 38(10): 963-970 [PMID: 17058158 DOI:10.1055/s-2006-944832

[4] Van Gossum A, Munoz-Navas M, Fernandez-Urien I, Carretero C, Gay G, Delvaux M, Lapalus MG, Ponchon T, Neuhaus H, Philipper M, Costamagna G, Riccioni ME, Spada C, Petruzziello L, Fraser C, Postgate A, Fitzpatrick A, Hagenmuller F, Keuchel M, Schoofs N, Devière J. Capsule Endoscopy versus Colonoscopy for the Detection of Polyps and Cancer. N Engl J Med 2009; 361:264-270 [PMID: 19605831 DOI 10.1056/ NEMJoa0806347

[5] Eliakim R, Yassin K, Niv Y, Metzger Y, Lachter J, Gal E, Sapoznikov B, Konikoff F, Leichtmann G, Fireman Z, Kopelman Y, Adler SN. Prospective multicenter performance evaluation of the second-generation colon capsule compared with colonoscopy. Endoscopy 2009; 41:1026–1031 [PMID: 19967618 DOI:10.1055/s-0029-1215360

[6] Spada C, Hassan C, Munoz-Navas M, Neuhaus H, Deviere J, Fockens P, Coron E, Gay G, Toth E, Riccioni ME, Carretero C, Charton JP, Van Gossum A, Wientjes CA, Sacher-Huvelin S, Delvaux M, Nemeth A, Petruzziello L, de Frias CP, Mayershofer R, Aminejab L, Dekker E, Galmiche JP, Frederic M, Johansson GW, Cesaro P, Costamagna G . Second-generation PillCam® Colon Capsule Compared with Colonoscopy. Gastrointest Endoscopy 2011; 74:581-589 DOI: 10.1016/j.gie.2011.03.1125

[7] Adler S.N., MetzgerY.C., Sompolinsky Y., Hassan C. Capsule Colonoscopy with Pillcam Colon 2 is Feasible as an Outpatient Procedure. UEGW 2011, Endoscopy 2011, 43 (Suppl I A215)

[8] Spada C, Hassan C, Galmiche J P, Neuhaus H, Dumonceau J M, Adler S, Epstein O, Gay G, Pennazio M, Rex DK, Benamouzig R, de Franchis R, Delvaux M, Devière J, Eliakim R, Fraser C, Hagenmuller F, Herrerias JM, Keuchel M, Macrae F, Munoz-Navas M, Ponchon T, Quintero E, Riccioni ME, Rondonott E, Marmo R, Sung JJ, Tajir H, Toth, Triantafyllou K, Van Gossum A, Costamagna G. Colon capsule endoscopy: European Society of Gastrointestinal Endoscopy (ESGE) Guideline. Endoscopy. 2012 May;44(5):527-36. Epub 2012 Mar 2. DOI http://dx.doi.org/10.1055/s-0031-1291717

[9] Inadomi JM, MD, Vijan S, MD, MS, Janz NK, PhD, et al. Adherence to Colorectal Cancer Screening. Arch Internal Medicine. 2012; 172(7):575-582 DOI:10.1001/archinternmed.2012.332

[10] Groth S, Krause H, Behrendt R, Hill H, Börner M, Bastürk M, Plathner N, Schütte F, Gauger U. Riemann JF, Altenhofen L, Rösch T. Capsule colonoscopy increases uptake of colorectal cancer screening. BMC Gastroenterology 2012, 12:80 DOI: 10.1186/1471-230X-12-80

[11] Adler SN, Metzger YC, Sompolinsky Y, Hassan C. Capsule Colonoscopy with PillCam COLON 2 is Feasible as an Out-of-Clinic Procedure. Gastroenterology 2012;142(5); Suppl:s53-s54

[12] Dafnis G, Granath F, Påhlman L, Ekbom A, Blomqvist P. Patient factors influencing the completion rate in colonoscopy. Dig Liver Dis. 2005 Feb;37(2):113-8

[13] Bowles CJ, Leicester R, Romaya C et al. A prospective study of colonoscopy practice in the UK today: are we adequately prepared for national colorectal cancer screening tomorrow? Gut 2004; 53: 277–283

[14] Lieberman DA, Weiss DG, Bond JH. Veterans Affairs Cooperative Study Group 380. et al. Use of colonoscopy to screen asymptomatic adults for colorectal cancer. N Engl J Med 2000; 343: 162–168

[15] Neerincx M, Terhaar sive Droste JS, Mulder CJ, Räkers M, Bartelsman JF, Loffeld RJ, Tuynman HA, Brohet RM, van der Hulst RW. Colonic work-up after incomplete colonoscopy: significant new findings during follow-up. Endoscopy. 2010 Sep;42(9): 730-5. Epub 2010 Jul 28.

[16] Pioche M, De Leusse A, Filoche B, Dalbies P-A, Adenis-Lamarre P, Jacob Pgaudin , J-L, Coulom P, Létard J-C, Borotto E, Huriez A, Cabaud J-M, Crampon D, Gincul R, Lévy P, Ben Soussan E, Garret M, Lapuelle J, Saurin J-C. Prospective, Multicenter Evaluation Of The Colon Pillcam Videocapsule In The Specific Indication Of Colonoscopy Failure Or Contra-Indication. Endoscopy 2011; 43 (Suppl I) A14

Chapter 12

Virtual Colonoscopy

Robert J. Richards and Jerome Zhengrong Liang

Additional information is available at the end of the chapter

http://dx.doi.org/10.5772/52544

1. Introduction

Colorectal carcinoma ranks as the third most commonly diagnosed cancer and the second leading cause of death from cancer in the United States [1]. It is estimated that more than 150,000 new cases are diagnosed with more than 50,000 dying from the disease yearly in the U.S. alone [1]. Similar to other cancers, it is often diagnosed at advanced stage, after the patient has developed symptoms. Many colon cancer deaths can be avoided because mostly they arise from adenomatous polyps, which may be detectable years before malignant transformation.

Since the first report of a complete examination of the entire colon using a flexible endoscope, optical colonoscopy (OC) has evolved to be the current gold standard for evaluation of the colon [2]. OC has several limitations and drawbacks as a population-based screening tool. It is an invasive procedure requiring sedation. An escort is usually required to take the patient home, which increases the cost of the procedure from a societal perspective. OC also carries a small but significant risk of perforation and death. The risk of colonic perforation is about 1 per 1,000 cases and death is approximately 1 in 5,000 cases [3-5]. Failure to reach the cecum (5-10%) and missed polyps (10-20%) also are known limitations of the current gold standard test [6-9].

Computed tomographic colonography (CTC), also known as "virtual colonoscopy" was first described more than a decade ago [10]. In the early 1990's, several pilot studies evaluated the feasibility of (CTC) [11]. The advantages of developing a computerized-based screening tool includes: increased accessibility, non-invasiveness, and no sedation required [12]. These advantages of CTC may help to increase compliance with current screening recommendation guidelines [13].

2. Technique

As advancements in scanner technology and three-dimensional (3D) post-processing helped develop this method to mature into a potential option in screening for colorectal cancer, the fundamentals of the examination remained the same. It is a minimally invasive, CT-based procedure that simulates conventional colonoscopy using 2D and 3D computerized reconstructions [10]. CTC utilizes computer virtual-reality techniques to navigate inside a three-dimensionalz (3D) patient-specific colon model reconstructed from abdominal CT images, looking for polyps.

CTC examination starts by inflating a cleansed colon with room air or carbon dioxide (CO_2) introduced through rectal catheter [14]. With the patient in a prone position, air or CO_2 is insufflated under gentle pressure to ensure adequate distention of the bowel. The insufflation of gas is usually associated with a mild degree of patient discomfort or pain [15]. Although not common, vaso-vagal reactions can occur, especially if with small bowel distention occurs [16].

Then abdominal CT slice images are taken in seconds (during a single breath hold) with sub millimeter resolution in both axial and transverse directions resulting in excellent contrast between the colon wall and the lumen. The sliced images are stacked together as a volume image, from which the colon model is constructed. Image segmentation is necessary for the construction of an accurate colon model. Computer graphics are heavily involved to navigate or fly through inside the 3D colon model. The patient is scanned in both a prone and supine view [17]. Using a second view significantly improves the ability to identify patients with polyps 0.5 cm in diameter or larger [18].

CTC can be performed in patients with prior abdominoperineal resection and sigmoid colostomy, although increased difficulties with CO2 retention and adequate bowel distention exist [19]. The prevalence of transient bacterium after CTC is low therefore it follows that patients with at risk cardiac lesions should not require antibiotic prophylaxis beforehand [20].

Most commonly used bowel preparations include sodium phosphates, magnesium citrate and polyethylene glycol (PEG) [21]. Typical oral preparations used for bowel cleansing are: 4 L of PEG solution; 90 ml of phosphosoda; or 300 ml of magnesium citrate. Polyp detection is comparable for all three preparations, although phosphosoda has a significantly higher patient compliance and the least residual stool [22]. Residual fluid coverage negatively affects the quality of CTC [23].

The use of fecal tagging agents and intravenous contrast is not standardized. CTC experts were surveyed regarding their practice patterns [24]. Thirty-eight percent performed fecal tagging regularly and 81% [21/26] believed intravenous contrast was not necessary [24].

Non-operator dependent false positives and false negatives occur with CTC. For example, inadequately tagged stool can have the same density as a polyp, however the two can sometimes be distinguished by comparing prone and supine views, since stool is

http://dx.doi.org/10.5772/52544

usually mobile and polyps are not. The rectal balloon is a potential blind spot for CTC, sometimes masking significant lesions [25, 26]. Also, poor colonic distention can result in a false negative reading [27].

3. Screening for colorectal cancer: CTC vs. OC

The primary aim of CTC is the detection of colorectal polyps and carcinomas, however; the precise role of CTC in screening asymptomatic patients is controversial [28]. Studies using patients with known adenomas generally report higher accuracy, while studies employing asymptomatic screening subjects report lower accuracy [28]. Two key areas have held back the widespread application of CTC as a screening test. These key areas are: [1] the variable sensitivity of CTC reported in mass screening programs (see Table) and [2], the expertise required to interpret the examination. These two areas are related [29]. Despite these drawbacks, the American College of Radiology, has endorsed the use of CTC as a screening tool for colo-rectal cancer stating that the sensitivity and specificity of CTC are high enough and comparable to those of OC [30]. In addition, CTC has received the endorsement of a multi-society task force that included the American Cancer Society and U. S. Multi-society Task Force on Colorectal Cancer [31].

Studies reveal a wide variation in performance measures (sensitivity and specificity) regarding polyp detection rates, especially for smaller polyps [10]. In an early feasibility study of 44 patients, CTC demonstrated reasonable sensitivity (83%) and specificity (100%) for polyps larger than 8 mm in size [32]. A second early study performed in 87 patients at high risk for colorectal neoplasia identified 49 patients with a total of 115 polyps and 3 carcinomas [33]. CTC identified all 3 cancers. The sensitivity was 91% for polyps that were 10 mm or more in diameter, 82% [33/40] that were 6 to 9 mm, and 55% [29/53] that were 5 mm or smaller [33]. There were 19 false positive findings of polyps and no false positive findings of cancer. In a larger study of 300 patients CTC demonstrated a sensitivity equal to 90% for polyps 10 mm or larger and 80.1% for polyps at least 5 mm in size [34]. The overall specificity for this study was 72.0% [34]. All 8 carcinomas in the study were detected by CTC.

Two later studies assessing the accuracy of CTC had varying results. Pickhardt et al. evaluated 1,233 asymptomatic patients with CTC and same-day OC [35]. The sensitivity of CTC for adenomatous polyps at least 10 mm in size was 93.8% and 88.7% for polyps at least 6 mm in size, which was comparable to OC. The specificity of CTC for adenomatous polyps at least 10 mm in size was 96.0% and 79.6% for polyps at least 6 mm in size. These encouraging results were followed a year later by less optimistic findings from a study by Cotton et al., that analyzed 600 participants undergoing both CTC and OC [36]. In the Cotton study, 104 of the participants (17.3%) had lesions sized at least 6 mm. The sensitivity of CTC for detecting 1 or more lesions sized at least 6 mm was only 39.0% and for lesions sized at least 10 mm, it was 55.0% (95% Cl, 39.9% - 70.0%) [36]. The specificity of CTC for detecting participants without any lesion sized at least 6 mm was 90.5% and without lesions sized at least 10 mm, 96.0% (95% Cl, 94.3% - 97.6%). CTC missed 2 of 8 cancers [36]. Lack of adequate radiologist training to read CTCs may have resulted in the low accuracy found in this study.

In a subsequent study of 2,531 asymptomatic patients, radiologists trained in CTC reported the accuracy of finding histologically confirmed adenomas [37]. The sensitivity for large adenomas [10 mm or larger) and medium-sized adenomas (6 – 9 mm) was 90% and 78% respectively [37]. CTC failed to detect a lesion measuring 10 mm or more in diameter in 10% of patients [37]. Pickhart et al. found that the positive predictive values (PPV) for polyps with threshold sizes 6 mm, 8 mm, and 10 mm are: 92.3%, 93.0%, and 93.1% respectively [38]. Others have also found that for significant adenomas, the PPV of CTC is high and ranges from 96 – 99% [37, 39].

Meta-analysis is a tool that attempts to summarize varying results across multiple studies. Meta-analysis of data suggests CTC has excellent per-patient average sensitivity and average specificity for detection of adenomatous polyps and cancer [40]. In one meta-analysis, 2,610 patients were included for study [41]. Large polyps (10 mm or greater) had a per-patient average sensitivity of 93% (95% CI,73% - 98%) and specificity of 97% 9(95% CI, 95% - 99%) [41]. The sensitivity and specificity decreased to 86% (95% CI: 75% - 93%) and 86% (95% CI, 76% - 93%), respectively, when the threshold was lowered to include medium sized polyps (6 mm to 9 mm). These findings are similar to another more recent meta-analysis using average risk patients that found a sensitivity of 87% and specificity of 97.6% for polyps at least 10 mm in size [42].

One of the problems of evaluating the test performance of CTC is the use of OC as the gold standard because OC has a miss-rate for polyps and cancer as well. In one study, Pickhardt et al. compared 1,233 asymptomatic adults who underwent same-day CTC and blinded segmental OC [43]. Polyps that were detected by CTC but initially missed by OC were considered missed polyps for OC. It was found that OC had a miss rate of 12% for adenomas 10 mm or greater. Of the missed polyps on OC, 14/15 (93.3%) non-rectal neoplasms were located on a fold. Five of 6 (83.3%) missed rectal lesions were located within 10 cm of the anal verge [43].

Another study analyzed 286 tandem colonoscopies [44]. The OC miss rates for adenomas 5 mm and larger and advanced adenomas (≥ 10 mm or high grade dysplasia) were: 11% and 9% respectively [44]. Therefore, OC does have a significant miss rate for adenomas 5 mm and larger and/or advanced adenomas. In fact, the OC miss-rate is similar to the CTC miss-rate for polyps 6-9 mm in size [27]. It should also be pointed out that in screening studies, CTC and OC have similar detection rates for advanced neoplastic polyps and cancer, 3.2% vs. 3.4% respectively [45]. OC detects significantly more adenomas less than 5 mm of size although the benefit of this remains to be seen [46]. In summary, CTC appears to have similar sensitivity to OC in detecting polyps 5 mm or greater when performed by readers with high experience [47].

The detection of flat adenomas are a major concern for colo-rectal cancer screening since these polyps are at a higher risk of harboring advanced pathology and are more difficult to detect by CTC as well as OC [48, 49]. In the general population, there is wide variation in the reported incidence of flat lesions, which may in part be due to the lack of a uniform definition of flat polyps. Various definitions of flat polyps have been used in CTC studies. For example, in one study flat polyps were defined as those having a height less than one-half of their width [50]. In other studies, a definition of 3 mm or less in height is used [51].

The sensitivity for flat polyps appears to be lower than non-flat polyps, however, Pickhardt et al. found that the sensitivity of CTC for detecting flat adenomas measuring 6 mm or greater was similar to that of non-flat polypoid lesions [50]. Others have found lower sensitivities for flat polyps ranging from 15% to 65% [52]. Regardless of reader skills, truly flat or depressed adenomas will most likely pose a challenge for CTC. Also, flat carpet lesions of the colon can be difficult to detect by CTC [53].

CTC readers may not report polyps less than 5 mm in size [54]. The justification for this is that small polyps are usually benign and rarely harbor cancer or have much prognostic significance. In a large OC screening study, advanced histology was found in only 1.7% of polyps sized 5 mm or less indicating the lack of reporting of these small polyps by CTC may be justified [55]. On the other hand, 6.6% of polyps sized 6 to 9 mm, had an advanced histology implying polyps of this size if found on CTC should be followed up with OC in the near future [55]. This last point is somewhat contentious and some radiologic guidelines suggest surveillance with CTC after a shortened interval as an acceptable option for polyps 6 – 9 mm in size [56].

We feel a reasonable algorithm for CTC screening might be: 1. follow-up screening in 5 years if no polyps are found: 2. Follow-up CTC or OC in 5 years for polyps smaller than 5 mm: 3. OC if polyps measuring 6 mm or greater are found [57]. This algorithm is consistent with clinical sentiment since 71% of primary care physicians and 86% of gastroenterologists would send patients with polyps 5 mm in size or greater for a follow-up OC [58]. If this approach were adopted, a referral rate for OC of about 8% - 14% would be expected in the general population [45, 59]. Using a 6 mm threshold however may be very costly. A decision-analysis estimated that to prevent one colon cancer death would require over 9,000 OCs, resulting in 10 additional perforations at an incremental cost of $327,853 dollars [60].

4. Other uses of CTC

4.1. After incomplete colonoscopy

Sometimes OC can not be completed to the cecum due to technical factors such as prior abdominal surgery, colon length and number of flexures [61]. An important use of CTC is examination of the colon after incomplete OC [62]. In a retrospective study, 88/546 patients had lesions 6 mm or greater on CTC after incomplete OC. OC was repeated if findings on CTC were significant. The PPV of CTC for masses, large polyps, and medium polyps were 90.9% and 91.7%, and 64.7% respectively [63].

It may be valuable to perform a low-dose diagnostic CT before rectal tube insertion in patients referred for incomplete colonoscopy. In one study of 262 patients referred for incomplete OC, colon perforation was found on the low-dose CT scans of two of the 262 patients (0.8%; 95% CI, 0.1-2.7%) [64]. One of these patients had no symptoms; the other had mild abdominal discomfort at the time of CTC. Therefore, the rate of occult colonic perforation after incomplete colonoscopy may warrant a spot CT prior to full examination.

4.2. For symptoms

CTC is being increasingly used for the radiological evaluation of colorectal symptoms. In symptomatic patients, CTC is equivalent to OC for diagnosing colon cancer and clinically significant polyps [65]. In a retrospective study of 1,177 older symptomatic patients, 59 invasive CRC were detected [66]. Three small colorectal cancers were missed by CTC. CTC has a high sensitivity (95%) and negative predictive value (99.7%) in excluding a CRC in patients with colorectal symptoms [66].

4.3. Inflammatory bowel disease and diverticulitis

CTC may be useful for diagnosing and managing patients with inflammatory bowel disease (IBD) [67]. CTC correctly identified acute and chronic IBD in 63.6%, and 100% of cases, respectively [68]. CTC was also helpful in assessing post-op strictures in Crohn's disease patients [69]. Perianastomotic narrowing or stenosis was detected by CTC in 11 of 15 patients. The sensitivity and specificity for perianastomatic narrowing were 73% and 100% respectively [69]. The risk of perforation, especially in patients with severe active colitis is a potential worry. Currently there is not enough data to measure the true risk in patients with severe active disease [70].

Examination of the colon is usually necessary after an adequate rest period for evaluation of patients with diverticulitis. CTC appears comparable to OC in the evaluation of these patients and is a reasonable alternative in follow-up of patients with symptomatic diverticular disease [71]. Diverticulosis may however, increase the chance of having a false positive test for polyps on CTC due to the appearance of inverted diverticula and fecoliths[72]. On the other hand, CTC may be helpful in diagnosing complications of diverticular disease and inflammatory bowel disease, such as colo-vesicular fistulae [73].

4.4. Detection of tumor for surgery

CTC is very useful in detecting colon cancer after incomplete colonoscopy and also for evaluating potential metastases [74-76]. CTC can help localize polyps or cancer prior to laparoscopic surgery and detect synchronous lesions beyond the reach of OC due to obstructing lesions [77, 78]. In fact, CTC is superior to OC in the localization of colonic tumors prior to surgery [79]. CTC is also a safe and useful method for preoperative examination of the proximal colon after metallic stent placement in patients with acute colon obstruction caused by cancer [80].

CTC is useful in surveillance after surgery for colo-rectal cancer, detecting local recurrence and metastasis [81-84]. In patients with ovarian cancer CTC may be helpful in detecting rectosigmoid wall involvement wall and predict the need for rectosigmoid resection [85]. The sensitivity, specificity, PPV and negative predictive value of CTC for the prediction of rectosigmoid resection in patients with ovarian cancer in one study were: 100%, 64.7%, 72.7% and 100%, respectively [85].

5. Reader experience and accuracy

Individual accuracy of reading polyps with CTC is highly variable among radiologists and depends largely on training and experience [86-88]. There is a significant learning curve involved in the interpretation of CTC studies, with performance improving with operator experience [89, 90]. Radiologists working in nonacademic centers may have less accurate results than would be expected from published data originating from experienced academic centers [91]. The steep learning curve involved with reading CTC has led some thought leaders to advise against widespread colorectal cancer screening programs with CTC outside of academic centers [29].

False negatives are a major concern, i.e. missing significant lesions. It appears that many false negatives are due to observer error and not due to the technical capabilities of CTC. For instance in one study, 53% of missed polyps (60 of 114) were attributed to observer-related errors, and 26% were attributed to errors classified as technical [92]. This implies that with improvements in reader skill the sensitivity of finding significant lesions would be acceptable and comparable to OC [90]. Technical factors that appear to be associated with higher accuracy include meticulous bowel preparation and inflation, multidetector CT, combined two and three-dimensional visualization [28, 93].

6. Radiation exposure

Radiation exposure at the time of CTC screening leads to a slight but increased risk of developing cancer at a future time [94]. Therefore, reducing radiation exposure is a major challenge for CTC screening.Currently, CTC scanning delivers a significant amount of X-ray radiation exposure to the patient [95]. In 2004, a survey of 28 institutions revealed the median effective dose of radiation was 5.1 mSv (range 1.2 mSv - 11.7 mSv) per position and the median mAs value was 67 mAs[96].

Given current CT technology, a simple and effective strategy to reduce radiation would be to lower the mAs level (i.e. deliver less X-ray photons to the body) during the data acquisition. This strategy would however, lead to a higher noise signal in the acquired data. Recent efforts on modeling a solution to avoid this noise artifact are aimed at minimizing the noise prior or during image reconstruction. Despite the great effort on this solution in the past decade, CTC still faces challenges at a mAs level lower than 50 [97].

A feasibility study examined low radiation doses from 10mAs to 40 mAs using adaptive statistical iterative reconstruction (ASIR) models [98]. Eighteen patients were scanned with a standard 50 mAs CTC dose in the supine position and a reduced dose of 25 mAs with 40%

ASIR in the prone position. No significant image quality differences were seen between standard-and low-dose images using 40% ASIR. The results of this pilot study show that the radiation dose during CTC can be reduced 50% below currently accepted low-dose techniques without significantly affecting image quality when ASIR is used [98]. Larger studies are needed to confirm this observation. Despite the increasing use of multi-slice scanners, which are slightly less dose-efficient, the median effective dose remained approximately constant between 1996 and 2004 [96]. Of 83 institutions, 62% used 64-detector row CT and 17 (50%) used dose modulation [99].

If the current CTC standards for radiation exposure are used for colorectal cancer screening, CTC is still be a viable screening tool, even after taking into account the increased risks of developing future cancers. Using a Monte Carlo simulation, it was found that for every 1 radiation-related cancer caused by CTC screening, 24 – 35 colorectal cancers would be prevented, implying a favorable risk to benefit ratio in favor of using CTC as a screening tool [100]. This model assumed using CTC every 5 years in patients aged 50 – 80 years old and using an estimated mean effective dose per CTC screening study of 8 mSv for women and 7 mSv for men.

An alternative solution to minimize the radiation is to use magnetic resonance imaging (MRI) instead of CT for virtual colonoscopy, i.e., MR colonography (MRC) [101]. However, this MRC alternative solution has several limitation compared to CTC. Currently it is more costly, more sensitive to motion and other artifacts, and has lower spatial resolution but with improvements with technology these disadvantages may be minimized.

7. Patient preferences

When asked if they would prefer CTC or OC, patients more often prefer CTC [102]. In one study, 696 asymptomatic patients at high risk for colorectal cancer screening underwent both CTC and OC [103]. Patients were asked using standardized forms about preparation inconvenience and discomfort, examination discomfort and examination preference. Overall, patients preferred CTC to OC (72.3% vs. 5.1%; $P < 0.001$). Reported discomfort however, was similar for CTC and OC ($P = 0.63$). In another study that evaluated patients with a history of diverticulitis, 74% preferred CTC preferred over OC [71]. Patients found colonoscopy more uncomfortable ($p < 0.03$), more painful ($p < 0.001$), and more difficult ($p < 0.01$) than CTC [71].

Other studies conflict with those mentioned above. Even though CTC is a less invasive alternative than OC, procedural pain is not uncommon. In several studies, the pain associated with CTC was higher than that associated with OC, albeit there is no sedation given for the former test [104]. Using a time-trade off technique, 295 patients reported statistically more pain and discomfort after CTC and showed preference for optical colonoscopy [105]. The pain during CTC however, is usually not so severe as to abort the test [33].

In a well-designed study, 111 patients underwent CTC followed immediately by OC [15]. The preference for either examination was evaluated after completion of both examinations. Of the 68 patients who favored one examination, 56 [82%) preferred CTC (P < 0.00001). CTC was regarded as "not painful" by 62 (57%) of 108 patients compared with 28 (26%) for colonoscopy [15].

Intuitively we may believe that CTC, being a noninvasive test, would be preferred to OC by most patients. However, when the risks of finding lesions that require follow-up and other factors are taken into account, patient preferences may change. In one study, OC was preferred over CTC as the need for a follow-up test increased, as the likelihood of missing cancers or polyps increased, and as the cost for CTC increased (the odds rato of preferring CTC to OC ranged from 0.65 to 0.80)[106]. Therefore, an informed decision regarding CTC vs. OC should include a discussion of the benefits, risks, costs and associated uncertainties of the tests. In summary, patients usually prefer CTC to OC but the preference is most likely dependent on a number of other factors such as insurance coverage, type of sedation used locally for OC, and the risk of finding a significant polyp on CTC thereby requiring a follow-up OC.

8. Extracolonic findings

Extracolonic findings are an important issue for CTC as they increase costs and patient risk by incurring addition tests. The frequency of extracolonic findings in the literature varies considerably as there are no standards for their reporting nor what constitutes a clinically significant extra-colonic finding. Some of the extracolonic lesions found are clinically important although most of them are incidental. In addition to increasing costs of CTC screening programs, they may cause undue worry and anxiety for the patient.

The prevalence of extracolonic findings can be as high as 40% - 75% and are increased with patient age [107-109]. Most extracolonic findings are incidental and not clinically important. The most common extracolonic findings causing further evaluation in one study were lung nodules and indeterminate kidney lesions adding a cost of $248 dollars per patient enrolled for CTC screening [110].

In general, significant extracolonic findings are found in about 10 - 23% of patients undergoing CTC [111-113]. Potentially important extracolonic findings were seen in 15.4% (89 of 577) of patients in one study, with a work-up rate of 7.8% (45 of 577)[114]. In another study only 4.4% - 6.0% of patients required follow-up radiologic testing for the extracolonic findings [109]. Another study showed that 10% of 681 patients screened for colon cancer had extracolonic findings of high clinical importance [115].

Although extracolonic finding add cost to CTC screening programs, they may benefit patients by diagnosing other potentially malignant lesions [112]. Unsuspected cancers (colonic and extra-colonic) are found in about 0.5% of screening cases [116]. In a large study, 36/10,286 patients (0.35%) undergoing a screening examination had an unsuspected extracolonic cancer which included renal cell carcinoma (n = 11), lung cancer (n = 8), non-Hodgkin lymphoma (n = 60, and a variety of other tumors (n = 11)[116). Other studies report a higher rate of 2.7% of extracolonic cancer detection [107].

9. Computer-Assisted Diagnosis (CAD)

An intensive area of research is the development of computer-assisted diagnosis (CAD) algorithms. CAD can assist radiologists as a second reader to improve accuracy [117, 118]. It has been shown that CAD can aid trained radiologists in the detection of significant polyps [119].CAD significantly improved polyp detection by 12% in one study, (from 48 to 60%) with only a moderate increase in interpretation time [120]. Another study demonstrated that using CAD in second-read mode increased accuracy in 13 of 19 readers 968%); CAD increased sensitivity of finding polyps but decreased specificity slightly [121]. In general, using CAD increases polyp detection but also increases false positives as well [122, 123].

Using CAD as a primary reader is feasible but early studies showed less sensitivity than human readers [124]. The sensitivity of CAD detected polyps 10 mm or greater was 64% (18/28) in one study [125]. In a later study of 1,186 patients undergoing both CTC and OC on the same day, CAD had a sensitivity of 89.3% (25/28; 95% CI: 71.8%-97.7%) for detecting adenomatous polyps at least 1 cm in size [126]. The false-positive rate was 2.1% (95% CI: 2.0% - 2.2%). CAD detected both of the carcinomas in the study group. In this study, CAD had a per-patient sensitivity comparable to that of OC for adenomas at least 8 mm in size [126]. Another study found a per-patient sensitivity of 96% was for CAD (in patients with a median polyp diameter of 6 mm) using external validation [127]. Several CAD polyp detection systems exist such as Polyp Enhanced Viewing (PEV) and the Summers computer-aided detection (CAD) system (National Institutes of Health (NIH)). These systems vary and have trade-offs in terms of sensitivity and specificity [128].

10. Safety

It is difficult to make a head-to-head comparison of the safety of CTC vs. OC since they are different technologies with varying risks. In one study, CTC screening was performed in 3,120 adults and compared to primary OC screening in 3,163 adults. There were seven colonic perforations in the OC group and none in the CTC group [45]. Colonic perforation has been reported with CTC but its occurrence is rare [129, 130]. Nine perforations out of 17,067 CTC examinations (0.052%) were reported in one study [131]. In another study of 11, 870 CTC studies, the perforation rate was 0.059% [132].

Possible factors that contribute to perforation are presence of an inguinal hernia containing colon (n = 4), severe diverticulosis (n = 3), and obstructive carcinoma (n = 1)[132, 133]. In cases of obstructing lesions, gas should be insufflated slowly [133]. Colonic pneumatosis is rarely seen (0.11%) in CTC studies and should not be confused with perforation [134, 135]. Overall, potentially serious adverse events related to CTC occur in less than 0.10% of patients [131].

11. Cost-effectiveness

With a 6-mm size threshold for polyps, the overall referral rate to optical colonoscopy is about 15% [114]. CTC is usually a less expensive test than OC, however the total costs may not be less if one considers all of the variables such as compliance rates and referral rates for OC after detecting lesions. Using a Markov model, screening by CTC costs $24,586 per life-year saved compared to $20,930 for OC screening [136]. CTC becomes a more cost-effective test as the compliance rate for screening increases or if the cost for CTC is 54% lower than OC. On the other hand in a recent analysis both CTC and OC were more costly and less effective than FOBT plus flexible sigmoidoscopy[137].

A Markov model was used to estimate the cost-effectiveness of CTC screening in an Italian population. In this study, colorectal cancer was reduced by 40.9% and 38.2%, with OC and CTC respectively. As compared to no screening, both CTC and OC were shown to be cost-saving with CTC being the less expensive option [138]. Since CTC can accurately detect and simultaneously screen for aortic aneurysms, cardiac atherosclerotic risk factors and osteoporosis, the benefits of CTC screening in an elderly population may be even more cost-effective than previously thought [139-141].

12. New directions – Noncathartic bowel preparations

One new hope for the future is for patients to undergo CTC without laxatives or the need for a purgative bowel preparation. Patients would only need to ingest fecal tagging agents such as Gastroview or barium, one to two days before the test [142]. A pilot study using a noncathartic bowel preparation (low fiber diet and fecal tagging) had disappointing results demonstrating that the lack of bowel cleansing made the examination subjectively harder to interpret and likely missed significant polyps [143]. A subsequent study however using a noncathartic bowel preparation was performed in a high risk population [144]. Subjects ingested 21.6 g of barium in nine divided doses. This study demonstrated that the sensitivity of CTC using a non-cathartic bowel preparation for polyps greater than 9 mm was over 90% [144].

Limited or non-cathartic bowel preparations may be especially useful in the frail or elderly patient. In a prospective study, 67 elderly patients with reduced functional status underwent CTC using a limited bowel preparation consisting of a low-residue diet for 3 days, 1 L of 2% oral diatrizoatemeglumine (Gastrografin) 24 hours before CTC, and 1 L of 2% oral Gastrografin over the 2 hours immediately before CTC [145]. No cathartic preparation was administered. All colonic segments were graded from 1 to 5 for image quality (1, unreadable; 2, poor; 3, equivocal; 4, good; 5, excellent). Overall image quality was rated good or excellent in 84% of the colonic segments. Colonic abnormalities were identified in 12 patients (18%), including four colonic tumors, two polyps, and seven colonic strictures [145].

Ref.	(%)Sensitivity	(%)Sensitivity	(%)Specificity	(N) Patients
	6 – 9 mm	1 cm or more		
33	82	91	79	87
34	80	90	72	300
35	89	94	79 – 96	1,233
36	39	55	91 – 96	600
37	78	90	90	2,531
41*	86	93	97	2,610
42*	76 – 83	83 – 88	91 – 98	4,086
* Meta-analysis				

Table 1. Sensitivity and specificity of polyps detected by CTC.

Author details

Robert J. Richards* and Jerome Zhengrong Liang

*Address all correspondence to: robert2841@yahoo.com

Stony Brook University, New York, USA

References

[1] Merrill RM, Anderson AE. Risk-Adjusted Colon and Rectal Cancer Incidence Rates in the United States. Diseases of the Colon & Rectum. 2011 Oct;54[10]:1301-6. PubMed PMID: WOS:000294727000017. English.

[2] Wolff WI, Shinya H. Colonofiberoscopy. Journal of the American Medical Association. 1971;217[11]:1509-&. PubMed PMID: WOS:A1971K270800002.

[3] Smith LE. Fiberoptic Colonoscopy - Complications of Colonoscopy and Polypectomy. Diseases of the Colon & Rectum. 1976;19[5]:407-12. PubMed PMID: WOS:A1976CA29600006.

[4] Stevenson GW, Wilson JA, Wilkinson J, Norman G, Goodacre RL. Pain Following Colonoscopy - Elimination with Carbon-Dioxide. Gastrointestinal Endoscopy. 1992 Sep-Oct;38[5]:564-7. PubMed PMID: WOS:A1992JT93000008.

[5] Weitzman ER, Zapka J, Estabrook B, Goins KV. Risk and reluctance: Understanding impediments to colorectal cancer screening. Preventive Medicine. 2001 Jun;32[6]: 502-13. PubMed PMID: WOS:000169145500007.

[6] Granqvist S. Distribution of Polyps in the Large Bowel in Relation to Age - A Colonoscopic Study. Scandinavian Journal of Gastroenterology. 1981;16[8]:1025-31. PubMed PMID: WOS:A1981MU13100013.

[7] Stryker SJ, Wolff BG, Culp CE, Libbe SD, Ilstrup DM, Maccarty RL. Natural-History of Untreated Colonic Polyps. Gastroenterology. 1987 Nov;93[5]:1009-13. PubMed PMID: WOS:A1987K557000012.

[8] Rex DK, Rahmani EY, Haseman JH, Lemmel GT, Kaster S, Buckley JS. Relative sensitivity of colonoscopy and barium enema for detection of colorectal cancer in clinical practice. Gastroenterology. 1997 Jan;112[1]:17-23. PubMed PMID: WOS:A1997WA90500005.

[9] Bressler B, Paszat LF, Vinden C, Li C, He JS, Rabeneck L. Colonoscopic miss rates for right-sided colon cancer: A population-based analysis. Gastroenterology. 2004 Aug; 127[2]:452-6. PubMed PMID: WOS:000223431200016.

[10] Aschoff AJ, Ernst AS, Brambs HJ, Juchems MS. CT colonography: an update. European Radiology. 2008 Mar;18[3]:429-37. PubMed PMID: WOS:000253006700001.

[11] Hara AK, Johnson CD, Reed JE, Ahlquist DA, Nelson H, Ehman RL, et al. Detection of colorectal polyps by computed tomographic colography: Feasibility of a novel technique. Gastroenterology. 1996 Jan;110[1]:284-90. PubMed PMID: WOS:A1996TN35200034.

[12] Blachar A, Sosna J. CT colonography (virtual colonoscopy): Technique, indications and performance. Digestion. 2007;76[1]:34-41. PubMed PMID: WOS: 000251437300005.

[13] Moawad FJ, Maydonovitch CL, Cullen PA, Barlow DS, Jenson DW, Cash BD. CT Colonography May Improve Colorectal Cancer Screening Compliance. American Journal of Roentgenology. 2010 Nov;195[5]:1118-23. PubMed PMID: WOS: 000283295300024.

[14] Shinners TJ, Pickhardt PJ, Taylor AJ, Jones DA, Olsen CH. Patient-controlled room air insufflation versus automated carbon dioxide delivery for CT colonography. American Journal of Roentgenology. 2006 Jun;186[6]:1491-6. PubMed PMID: WOS: 000237759300004.

[15] Svensson MH, Svensson E, Lasson A, Hellstrom M. Patient acceptance of CT colonography and conventional colonoscopy: Prospective comparative study in patients

with or suspected of having colorectal disease. Radiology. 2002 Feb;222[2]:337-45. PubMed PMID: WOS:000173502500008.

[16] Neri E, Caramella D, Vannozzi F, Turini F, Cerri F, Bartolozzi C. Vasovagal reactions in CT colonography. Abdominal Imaging. 2007 Sep;32[5]:552-5. PubMed PMID: WOS:000250204200002.

[17] Chen SC, Lu DSK, Hecht JR, Kadell BM. CT colonography: Value of scanning in both the supine and prone positions. American Journal of Roentgenology. 1999 Mar; 172[3]:595-9. PubMed PMID: WOS:000078729000004.

[18] Fletcher JG, Johnson CD, Welch TJ, MacCarty RL, Ahlquist DA, Reed JE, et al. Optimization of CT colonography technique: Prospective trial in 180 patients. Radiology. 2000 Sep;216[3]:704-11. PubMed PMID: WOS:000088964900014. English.

[19] Lee JH, Park SH, Lee SS, Kim AY, Kim JC, Yu CS, et al. CT Colonography in Patients Who Have Undergone Sigmoid Colostomy: A Feasibility Study. American Journal of Roentgenology. 2011 Oct;197[4]:W653-W7. PubMed PMID: WOS:000295081000013. English.

[20] Ridge CA, Carter MR, Browne LP, Ryan R, Hegarty C, Schaffer K, et al. CT colonography and transient bacteraemia: implications for antibiotic prophylaxis. European Radiology. 2011 Feb;21[2]:360-5. PubMed PMID: WOS:000287079300018.

[21] Borden ZS, Pickhardt PJ, Kim DH, Lubner MG, Agriantonis DJ, Hinshaw JL. Bowel Preparation for CT Colonography: Blinded Comparison of Magnesium Citrate and Sodium Phosphate for Catharsis. Radiology. 2010 Jan;254[1]:138-44. PubMed PMID: WOS:000273820400018.

[22] Hara AK, Blevins M, Chen MH, Dachman AH, Kuo MD, Menias CO, et al. ACRIN CT Colonography Trial: Does Reader's Preference for Primary Two-dimensional versus Primary Three-dimensional Interpretation Affect Performance? Radiology. 2011 May;259[2]:435-41. PubMed PMID: WOS:000289667300016.

[23] Deshpande KK, Summers RM, Van Uitert RL, Franaszek M, Brown L, Dwyer AJ, et al. Quality assessment for CT colonography: Validation of automated measurement of colonic distention and residual fluid. American Journal of Roentgenology. 2007 Dec;189[6]:1457-63. PubMed PMID: WOS:000251172000031.

[24] Barish MA, Soto JA, Ferrucci JT. Consensus on current clinical practice of virtual colonoscopy. American Journal of Roentgenology. 2005 Mar;184[3]:786-92. PubMed PMID: WOS:000227286100012.

[25] Choi EK, Park SH, Kim DY, Ha HK. Malignant rectal polyp overlooked on CT colonography because of retention balloon: Opposing crescent appearance as sign of compressed polyp. American Journal of Roentgenology. 2007 Jul;189[1]:W1-W3. PubMed PMID: WOS:000247588100040.

[26] Pickhardt PJ, Choi JR. Adenomatous polyp obscured by small-caliber rectal catheter at low-dose CT colonography: A rare diagnostic pitfall. American Journal of Roentgenology. 2005 May;184[5]:1581-3. PubMed PMID: WOS:000228875300037.

[27] Cornett D, Barancin C, Roeder B, Reichelderfer M, Frick T, Gopal D, et al. Findings on optical colonoscopy after positive CT colonography exam. American Journal of Gastroenterology. 2008 Aug;103[8]:2068-74. PubMed PMID: WOS:000258278200027.

[28] Fletcher JG, Booya F, Johnson CD, Ahlquist D. CT colonography: unraveling the twists and turns. Current Opinion in Gastroenterology. 2005 Jan;21[1]:90-8. PubMed PMID: WOS:000225874600016.

[29] Dachman AH, Yoshida H. Virtual colonoscopy: past, present, and future. Radiologic Clinics of North America. 2003 Mar;41[2]:377-+. PubMed PMID: WOS: 000181611900012.

[30] El-Maraghi RH, Kielar AZ. CT Colonography Versus Optical Colonoscopy for Screening Asymptomatic Patients for Colorectal Cancer: A Patient, Intervention, Comparison, Outcome (PICO) Analysis. Academic Radiology. 2009 May;16[5]:564-71. PubMed PMID: WOS:000265229500009.

[31] Johnson CD. CT Colonography: Coming of Age. American Journal of Roentgenology. 2009 Nov;193[5]:1239-42. PubMed PMID: WOS:000270956700006.

[32] Dachman AH, Kuniyoshi JK, Boyle CM, Samara Y, Hoffmann KR, Rubin DT, et al. CT colonography with three-dimensional problem solving for detection of colonic polyps. American Journal of Roentgenology. 1998 Oct;171[4]:989-95. PubMed PMID: WOS:000076117300016. English.

[33] Fenlon HM, Nunes DP, Schroy PC, Barish MA, Clarke PD, Ferrucci JT. A comparison of virtual and conventional colonoscopy for the detection of colorectal polyps. New England Journal of Medicine. 1999 Nov;341[20]:1496-503. PubMed PMID: WOS: 000083625800003. English.

[34] Yee J, Akerkar GA, Hung RK, Steinauer-Gebauer AM, Wall SD, McQuaid KR. Colorectal neoplasia: Performance characteristics of CT colonography for detection in 300 patients. Radiology. 2001 Jun;219[3]:685-92. PubMed PMID: WOS:000168864800015. English.

[35] Pickhardt PJ, Choi JR, Hwang I, Butler JA, Puckett ML, Hildebrandt HA, et al. Computed tomographic virtual colonoscopy to screen for colorectal neoplasia in asymptomatic adults. New England Journal of Medicine. 2003 Dec;349[23]:2191-200. PubMed PMID: WOS:000186921700005. English.

[36] Cotton PB, Durkalski VL, Benoit PC, Palesch YY, Mauldin PD, Hoffman B, et al. Computed tomographic colonography (virtual colonoscopy) - A multicenter comparison with standard colonoscopy for detection of colorectal neoplasia. Jama-Journal of the American Medical Association. 2004 Apr;291[14]:1713-9. PubMed PMID: WOS: 000220788700028. English.

[37] Johnson CD, Chen MH, Toledano AY, Heiken JP, Dachman A, Kuo MD, et al. Accuracy of CT colonography for detection of large adenomas and cancers. New England Journal of Medicine. 2008 Sep;359[12]:1207-17. PubMed PMID: WOS: 000259259900004. English.

[38] Pickhardt PJ, Wise SM, Kim DH. Positive predictive value for polyps detected at screening CT colonography. European Radiology. 2010 Jul;20[7]:1651-6. PubMed PMID: WOS:000278522800017.

[39] Iafrate F, Hassan C, Ciolina M, Lamazza A, Baldassari P, Pichi A, et al. High positive predictive value of CT colonography in a referral centre. European Journal of Radiology. 2011 Dec;80[3]:E289-E92. PubMed PMID: WOS:000296763300018. English.

[40] Halligan S, Taylor SA. CT colonography: Results and limitations. European Journal of Radiology. 2007 Mar;61[3]:400-8. PubMed PMID: WOS:000245141800005.

[41] Halligan S, Altman DG, Taylor SA, Mallett S, Deeks JJ, Bartram CI, et al. CT colonography in the detection of colorectal polyps and cancer: Systematic review meta-analysis and proposed minimum data set for study level reporting. Radiology. 2005 Dec; 237[3]:893-904. PubMed PMID: WOS:000233380100018.

[42] de Haan MC, van Gelder RE, Graser A, Bipat S, Stoker J. Diagnostic value of CT-colonography as compared to colonoscopy in an asymptomatic screening population: a meta-analysis. European Radiology. 2011 Aug;21[8]:1747-63. PubMed PMID: WOS: 000292311000023.

[43] Pickhardt PJ, Nugent PA, Mysliwiec PA, Choi JR, Schindler WR. Location of adenomas missed by optical colonoscopy. Annals of Internal Medicine. 2004 Sep;141[5]: 352-9. PubMed PMID: WOS:000223733800003.

[44] Heresbach D, Barrioz T, Lapalus MG, Coumaros D, Bauret P, Potier P, et al. Miss rate for colorectal neoplastic polyps: a prospective multicenter study of back-to-back video colonoscopies. Endoscopy. 2008 Apr;40[4]:284-90. PubMed PMID: WOS: 000255123500003.

[45] Kim DH, Pickhardt PJ, Taylor AJ, Leung WK, Winter TC, Hinshaw JL, et al. CT colonography versus colonoscopy for the detection of advanced neoplasia. New England Journal of Medicine. 2007 Oct;357[14]:1403-12. PubMed PMID: WOS: 000249892900006. English.

[46] Benson M, Dureja P, Gopal D, Reichelderfer M, Pfau PR. A Comparison of Optical Colonoscopy and CT Colonography Screening Strategies in the Detection and Recovery of Subcentimeter Adenomas. American Journal of Gastroenterology. 2010 Dec; 105[12]:2578-85. PubMed PMID: WOS:000284940900008.

[47] Graser A, Stieber P, Nagel D, Schafer C, Horst D, Becker CR, et al. Comparison of CT colonography, colonoscopy, sigmoidoscopy and faecal occult blood tests for the detection of advanced adenoma in an average risk population. Gut. 2009 Feb;58[2]: 241-8. PubMed PMID: WOS:000262369800018.

[48] Lostumbo A, Suzuki K, Dachman AH. Flat lesions in CT colonography. Abdominal Imaging. 2010 Oct;35[5]:578-83. PubMed PMID: WOS:000282424100011.

[49] MacCarty RL, Johnson CD, Fletcher JG, Wilson LA. Occult colorectal polyps on CT colonography: Implications for surveillance. American Journal of Roentgenology. 2006 May;186[5]:1380-3. PubMed PMID: WOS:000237003300029.

[50] Pickhardt PJ, Nugent PA, Choi JR, Schindler WR. Flat colorectal lesions in asymptomatic adults: Implications for screening with CT virtual colonoscopy. American Journal of Roentgenology. 2004 Nov;183[5]:1343-7. PubMed PMID: WOS: 000224685700027.

[51] Pickhardt PJ, Kim DH, Robbins JB. Flat (Nonpolypoid) Colorectal Lesions Identified at CT Colonography in a US Screening Population. Academic Radiology. 2010 Jun; 17[6]:784-90. PubMed PMID: WOS:000277945700015.

[52] Fidler JL, Johnson CD, MacCarty RL, Welch TJ, Hara AK, Harmsen WS. Detection of flat lesions in the colon with CT colonography. Abdominal Imaging. 2002 May-Jun; 27[3]:292-300. PubMed PMID: WOS:000175176000010.

[53] Galdino GM, Yee J. Carpet lesion on CT colonography: A potential pitfall. American Journal of Roentgenology. 2003 May;180[5]:1332-4. PubMed PMID: WOS: 000182423300023.

[54] Rex DK, Overhiser AJ, Chen SC, Cummings OW, Ulbright TM. Estimation of Impact of American College of Radiology Recommendations on CT Colonography Reporting for Resection of High-Risk Adenoma Findings. American Journal of Gastroenterology. 2009 Jan;104[1]:149-53. PubMed PMID: WOS:000262265800025.

[55] Lieberman D, Moravec M, Holub J, Michaels L, Eisen G. Polyp size and advanced histology in patients undergoing colonoscopy screening: Implications for CT colonography. Gastroenterology. 2008 Oct;135[4]:1100-5. PubMed PMID: WOS: 000259982800016.

[56] Pickhardt PJ, Taylor AJ, Kim DH, Reichelderfer M, Gopal DV, Pfau PR. Screening for colorectal neoplasia with CT colonography: Initial experience from the 1st year of coverage by third-party payers. Radiology. 2006 Nov;241[2]:417-25. PubMed PMID: WOS:000241519400012.

[57] Macari M, Bini EJ, Jacobs SL, Lui YW, Laks S, Milano A, et al. Significance of missed polyps at CT colonography. American Journal of Roentgenology. 2004 Jul;183[1]: 127-34. PubMed PMID: WOS:000222163900027.

[58] Shah JP, Hynan LS, Rockey DC. Management of Small Polyps Detected by Screening CT Colonography: Patient and Physician Preferences. American Journal of Medicine. 2009 Jul;122[7]. PubMed PMID: WOS:000267341000017.

[59] Edwards JT, Mendelson RM, Fritschi L, Foster NM, Wood C, Murray D, et al. Colorectal neoplasia screening with CT colonography in average-risk asymptomatic sub-

jects: Community-based study. Radiology. 2004 Feb;230[2]:459-64. PubMed PMID: WOS:000188463700023.

[60] Pickhardt PJ, Hassan C, Laghi A, Zullo A, Kim DH, Iafrate F, et al. Clinical Management of Small [6- to 9-mm) Polyps Detected at Screening CT Colonography: A Cost-Effectiveness Analysis. American Journal of Roentgenology. 2008 Nov;191[5]: 1509-16. PubMed PMID: WOS:000260246700035.

[61] Hanson ME, Pickhardt PJ, Kim DH, Pfau PR. Anatomic factors predictive of incomplete colonoscopy based on findings at CT colonography. American Journal of Roentgenology. 2007 Oct;189[4]:774-9. PubMed PMID: WOS:000249595800005.

[62] Dachman AH. Diagnostic performance of virtual colonoscopy. Abdominal Imaging. 2002 May-Jun;27[3]:260-7. PubMed PMID: WOS:000175176000006.

[63] Copel L, Sosna J, Kruskal JB, Raptopoulos V, Farrell RJ, Morrin MM. CT colonography in 546 patients with incomplete colonoscopy. Radiology. 2007 Aug;244[2]:471-8. PubMed PMID: WOS:000248821400017.

[64] Hough DM, Kuntz MA, Fidler JL, Johnson CD, Petersen BT, Kofler JM, et al. Detection of Occult Colonic Perforation Before CT Colonography After Incomplete Colonoscopy: Perforation Rate and Use of a Low-Dose Diagnostic Scan Before CO2 Insufflation. American Journal of Roentgenology. 2008 Oct;191[4]:1077-81. PubMed PMID: WOS:000259364100018.

[65] Bose M, Bell J, Jackson L, Casey P, Saunders J, Epstein O. Virtual vs. optical colonoscopy in symptomatic gastroenterology out-patients: the case for virtual imaging followed by targeted diagnostic or therapeutic colonoscopy. Alimentary Pharmacology & Therapeutics. 2007 Sep;26[5]:727-36. PubMed PMID: WOS:000248666200010.

[66] Badiani S, Hernandez ST, Karandikar S, Roy-Choudhury S. CT Colonography to exclude colorectal cancer in symptomatic patients. European Radiology. 2011 Oct; 21[10]:2029-38. PubMed PMID: WOS:000294471100001. English.

[67] Tarjan Z, Zagoni T, Gyorke T, Mester A, Karlinger K, Mako EK. Spiral CT colonography in inflammatory bowel disease. European Journal of Radiology. 2000 Sep;35[3]: 193-8. PubMed PMID: WOS:000089513600006.

[68] Andersen K, Vogt C, Blondin D, Beck A, Heinen W, Aurich V, et al. Multi-detector CT-colonography in inflammatory bowel disease: Prospective analysis of CT-findings to high-resolution video colonoscopy. European Journal of Radiology. 2006 Apr; 58[1]:140-6. PubMed PMID: WOS:000236771700017.

[69] Biancone L, Fiori R, Tosti C, Marinetti T, Catarinacci T, De Nigris F, et al. Virtual colonoscopy compared for stricturing postoperative with conventional colonoscopy recurrence in Crohn's disease. Inflammatory Bowel Diseases. 2003 Nov;9[6]:343-50. PubMed PMID: WOS:000186618800001.

[70] Coady-Fariborzian L, Angel LP, Procaccino JA. Perforated colon secondary to virtual colonoscopy: Report of a case. Diseases of the Colon & Rectum. 2004 Jul;47[7]:1247-9. PubMed PMID: WOS:000222364600025.

[71] Hjern F, Jonas E, Holmstrom B, Josephson T, Mellgren A, Johansson C. CT colonography versus colonoscopy in the follow-up of patients after diverticulitis - A prospective, comparative study. Clinical Radiology. 2007 Jul;62[7]:645-50. PubMed PMID: WOS:000247912900006.

[72] Lefere P, Gryspeerdt S, Baekelandt M, Dewyspelaere J, van Holsbeeck B. Diverticular disease in CT colonography. European Radiology. 2003 Dec;13:L62-L74. PubMed PMID: WOS:000187789400011.

[73] Nadir I, Ozin Y, Kilic ZMY, Oguz D, Ulker A, Arda K. Colovesical fistula as a complication of colonic diverticulosis: diagnosis with virtual colonoscopy. Turkish Journal of Gastroenterology. 2011 Feb;22[1]:86-8. PubMed PMID: WOS:000289710100016.

[74] Neri E, Giusti P, Battolla L, Vagli P, Boraschi P, Lencioni R, et al. Colorectal cancer: Role of CT colonography in preoperative evaluation after incomplete colonoscopy. Radiology. 2002 Jun;223[3]:615-9. PubMed PMID: WOS:000175757300004.

[75] Kim JH, Kim WH, Kim TI, Kim NK, Lee KY, Kim MJ, et al. Incomplete colonoscopy in patients with occlusive colorectal cancer: Usefulness of CT colonography according to tumor location. Yonsei Medical Journal. 2007 Dec;48[6]:934-41. PubMed PMID: WOS:000252239900004.

[76] Mainenti PP, Romano M, Imbriaco M, Camera L, Pace L, D'Antonio D, et al. Added value of CT colonography after a positive conventional colonoscopy: impact on treatment strategy. Abdominal Imaging. 2005 Jan-Feb;30[1]:42-7. PubMed PMID: WOS: 000226002300006.

[77] Baca B, Selcuk D, Kilic IE, Erdamar S, Salihoglu Z, Hamzaoglu I, et al. The contributions of virtual colonoscopy to laparoscopic colorectal surgery. Hepato-Gastroenterology. 2007 Oct-Nov;54[79]:1976-82. PubMed PMID: WOS:000251892700019.

[78] Fenlon HM, McAneny DB, Nunes DP, Clarke PD, Ferrucci JT. Occlusive colon carcinoma: Virtual colonoscopy in the preoperative evaluation of the proximal colon. Radiology. 1999 Feb;210[2]:423-8. PubMed PMID: WOS:000078277900021.

[79] Neri E, Turini F, Cerri F, Faggioni L, Vagli P, Naldini G, et al. Comparison of CT colonography vs. conventional colonoscopy in mapping the segmental location of colon cancer before surgery. Abdominal Imaging. 2010 Oct;35[5]:589-95. PubMed PMID: WOS:000282424100013.

[80] Cha EY, Park SH, Lee SS, Kim JC, Yu CS, Lim SB, et al. CT Colonography after Metallic Stent Placement for Acute Malignant Colonic Obstruction. Radiology. 2010 Mar; 254[3]:774-82. PubMed PMID: WOS:000274796200018.

[81] Choi YJ, Park SH, Lee SS, Choi EK, Yu CS, Kim HC, et al. CT Colonography for follow-up after surgery for colorectal cancer. American Journal of Roentgenology. 2007 Aug;189[2]:283-9. PubMed PMID: WOS:000248624400008.

[82] Fletcher JG, Johnson CD, Krueger WR, Ahlquist DA, Nelson H, Ilstrup D, et al. Contrast-enhanced CT colonography in recurrent colorectal carcinoma: Feasibility of simultaneous evaluation for metastatic disease, local recurrence, and metachronous neoplasia in colorectal carcinoma. American Journal of Roentgenology. 2002 Feb; 178[2]:283-90. PubMed PMID: WOS:000173486500003.

[83] Kim HJ, Park SH, Pickhardt PJ, Yoon SN, Lee SS, Yee J, et al. CT Colonography for Combined Colonic and Extracolonic Surveillance after Curative Resection of Colorectal Cancer. Radiology. 2010 Dec;257[3]:697-704. PubMed PMID: WOS: 000284469300014.

[84] Neri E, Vagli P, Turini F, Cerri F, Faggioni L, Angeli S, et al. Post-surgical follow-up of colorectal cancer: role of contrast-enhanced CT colonography. Abdominal Imaging. 2010 Dec;35[6]:669-75. PubMed PMID: WOS:000284153500006.

[85] Kato K, Funatsu H, Suzuka K, Osaki T, Imarnura A, Takano H, et al. CT colonography to detect rectosigmoid involvement in patients with primary ovarian cancer. European Journal of Gynaecological Oncology. 2008;29[5]:462-7. PubMed PMID: WOS: 000259328800009.

[86] Fletcher JG, Chen MH, Herman BA, Johnson CD, Toledano A, Dachman AH, et al. Can Radiologist Training and Testing Ensure High Performance in CT Colonography? Lessons From the National CT Colonography Trial. American Journal of Roentgenology. 2010 Jul;195[1]:117-25. PubMed PMID: WOS:000278998200015.

[87] Gluecker T, Meuwly JY, Pescatore P, Schnyder P, Delarive J, Jornod P, et al. Effect of investigator experience in CT colonography. European Radiology. 2002 Jun;12[6]: 1405-9. PubMed PMID: WOS:000176197400019.

[88] Halligan S, Burling D, Atkin W, Bartram C, Fenlon H, Laghi A, et al. Effect of directed training on reader performance for CT colonography: Multicenter study. Radiology. 2007 Jan;242[1]:152-61. PubMed PMID: WOS:000243842500020.

[89] Nio CY, de Vries AH, Stoker J. Perceptive errors in CT colonography. Abdominal Imaging. 2007 Sep;32[5]:556-70. PubMed PMID: WOS:000250204200003.

[90] Slater A, Taylor SA, Tam E, Gartner L, Scarth J, Peiris C, et al. Reader error during CT colonography: causes and implications for training. European Radiology. 2006 Oct;16[10]:2275-83. PubMed PMID: WOS:000240362400016.

[91] Burling D, Halligan S, Atchley J, Dhingsar R, Guest P, Hayward S, et al. CT colonography: interpretative performance in a non-academic environment. Clinical Radiology. 2007 May;62[5]:424-9. PubMed PMID: WOS:000246266100004.

[92] Doshi T, Rusinak D, Halvorsen RA, Rockey DC, Suzuki K, Dachman AH. CT colonography: False-negative interpretations. Radiology. 2007 Jul;244[1]:165-73. PubMed PMID: WOS:000247436500019.

[93] Gluecker TM, Fletcher JG, Welch TJ, MacCarty RL, Harmsen WS, Harrington JR, et al. Characterization of lesions missed on interpretation of CT colonography using a 2D search method. American Journal of Roentgenology. 2004 Apr;182[4]:881-9. PubMed PMID: WOS:000220382800017.

[94] Brenner DJ, Hall EJ. Current concepts - Computed tomography - An increasing source of radiation exposure. New England Journal of Medicine. 2007 Nov;357[22]: 2277-84. PubMed PMID: WOS:000251176400009.

[95] Brenner DJ, Georgsson MA. Mass screening with CT colonography: Should the radiation exposure be of concern? Gastroenterology. 2005 Jul;129[1]:328-37. PubMed PMID: WOS:000230423100033.

[96] Jensch S, van Gelder RE, Venema HW, Reitsma JB, Bossuyt PMM, Lameris JS, et al. Effective radiation doses in CT colonography: results of an inventory among research institutions. European Radiology. 2006 May;16[5]:981-7. PubMed PMID: WOS: 000236751800003.

[97] Fisichella VA, Bath M, Johnsson AA, Jaderling F, Bergsten T, Persson U, et al. Evaluation of image quality and lesion perception by human readers on 3D CT colonography: comparison of standard and low radiation dose. European Radiology. 2010 Mar; 20[3]:630-9. PubMed PMID: WOS:000274544800014.

[98] Flicek KT, Hara AK, Silva AC, Wu Q, Peter MB, Johnson CD. Reducing the Radiation Dose for CT Colonography Using Adaptive Statistical Iterative Reconstruction: A Pilot Study. American Journal of Roentgenology. 2010 Jul;195[1]:126-31. PubMed PMID: WOS:000278998200016.

[99] Liedenbaum MH, Venema HW, Stoker J. Radiation dose in CT colonography-trends in time and differences between daily practice and screening protocols. European Radiology. 2008 Oct;18[10]:2222-30. PubMed PMID: WOS:000259141900024.

[100] de Gonzalez AB, Kim KP, Knudsen AB, Lansdorp-Vogelaar I, Rutter CM, Smith-Bindman R, et al. Radiation-Related Cancer Risks From CT Colonography Screening: A Risk-Benefit Analysis. American Journal of Roentgenology. 2011 Apr;196[4]:816-23. PubMed PMID: WOS:000288650600038.

[101] Saar B, Heverhagen JT, Obst T, Berthold LD, Kopp I, Klose KJ, et al. Magnetic resonance colonography and virtual magnetic resonance colonoscopy with the 1.0-T system - A feasibility study. Investigative Radiology. 2000 Sep;35[9]:521-6. PubMed PMID: WOS:000089025900001.

[102] Angtuaco TL, Banaad-Omiotek GD, Howden CW. Differing attitudes toward virtual and conventional colonoscopy for colorectal cancer screening: Surveys among pri-

mary care physicians and potential patients. American Journal of Gastroenterology. 2001 Mar;96[3]:887-93. PubMed PMID: WOS:000167596300049.

[103] Gluecker TM, Johnson CD, Harmsen WS, Offord KP, Harris AM, Wilson LA, et al. Colorectal cancer screening with CT colonography, colonoscopy, and double-contrast barium enema examination: Prospective assessment of patient perceptions and preferences. Radiology. 2003 May;227[2]:378-84. PubMed PMID: WOS: 000182534900011.

[104] Boellaard TN, van der Paardt MP, Eberl S, Hollmann MW, Stoker J. A randomized double-blind placebo-controlled trial to evaluate the value of a single bolus intravenous alfentanil in CT colonography. Bmc Gastroenterology. 2011 Nov;11:8. PubMed PMID: WOS:000301040200001. English.

[105] Akerkar GA, Yee J, Hung R, McQuaid K. Patient experience and preferences toward colon cancer screening: a comparison of virtual colonoscopy and conventional colonoscopy. Gastrointestinal Endoscopy. 2001 Sep;54[3]:310-5. PubMed PMID: WOS: 000170784600006.

[106] Howard K, Salkeld G, Pignone M, Hewett P, Cheung P, Olsen J, et al. Preferences for CT Colonography and Colonoscopy as Diagnostic Tests for Colorectal Cancer: A Discrete Choice Experiment. Value in Health. 2011 Dec;14[8]:1146-52. PubMed PMID: WOS:000299081900023. English.

[107] Xiong T, Richardson M, Woodroffe R, Halligan S, Morton D, Lilford RJ. Incidental lesions found on CT colonography: their nature and frequency. British Journal of Radiology. 2005 Jan;78[925]:22-9. PubMed PMID: WOS:000226885900008.

[108] Yee J, Kumar NN, Godara S, Casamina JA, Hom R, Galdino G, et al. Extracolonic abnormalities discovered incidentally at CT colonography in a male population. Radiology. 2005 Aug;236[2]:519-26. PubMed PMID: WOS:000230670200020.

[109] Macari M, Nevsky G, Bonavita J, Kim DC, Megibow AJ, Babb JS. CT Colonography in Senior versus Nonsenior Patients: Extracolonic Findings, Recommendations for Additional Imaging, and Polyp Prevalence. Radiology. 2011 Jun;259[3]:767-74. PubMed PMID: WOS:000290898100016.

[110] Kimberly JR, Phillips KC, Santago P, Perumpillichira J, Bechtold R, Pineau B, et al. Extracolonic Findings at Virtual Colonoscopy: An Important Consideration in Asymptomatic Colorectal Cancer Screening. Journal of General Internal Medicine. 2009 Jan;24[1]:69-73. PubMed PMID: WOS:000261969900012.

[111] Hara AK, Johnson CD, MacCarty RL, Welch TJ. Incidental extracolonic findings at CT colonography. Radiology. 2000 May;215[2]:353-7. PubMed PMID: WOS: 000086578500007. English.

[112] Edwards JT, Wood CJ, Mendelson RM, Forbes GM. Extracolonic findings at virtual colonoscopy: Implications for screening programs. American Journal of Gastroenterology. 2001 Oct;96[10]:3009-12. PubMed PMID: WOS:000171445900035.

[113] Hellstrom M, Svensson MH, Lasson A. Extracolonic and incidental findings on CT colonography (virtual colonoscopy). American Journal of Roentgenology. 2004 Mar; 182[3]:631-8. PubMed PMID: WOS:000189126100018.

[114] Kim DH, Pickhardt PJ, Hanson ME, Hinshaw JL. CT Colonography: Performance and Program Outcome Measures in an Older Screening Population. Radiology. 2010 Feb;254[2]:493-500. PubMed PMID: WOS:000273824600021.

[115] Gluecker TM, Johnson CD, Wilson LA, MacCarty RL, Welch TJ, Vanness DJ, et al. Extracolonic findings at CT colonography: Evaluation of prevalence and cost in a screening population. Gastroenterology. 2003 Apr;124[4]:911-6. PubMed PMID: WOS:000182002700011.

[116] Pickhardt PJ, Kim DH, Meiners RJ, Wyatt KS, Hanson ME, Barlow DS, et al. Colorectal and Extracolonic Cancers Detected at Screening CT Colonography in 10 286 Asymptomatic Adults. Radiology. 2010 Apr;255[1]:83-8. PubMed PMID: WOS: 000275863000012.

[117] Linguraru MG, Panjwani N, Fletcher J, Summers R. Automated image-based colon cleansing for laxative-free CT colonography computer-aided polyp detection. Medical Physics. 2011 Dec;38[12]:6633-42. PubMed PMID: WOS:000298250100031. English.

[118] Taylor SA, Brittenden J, Lenton J, Lambie H, Goldstone A, Wylie PN, et al. Influence of Computer-Aided Detection False-Positives on Reader Performance and Diagnostic Confidence for CT Colonography. American Journal of Roentgenology. 2009 Jun; 192[6]:1682-9. PubMed PMID: WOS:000266177400033.

[119] Summers RM, Jerebko AK, Franaszek M, Malley JD, Johnson CD. Colonic polyps: Complementary role of computer-aided detection in CT Colonography. Radiology. 2002 Nov;225[2]:391-9. PubMed PMID: WOS:000178822500013.

[120] Burling D, Moore A, Marshall M, Weldon J, Gillen C, Baldwin R, et al. Virtual colonoscopy: effect of computer-assisted detection (CAD) on radiographer performance. Clinical Radiology. 2008 May;63[5]:549-56. PubMed PMID: WOS:000255546700010.

[121] Dachman AH, Obuchowski NA, Hoffmeister JW, Hinshaw JL, Frew MI, Winter TC, et al. Effect of Computer-aided Detection for CT Colonography in a Multireader, Multicase Trial. Radiology. 2010 Sep;256[3]:827-35. PubMed PMID: WOS: 000282335300017.

[122] Bogoni L, Cathier P, Dundar M, Jerebko A, Lakare S, Liang J, et al. Computer-aided detection (CAD) for CT colonography: a tool to address a growing need. British Journal of Radiology. 2005;78:S57-S62. PubMed PMID: WOS:000230400000008.

[123] Nappi JJ, Nagata K. Sources of false positives in computer-assisted CT colonography. Abdominal Imaging. 2011 Apr;36[2]:153-64. PubMed PMID: WOS:000289296700007.

[124] Summers RM, Beaulieu CF, Pusanik LM, Malley JD, Jeffrey RB, Glazer DI, et al. Automated polyp detector for CT colonography: Feasibility study. Radiology. 2000 Jul; 216[1]:284-90. PubMed PMID: WOS:000087829500042.

[125] Summers RM, Johnson CD, Pusanik LM, Malley JD, Youssef AM, Reed JE. Automated polyp detection at CT colonography: Feasibility assessment in a human population. Radiology. 2001 Apr;219[1]:51-9. PubMed PMID: WOS:000167667400008. English.

[126] Summers RM, Yao JH, Pickhardt PJ, Franaszek M, Bitter I, Brickman D, et al. Computed tomographic virtual colonoscopy computer-aided polyp detection in a screening population. Gastroenterology. 2005 Dec;129[6]:1832-44. PubMed PMID: WOS: 000234079300005.

[127] Halligan S, Taylor SA, Dehmeshki J, Amin H, Ye X, Tsang J, et al. Computer-assisted detection for CT colonography: external validation. Clinical Radiology. 2006 Sep; 61[9]:758-63. PubMed PMID: WOS:000240366600006.

[128] Fletcher JG, Booya F, Summers RM, Roy D, Guendel L, Schmidt B, et al. Comparative performance of two polyp detection systems on CT colonography. American Journal of Roentgenology. 2007 Aug;189[2]:277-82. PubMed PMID: WOS:000248624400007.

[129] Bassett JT, Liotta RA, Barlow D, Lee D, Jensen D. Colonic perforation during screening CT colonography using automated CO2 insufflation in an asymptomatic adult. Abdominal Imaging. 2008 Sep;33[5]:598-600. PubMed PMID: WOS:000258540200015.

[130] Belo-Oliveira P, Curvo-Semedo L, Rodrigues H, Belo-Soares P, Caseiro-Alves F. Sigmoid colon perforation at CT colonography secondary to a possible obstructive mechanism: Report of a case. Diseases of the Colon & Rectum. 2007 Sep;50[9]: 1478-80. PubMed PMID: WOS:000249203900025.

[131] Burling D, Halligan S, Slater A, Noakes MJ, Taylor SA. Potentially serious adverse events at CT colonography in symptomatic patients: National survey of the United Kingdom. Radiology. 2006 May;239[2]:464-71. PubMed PMID: WOS: 000237090800019.

[132] Sosna J, Blachar A, Amitai M, Barmeir E, Peled N, Goldberg SN, et al. Colonic perforation at CT colonography: Assessment of risk in a multicenter large cohort. Radiology. 2006 May;239[2]:457-63. PubMed PMID: WOS:000237090800018.

[133] Kamar M, Portnoy O, Bar-Dayan A, Amitai M, Munz Y, Ayalon A, et al. Actual colonic perforation in virtual colonoscopy: Report of a case. Diseases of the Colon & Rectum. 2004 Jul;47[7]:1242-4. PubMed PMID: WOS:000222364600023.

[134] Pickhardt PJ, Kim DH, Taylor AJ. Asymptomatic pneumatosis at CT colonography: A benign self-limited imaging finding distinct from perforation. American Journal of Roentgenology. 2008 Feb;190[2]:W112-W7. PubMed PMID: WOS:000252932100041.

[135] Shimada R, Hayama T, Yamazaki N, Akahane T, Horiuchi A, Shibuya H, et al. Intestinal Pneumatosis in Which CT Colonography Was of Significant Diagnostic Value: Case Report. International Surgery. 2011 Jul-Sep;96[3]:217-9. PubMed PMID: WOS: 000299134000006.

[136] Sonnenberg A, Delco F, Bauerfeind P. Ts virtual colonoscopy a cost-effective option to screen for colorectal cancer? American Journal of Gastroenterology. 1999 Aug; 94[8]:2268-74. PubMed PMID: WOS:000081868900044.

[137] Vanness DJ, Knudsen AB, Lansdorp-Vogelaar I, Rutter CM, Gareen IF, Herman BA, et al. Comparative Economic Evaluation of Data from the ACRIN National CT Colonography Trial with Three Cancer Intervention and Surveillance Modeling Network Microsimulations. Radiology. 2011 Nov;261[2]:487-98. PubMed PMID: WOS: 000296524600018. English.

[138] Hassan C, Zullo A, Laghi A, Reitano I, Taggi F, Cerro P, et al. Colon cancer prevention in Italy: Cost-effectiveness analysis with CT colonography and endoscopy. Digestive and Liver Disease. 2007 Mar;39[3]:242-50. PubMed PMID: WOS: 000245460900007.

[139] Pickhardt PJ, Hassan C, Laghi A, Kim DH. CT Colonography to Screen for Colorectal Cancer and Aortic Aneurysm in the Medicare Population: Cost-Effectiveness Analysis. American Journal of Roentgenology. 2009 May;192[5]:1332-40. PubMed PMID: WOS:000265387300027.

[140] Pickhardt PJ, Lee LJ, del Rio AM, Lauder T, Bruce RJ, Summers RM, et al. Simultaneous Screening for Osteoporosis at CT Colonography: Bone Mineral Density Assessment Using MDCT Attenuation Techniques Compared With the DXA Reference Standard. Journal of Bone and Mineral Research. 2011 Sep;26[9]:2194-203. PubMed PMID: WOS:000294444300019.

[141] Davila JA, Johnson CD, Behrenbeck TR, Hoskin TL, Harmsen WS. Assessment of cardiovascular risk status at CT colonography. Radiology. 2006 Jul;240[1]:110-5. PubMed PMID: WOS:000238481000014.

[142] Callstrom MR, Johnson CD, Fletcher JG, Reed JE, Ahlquist DA, Harmsen WS, et al. CT colonography without cathartic preparation: Feasibility study. Radiology. 2001 Jun;219[3]:693-8. PubMed PMID: WOS:000168864800016.

[143] Dachman AH, Dawson DO, Lefere P, Yoshida H, Khan NU, Cipriani N, et al. Comparison of routine and unprepped CT colonography augmented by low fiber diet and stool tagging: a pilot study. Abdominal Imaging. 2007 Feb;32[1]:96-104. PubMed PMID: WOS:000246405800015.

[144] Johnson CD, Manduca A, Fletcher JG, MacCarty RL, Carston MJ, Harmsen WS, et al. Noncathartic CT Colonography with stool tagging: Performance with and without electronic stool subtraction. American Journal of Roentgenology. 2008 Feb;190[2]: 361-6. PubMed PMID: WOS:000252932100014.

[145] Keeling AN, Slattery MM, Leong S, McCarthy E, Susanto M, Lee MJ, et al. Limited-Preparation CT Colonography in Frail Elderly Patients: A Feasibility Study. American Journal of Roentgenology. 2010 May;194[5]:1279-87. PubMed PMID: WOS: 000276906400019.